Pulmonary Medicine: An Evidence-Based Approach

Pulmonary Medicine: An Evidence-Based Approach

Edited by Michael Glass

AMERICAN
MEDICAL PUBLISHERS
www.americanmedicalpublishers.com

American Medical Publishers,
41 Flatbush Avenue,
1st Floor, New York,
NY 11217, USA

Visit us on the World Wide Web at:
www.americanmedicalpublishers.com

ISBN: 978-1-63927-465-9

Cataloging-in-Publication Data

Pulmonary medicine : an evidence-based approach / edited by Michael Glass.
p. cm.
Includes bibliographical references and index.
ISBN 978-1-63927-465-9
1. Lungs--Diseases. 2. Lungs--Diseases--Treatment. 3. Evidence-based medicine.
4. Respiratory organs--Diseases. I. Glass, Michael.
RC756 .P853 2022
616.24--dc23

Table of Contents

Preface

Every book is initially just a concept; it takes months of research and hard work to give it the final shape in which the readers receive it. In its early stages, this book also went through rigorous reviewing. The notable contributions made by experts from across the globe were first molded into patterned chapters and then arranged in a sensibly sequential manner to bring out the best results.

Pulmonary medicine also known as pulmonology is the specialty of medicine that deals with the diseases of respiratory tract. Pulmonary medicine is a branch of internal medicine and is concerned with a patient that needs life support and mechanical ventilation. Pulmonary medicine helps in the treatment of various diseases such as asthma, chronic obstructive pulmonary diseases, pneumonia, tuberculosis and chest infections. It treats the disease using various medication methods that includes inhalation using bronchodilators and steroids or in the oral form by using antibiotics and leukotriene antagonists. When the respiratory disease is severe, oxygen therapy is often given. When this is inadequate, the patient is treated with mechanical ventilation. This book provides comprehensive insights into the field of pulmonary medicine. It aims to shed light on some of the unexplored aspects and the recent researches in this field. Those in search of information to further their knowledge will be greatly assisted by this book.

It has been my immense pleasure to be a part of this project and to contribute my years of learning in such a meaningful form. I would like to take this opportunity to thank all the people who have been associated with the completion of this book at any step.

Editor

1

Challenging the diagnosis of Cystic Fibrosis in a patient carrying the 186-8T/C allelic variant in the CF Transmembrane Conductance Regulator gene

Sara Caldrer[1,2*], Genny Verzè[1,2], Jan Johansson[1], Claudio Sorio[1], Chiara Angiari[2], Mario Buffelli[3], Baroukh Maurice Assael[2] and Paola Melotti[2*]

Abstract

Background: This report describe for the first time a clinical case with a CFTR allelic variant 186-8T/C (c.54-8 T/C) in intron 1 of CFTR and underline the importance of applying a combination of genetic and functional tests to establish or exclude a diagnosis of Cystic Fibrosis. In this case the diagnostic algorithm proposed for CF has been successfully applied at our Center and previous CF diagnosis assigned in a different Center was not confirmed.

Case presentation: A 38 year-old Italian woman had been treated as affected by CF since 2010, following diagnosis based on sweat tests (reported values of 73 and 57 mEq/L) and a clinical history consistent with CF. No mutations were identified by first level of genetic analysis. Afterwards the patient referred to our center for assessing the relevance of these findings. The genetic variant 186-8T/C (c.54-8 T/C) in intron 1 of the CFTR gene was detected by sequencing. Low-level interstitial-alveolar infiltration was recorded by high-resolution computerized tomography. Lung function was normal and sputum and Broncho Alveolar Lavage cultures resulted bacteriologically negative. Sweat chloride levels was re-assessed and resulted with values of 57 and 35 mEq/L, with a borderline range between 40 and 60 mEq/L. Nasal Potential Difference measurements resulted in three reliable measurements consistent with a non-CF phenotype. Differential diagnosis with ciliary dyskinesia was excluded, as was exon 2 skipping of CFTR gene that might have caused a CFTR functional defect. Furthermore, single cell fluorescence analysis in response to cAMP agonists performed in patient's monocytes overlapped those obtained in healthy donors.

Conclusion: We concluded that this patient was not affected by CF. This case highlights the need for referrals to highly specialized centers and the importance of combined functional and genetic tests in making a correct diagnosis. Moreover, we confirmed a correlation between NPD tracings and cell depolarization in monocytes providing a rationale for proposing the use of leukocytes as a potential support for CF diagnosis.

Keywords: Cystic Fibrosis, Cystic Fibrosis Conductance Transmembrane Regulator, Mutation analysis, Nasal potential difference measurements, Cystic fibrosis conductance transmembrane regulator function

Background

Cystic Fibrosis (CF) is the most commonly occurring severe disease with autosomal recessive inheritance in Caucasians, with an incidence of approximately 1 in 3000, and among sufferers clinical manifestations vary considerably. Mutations in the CF Transmembrane Conductance Regulator (CFTR) gene bring about the disease. Up to now around 1900 mutations in the CFTR gene have been identified (www.genet.sickkids.on.ca). Most of them are somewhat rare and this means that genetic test results are not always sufficient for CF diagnosis [1] and, in addition, a single genotype may result in different clinical symptoms. CF is usually associated with exocrine pancreatic insufficiency, gradual loss of pulmonary function and lung tissue destruction, but it can also be associated with sufficient residual pancreatic function and a much milder clinical picture [2]. CFTR related disorders [3] include a range

* Correspondence: saracaldrer@gmail.com; paola.melotti@ospedaleuniverona.it
[1]Department of Pathology and Diagnostics, General Pathology Section, University of Verona School of Medicine, Verona, Italy
[2]Cystic Fibrosis Center, Azienda Ospedaliera di Verona, Verona, Italy
Full list of author information is available at the end of the article

of mild conditions caused by CFTR dysfunction, associated with limited deterioration over time and clinical manifestations in at least one organ in the presence of normal or borderline sweat chloride values. The borderline range is between 60 and 40 or 30 mmol/L depending on age and international guidelines [4,5] with the lowest threshold for normal values only during the first year of age [4,5] or always according to De Boeck et al. [4,5]. Sometimes CF diagnosis is challenging and requires, in addition to sweat test and genetic analysis, the use of sophisticated diagnostic tools [6,7]. They aim at testing CFTR function as ion channel *in vivo* or *ex vivo* as under the inferior turbinate of the nose or in rectal biopsies by Nasal Potential Difference (NPD) measurements or intestinal current measurements (ICM), respectively. Both these tests need standardization and validation, and recently European Standard Operative Procedures have been developed by the European Cystic Fibrosis Society Diagnostic Network Working Group for use as a diagnostic aid. Other methods measuring *ex vivo* the functional properties of CFTR in patients' tissues utilizing nasal epithelium [8], leukocytes [9] or intestinal organoids [10] have been proposed.

Case presentation

Here we report the clinical case of a 38 year-old Italian woman who, since 2010, had been treated as affected by CF in a European CF Center. This had followed diagnosis based on repeated sweat tests (chloride 60 and 74 mEq/L, normal values <50 mEq/L) and a clinical history consistent with CF (chronic sinusitis, recurrent bronchitis, gallstones). Chronic sinusitis was associated with deviation of the nasal septum treated surgically. Low-level infiltrative interstitial lung damage was evident from High Resolution Computerized Tomography (HRCT), bronchiectasis were absent. No mutations were identified by genetic analysis performed where the patient was diagnosed as CF. Subsequently the CFTR allelic variant 186-8T/C (c.54-8 T/C) in intron 1 of CFTR gene was identified by gene sequencing in an Italian CF Center where genetic analysis was performed by reverse dot blot (INNO-LIPA CFTR19, CFTR17 + TN Update, CFTR Italian Regional), sequencing and Multiplex ligation-dependent probe amplification (MLPA). To our knowledge, this is the first time this allelic variant has been reported. The patient was then referred to our center for assessment of the relevance of these findings. We then applied a diagnostic algorithm (Figure 1) based on established guidelines [4], where it is advised to continue the diagnostic work up if symptoms in a patient persist, as well as when symptoms have resolved but are highly suspicious for CF such as pancreatitis or Pseudomonas aeruginosa-associated lung disease. Wherever the algorithm ends with "CF unlikely" it is advised to investigate for alternative diagnoses such as

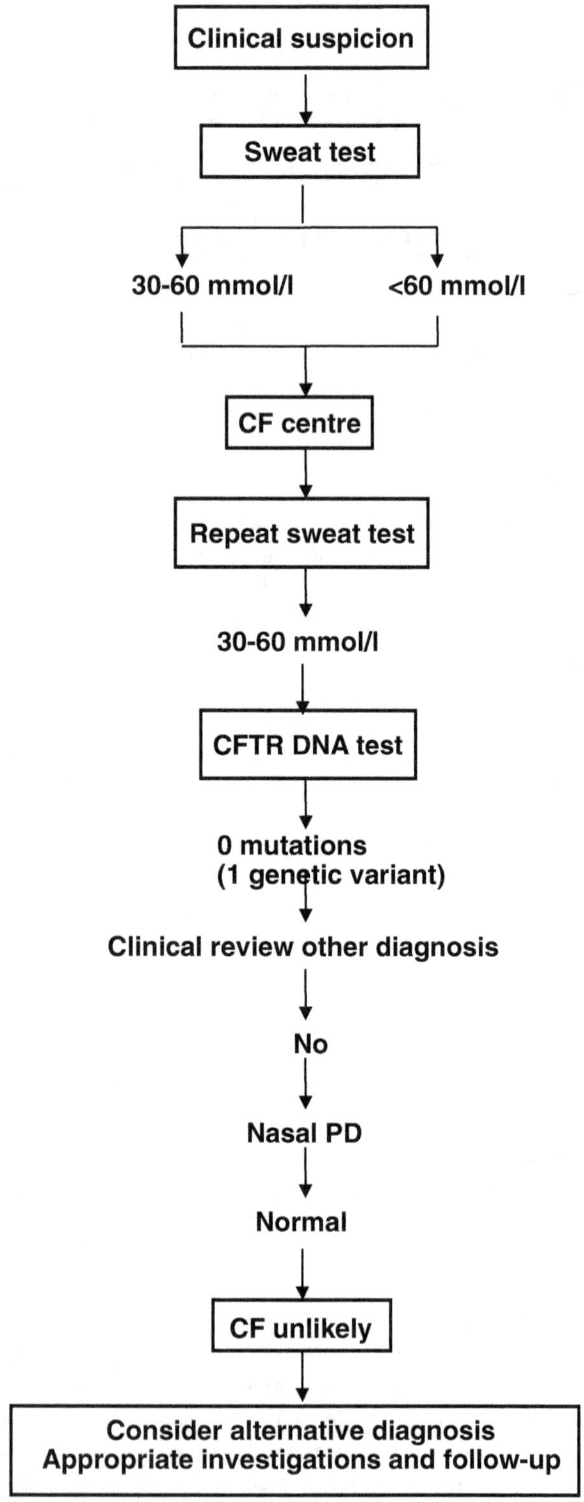

Figure 1 Diagnostic algorithm: diagram describing the diagnostic algorithm utilized for the case described and based on the proposals from De Boeck et al. [4].

primary ciliary dyskinesia, humoral immunodeficiency, Shwachman syndrome. For patients with CFTR dysfunction, the physician needs to decide the most appropriate diagnostic label (non-classic CF or other WHO diagnostic definitions in patients with very limited symptoms). Patients with a borderline sweat test (30–60 mmol/l), only one CFTR mutation identified, and an inconclusive nasal potential difference (PD) cannot at present be classified correctly. They are at least CF carriers. In the presence of persistent symptoms they need structured follow up at an appropriate facility (for some patients this may be the CF centre) and symptomatic treatment. Genetic counseling is important in these patients and their families. CFTR DNA test: screening test to search for the most frequent mutations in the population from which the patient originates. Mutation scanning of CFTR gene: this test is only necessary in some patients in whom the diagnosis cannot be supported by other means. The tests in the grey area are optional because two clearly positive sweat tests are sufficient to support the diagnosis of CF in a compatible clinical setting. However, in most CF centres the CFTR DNA test will be performed to confirm the diagnosis, to allow for further cascade screening if necessary, and at times for research purposes. Consult genetic lab: in patients with an elevated sweat chloride level it would be unusual but not impossible not to find any mutation. In case of doubt about the diagnosis, a mutation scanning of the complete gene can be done. A falsely positive sweat test and the possibility of CF heterogeneity also need to be considered.

In the case here presented NPD was measured in accordance with a standardized protocol [6] and normal tracings were obtained. Three repeated measurements were consistent with a non-CF phenotype. The Wilschanski index [7] was calculated and results ranged from 0.06 to 0.24, with non-CF values < 0.82 in our Center (Figure 2). Two consecutive sweat tests were carried out 3 months apart (on May and July) in accordance with the Gibson and Cooke method [11] and chloride values of 35 mEq/L and 57 mEq/L were obtained respectively. The previously reported sweat test was performed only in the summer following an unspecified method with a local cut-off for normal value. These might be reasons for discrepancies with test results from our Center, along with patient's diet and hydration levels. It is known that Normal and borderline sweat tests were obtained in CF patients in the presence of specific CFTR genotypes: the most representative includes mutations 3849 + 10 kb C > T, D1152H and R117H [12,13]. Lung function was normal (forced vital capacity and forced expiratory volume in the first second were both 103% and forced expiratory flow at 25-75% was 113% of predicted values) and lung infection was excluded by several sputum cultures and Broncho Alveolar Lavage (BAL). We have no data available about eventual differential cell count in BALFs. However normal pulmonary function tests and negative sputum/BAL cultures are reported in some CF patients.

We then considered primary ciliary dyskinesia as a possible, alternative diagnosis. However televideo microscopic technique carried out in a specialized center displayed normal ciliary beat and the saccharin test showed normal ciliary mucus transport, allowing the exclusion of this disease.

We decided to investigate CFTR-channel function using NPD analysis and additional ex-vivo and molecular assays, aimed at supporting the previous findings, were carried out in parallel. Ferec et al. previously reported a possible exon 2 splicing in the genetic 186-13C > G variant detected in-trans with F508del in a 13 year old child with

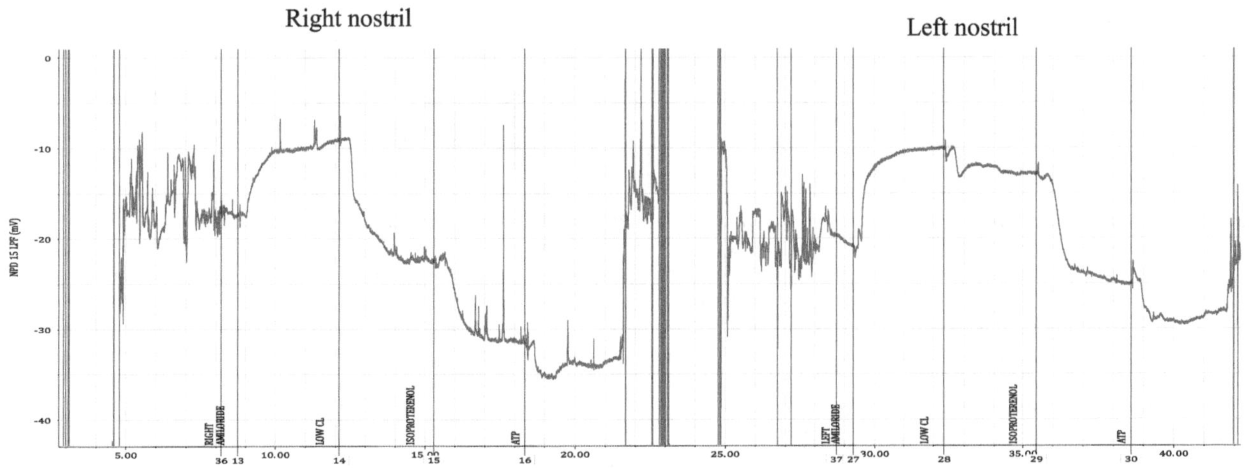

Figure 2 NDP measurements. The agents indicated at the bottom were added at the times (minutes) shown on the x-axis. On the y-axis, PD is expressed in mV. The graph on the left was obtained from right nostril measurements; the right one was obtained from left nostril measurements. Baseline NPD value was -21 mV. After the addition of amiloride PD increased to 13 mV, falling to 2.8 mV after exposure to 0 Cl- and isoproterenol. NDP measurements were repeated three times and readings were always consistent with a non-CF phenotype.

pancreatic sufficiency where nasal polyposis was the main symptom [14]. Although the T to C substitution is conservative, in this case we aimed to exclude the possibility that the genetic variant 186-8T/C could affect the splicing. For this reason, CFTR mRNA from blood cells was analyzed by RT-PCR, using exon 2 spanning primers or with primers designed to amplify fragments of different lengths depending on the presence or absence of exon 2 (Figure 3A). In all cases patient mRNA amplification products were identified as being the same as in a healthy donor (Figure 3B). Therefore we concluded that 186-8T/C mutation does not cause changes in the CFTR cDNA sequence despite its localization in intron 1 at position −8. However, the substitution of T with C is unlikely to be able to affect splicing since it is conservative in this polypyrimidine-rich, intronic region.

Further CFTR protein function testing was carried out using single cell fluorescence analysis in monocytes. To summarize: the potential-sensitive probe bis-(1,3-diethylthiobarbituric acid) trimethine oxonol (DiSBAC2 (3) Invitrogen, USA) was used to monitor CFTR-dependent membrane-potential (Vm) changes. We previously defined the CF index as an outcome of this assay and it was shown to be positive in healthy subjects and negative in CF patients [9]. In the genetic variant 186-8T/C the CF index was positive (mean: +43 ± 12; n = 2), a result that overlaps those obtained in monocytes/leukocytes from healthy donors (Figures 4A and 3B).

Doubts about the original CF diagnosis might also arise from the presence of interstitial infiltration in the lung in the absence of bronchiectasis and of CFTR dysfunction-causing mutations in this patient. Since at our center the patient had normal/ borderline sweat test values we did not investigate for eventual differential diagnosis with diseases associated with a raise in electrolyte levels [15].

In the case reported, the application at our Center of the CF diagnostic algorithm [4] was successful and the previous CF-diagnosis was not confirmed (Figure 1). Our interpretation of NPD data seems in agreement with the recommendation provided by Boucher [16] who underlined the importance to correctly evaluate sodium transport to establish a correct diagnosis when NPD are required. Based on a French study he proposed bronchiectasis to be a multiple hits process or a continuum of ion transport dysfunction measured by NPD according to presence of zero, one or two mutations or genetic variants. Diffuse bronchiectasis are a possible phenotype of CFTR related disorders. In this patients no bronchiectasis were evident by HRCT and low-level infiltrative interstitial lung damage in conjunction with recurrent bronchitis are still of unknown origin.

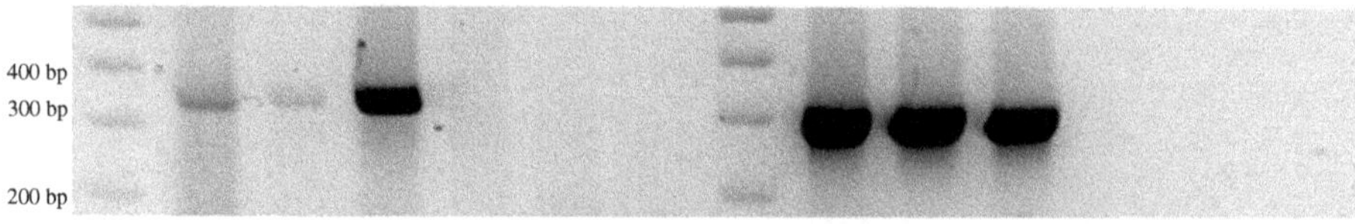

Figure 3 Search for CFTR exon 2 skipping by reverse-transcriptase PCR amplification of mRNA from monocytes. (A) *RT-PCR design*: mRNA from monocytes was analyzed by RT-PCR using primers designed to amplify fragments of different length, depending on the presence or absence of exon 2, to better define if the genetic variant 186-8T/C had caused alternative splicing in this subject. Total RNA was purified and reverse-transcribed with random primers. PCR was then carried out for 35 cycles (30" at 94°C, 30" at 60°C, 30" at 72°C) using the forward primer, Ex 1–4 Forward 5'-AAAGGCCAGCGTTGTCT-3' (black arrow) or W/O exon 2 Forward primer 5'-ACTTTTTTTCAGAGAATGGGATAGAG-3' (gray arrow), and the reverse primer, Exon 1–4 5'-GCGATAGAGCGTTCCTC-3' (black arrow). The exon-spanning primer "W/O exon 2 Forward primer" is localized between the exons 1 and 3 coding sequence, and thus works properly only in the absence of exon 2. Amplified fragment lengths using Exon1-4 Forward and Reverse primers (black arrows) were expected to be 339 bp. Therefore, in the case of exon 2 skipping, we would expect a shorter PCR-product (228 bp). With the exon-spanning Forward primer (W/O Exon 2; grey arrow) we expected an amplified product of a length of 207 bp. **(B)** *PCR-amplification products*: We compared the PCR-amplified products obtained from the patient (186–8 T/C), with a healthy subject heterozygous for the common F508del mutation, and with a healthy subject (no mutations) as internal control. The amplification product obtained from the subject carrying the 186-8T/C variant, using Exon 1–4 Forw/Rev primers, was undistinguishable from controls, moreover, using the exon2-spanning primer no amplification products were observed in the samples from any of the subjects (Negative Controls-NC). As control we amplified a portion (290 bp) of the housekeeping gene actin; this PCR was then carried out for 25 cycle.

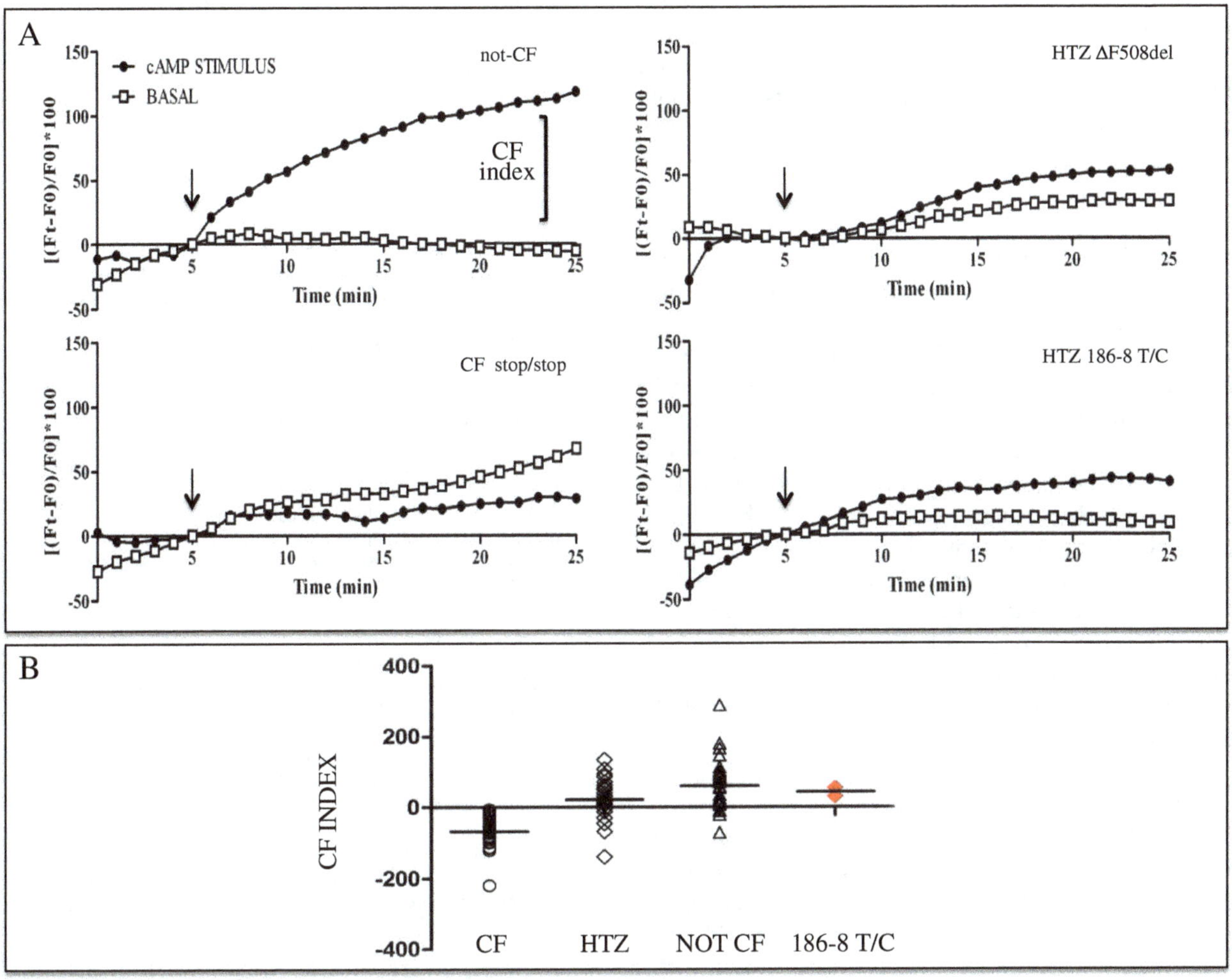

Figure 4 Diagnostic algorithm. (A) *Monocyte cell membrane depolarization assay.* Single cell fluorescence assay was performed as described[10]. Measurements of the cell membrane depolarization were obtained in a extracellular environment lacking chloride-ion and were measured at two different conditions: under basal conditions (empty boxes), or with a stimulus-cocktail consisting of 8-Br-cAMP, Forkolin and IBMX (filled boxes) added at the 5th minute. Percentage of DiSBAC2(3) fluorescence variation (ΔF) is shown over time according to the equation: $\Delta Ft = [(Ft-F0)/F0] *100$, where Ft and F0 are the fluorescence values at time t and at the time t0 (5th minute). The difference between the maximum fluorescence values obtained on stimulation (filled boxes) and the matching fluorescence under basal conditions (empty boxes) represents the CF index. We defined the CF index outcome for this assay being a positive value in healthy subjects and a negative value in CF patients. A typical non-CF pattern, where a higher signal can be observed after stimulation, is represented at the top-left panel, with a CF index of +116. On the other hand, when monocytes from a subject carrying a non-sense mutation on both alleles were used, the opposite trend was observed (bottom-left panel), with a negative CF index of −25,2. With the monocytes from the patient (186-8T/C) a positive CF index was obtained (43 ± 12; n = 2; right-bottom panel), with a response to the cAMP-analogue similar to those obtained from the other HTZ subject (CF = +22; right-up panel). **(B)** *CF index.* Plotting of the CF index values obtained from the subject in comparison with recording from patients and controls performed in our laboratory using the same experimental setting. Number of Samples: CF subjects n = 40, HTZ subjects n = 28 and non CF subjects n = 31. Analysis of the 186–8 T/C subject was repeated twice (technical duplicate).

It is important to consider the negative impact of a wrong diagnosis of CF for a patient and relatives in terms of medical, psychological, social and insurance implications. It is indeed a chronic progressive disease compromising quality and expectancy of life. Considering its autosomal recessive inheritance also for genetic counselling it is very relevant to avoid wrong diagnosis, in particular in this case having no disease causing mutations identified.

This outlines how important is for the CF community to have access to clinical and electrophysiological information on rare mutations; it can lead to further improvements in diagnostic procedure and genetic counseling. A large number of genetic variants of uncertain functional significance have been identified due to the extensive sequencing being carried out, diluting the practical application of this valuable information [17,18]. Besides CFTR, several modifier genes have also been described as being able to influence CF phenotype [19]. CFTR functional tests are under development [20] but need to be validated and standardized assays are available only for NPD and intestinal current measurements [21]. Both these measurements are minimally invasive and can be used in selected cases.

Conclusion

In the clinical case reported here, sweat tests and genetic analysis were inconclusive and CFTR functional testing, in accordance with a standard method (NPD), was carried out. In addition, we evaluated a possible exon skipping and CFTR function in leukocytes. None of the results obtained at our Center were consistent with CF diagnosis. An innovative approach using leukocytes was also applied, being potentially more convenient than currently available and standardized approaches. Validation with a large group of subjects is in progress and research to develop simpler, more feasible functional assays in leukocytes and epithelial cells are underway in our and in other Centres, with the aim of providing additional tools for testing genetic variants of uncertain clinical relevance as well as the effects of drugs targeting the basic CF defect.

Consent

Written informed consent for publication of their clinical details and/or clinical images was obtained from the patient/parent/guardian/relative of the patient. A copy of the consent form is available for review by the Editor of this journal.

Abbreviations

CF: Cystic Fibrosis; CFTR CF: Transmembrane Conductance Regulator gene; HRCT: High Resolution Computerized Tomography; NDP: Nasal potential difference; (DiSBAC2(3): bis-(1,3-diethylthiobarbituric acid) trimethine oxonol; BAL: Broncho Alveolar Lavage.

Competing interests

The authors declare that they have no competing interests.

Authors' contributions

PM, and BA are clinicians responsible for the patient at the Cystic Fibrosis Center of Verona and had performed clinical trials. SC, GV, JJ, CA have performed the cellular studies. CS and MB read and commented the manuscript and are the responsible of the two laboratories that had performed these experiments. Authors read and approved the final manuscript.

Acknowledgements

SC is supported by the Italian CF Research Foundation (grant#06/2010), the work is supported by FFC grant#06/2010, adopted by Delegazione FFC di V.C.O. Verbania, Associazione Trentina FC Onlus Gruppo di Sostegno FFC in ricordo di Silvia Sommavilla, Consorzio Promotre s.c.r.l., Antonio Guadagnin e Figlio, Alessandra Boccanera and FFC #26/2011, adopted by Donatori SMS Solidale 2011, Delegazione FFC di Varese, Associazione Trentina FC onlus and by Lega Italiana Fibrosi Cistica- Associazione Veneta Onlus.

Author details

[1]Department of Pathology and Diagnostics, General Pathology Section, University of Verona School of Medicine, Verona, Italy. [2]Cystic Fibrosis Center, Azienda Ospedaliera di Verona, Verona, Italy. [3]Department of Neurological Sciences, Physiology Section, University of Verona School of Medicine, Verona, Italy.

References

1. Fanen P, Ghanem N, Vidaud M, Besmond C, Martin J, Costes B, Plassa F, Goossens M: **Molecular characterization of cystic fibrosis: 16 novel mutations identified by analysis of the whole cystic fibrosis conductance transmembrane regulator (CFTR) coding regions and splice site junctions.** *Genomics* 1992, **13**(3):770–776.
2. **Classification of cystic fibrosis and related disorders.** *J Cyst Fibros* 2002, **1**(1):5–8.
3. Bombieri C, Claustres M, De Boeck K, Derichs N, Dodge J, Girodon E, Sermet I, Schwarz M, Tzetis M, Wilschanski M, Bareil C, Bilton D, Castellani C, Cuppens H, Cutting GR, Drevínek P, Farrell P, Elborn JS, Jarvi K, Kerem B, Kerem E, Knowles M, Macek M Jr, Munck A, Radojkovic D, Seia M, Sheppard DN, Southern KW, Stuhrmann M, Tullis E, Zielenski J, Pignatti PF, Ferec C: **Recommendations for the classification of diseases as CFTR-related disorders.** *J Cystic Fibrosis* 2011, **10**:S86–S102.
4. De Boeck K, Wilschanski M, Castellani C, Taylor C, Cuppens H, Dodge J, Sinaasappel M: **Cystic fibrosis: terminology and diagnostic algorithms.** *Thorax* 2006, **61**(7):627–635.
5. Farrell PM, Rosenstein BJ, White TB, Accurso FJ, Castellani C, Cutting GR, Durie PR, LeGrys VA, Massie J, Parad RB, Rock MJ, Campbell PW III: **Guidelines for Diagnosis of Cystic Fibrosis in Newborns through Older Adults: Cystic Fibrosis Foundation Consensus Report.** *J Pediatr* 2008, **153**(2):S4–S14.
6. Bronsveld I, Sinaasappel M, Southern KW, Sermet-Gaudelus I, Leal T, Melotti P, Ballmann M, Hjelte L, Middleton PG, De Boeck K, Wilschnski M: **Evaluation of European protocols for measuring nasal potential differences.** *J Cystic Fibrosis* 2009, **8**(Supplement 2(0)):S10.
7. Wilschanski M, Famini H, Strauss-Liviatan N, Rivlin J, Blau H, Bibi H, Bentur L, Yahav Y, Springer H, Kramer MR, Klar A, Ilani A, Kerem B, Kerem E: **Nasal potential difference measurements in patients with atypical cystic fibrosis.** *Eur Respir J* 2001, **17**(6):1208–1215.
8. Canani RB, Terrin G, Elce A, Pezzella V, Heinz-Erian P, Pedrolli A, Centenari C, Amato F, Tomaiuolo R, Calignano A, Troncone R, Castaldo G: **Genotype-dependency of butyrate efficacy in children with congenital chloride diarrhea.** *Orphanet J Rare Dis* 2013, **8**(1):194.
9. Sorio C, Buffelli M, Angiari C, Ettorre M, Johansson J, Vezzalini M, Viviani L, Ricciardi M, Verze G, Assael BM, Melotti P: **Defective CFTR expression and function are detectable in blood monocytes: development of a new blood test for cystic fibrosis.** *PLoS One* 2011, **6**(7):e22212.
10. Dekkers JF, Wiegerinck CL, de Jonge HR, Bronsveld I, Janssens HM, de Winter-de Groot KM, Brandsma AM, de Jong NW, Bijvelds MJ, Scholte BJ, Nieuwenhuis EES, van den Brink S, Clevers H, van der Ent CK, Middendorp S, Beekman JM: **A functional CFTR assay using primary cystic fibrosis intestinal organoids.** *Nat Med* 2013, **19**(7):939–945.
11. Gibson LE, Cooke RE: **A test for concentration of electrolytes in sweat in cystic fibrosis of the pancreas utilizing pilocarpine by iontophoresis.** *Pediatrics* 1959, **23**(3):545–549.
12. Highsmith WE, Burch LH, Zhou Z, Olsen JC, Boat TE, Spock A, Gorvoy JD, Quittel L, Friedman KJ, Silverman LM, Boucher RC, Knowles MR: **A novel mutation in the cystic fibrosis gene in patients with pulmonary disease but normal sweat chloride concentrations.** *N Engl J Med* 1994, **331**(15):974–980.
13. **Correlation between genotype and phenotype in patients with cystic fibrosis. The Cystic Fibrosis Genotype-Phenotype Consortium.** *N Engl J Med* 1993, **329**(18):1308–1313.
14. Ferec C, Quere I, Audrezt MP, Verlingue C, Guillermit H, Mercier B: **Mutation Details for c.54-13C>G.** In *Cystic Fibrosis Mutation Database NEWSLETTER #50.* 1992nd edition. 1992.
15. Casaulta C, Stirnimann A, Schoeni MH, Barben J: **Sweat test in patients with glucose-6-phosphate-1-dehydrogenase deficiency.** *Arch Dis Child* 2008, **93**(10):878–879.
16. Boucher RC: **Bronchiectasis: a continuum of ion transport dysfunction or multiple hits?** *Am J Respir Crit Care Med* 2010, **181**(10):1017–1019.

17. Modiano G, Bombieri C, Ciminelli BM, Belpinati F, Giorgi S, Georges M, Scotet V, Pompei F, Ciccacci C, Guittard C, Pierre Audrézet M, Begnini A, Toepfer M, Macek M Jr, Ferec C, Claustres M, Pignatti PF: **A large-scale study of the random variability of a coding sequence: a study on the CFTR gene.** *Eur J Hum Genet* 2005, **13**(2):184–192.
18. Spinelli E, Seia M, Melotti P, Marchina E, Padoan R: **CFTR mutation in an Arab patient: clinical and functional features of 875 + 1G- > A/875 + 1G- > A genotype.** *J Cyst Fibros* 2009, **8**(4):282–284.
19. Cutting GR: **Modifier genes in Mendelian disorders: the example of cystic fibrosis.** *Ann N Y Acad Sci* 2010, **1214**:57–69.
20. Stumpf A, Almaca J, Kunzelmann K, Wenners-Epping K, Huber SM, Haberle J, Falk S, Duebbers A, Walte M, Oberleithner H, Schillers H: **IADS, a decomposition product of DIDS activates a cation conductance in Xenopus oocytes and human erythrocytes: new compound for the diagnosis of cystic fibrosis.** *Cell Physiol Biochem* 2006, **18**(4–5):243–252.
21. Derichs N, Sanz J, Von Kanel T, Stolpe C, Zapf A, Tummler B, Gallati S, Ballmann M: **Intestinal current measurement for diagnostic classification of patients with questionable cystic fibrosis: validation and reference data.** *Thorax* 2010, **65**(7):594–599.

2

Prognostic value of extravascular lung water assessed with lung ultrasound score by chest sonography in patients with acute respiratory distress syndrome

Zhen Zhao[1], Li Jiang[1*], Xiuming Xi[1], Qi Jiang[1], Bo Zhu[1], Meiping Wang[1], Jin Xing[2] and Dan Zhang[2]

Abstract

Background: The prognostic value of extravascular lung water indices (EVLWI) has been widely investigated, which is determined by lung ultrasound B-lines. However, the clinical value of lung ultrasound B-lines for determining prognosis/intensive care unit (ICU) outcomes in patients with acute respiratory distress syndrome (ARDS) has been rarely reported.

Methods: Twenty-one ARDS patients admitted to the ICU of Fu Xing Hospital underwent both lung ultrasonography and pulse index continuous cardiac output (PiCCO) monitoring on the first, second, and third days after diagnosis. The correlation between lung ultrasound score (LUS) and EVLWI measured by the PiCCO system was investigated. The prognostic clinical value of lung ultrasonography in ARDS patients was explored. Chest ultrasound was performed using the 12 regions method. The comprehensive score of lung ultrasound was determined according to the level of lung aeration.

Results: With ICU mortality as the end point, 21 patients were divided into a survivor group (8 patients, 39.1 %) and a non-survivor group (13 patients, 61.9 %). Significant positive linear correlations were found between LUS and EVLWI, including predicted body weight ($r^2 = 0.906$), sequential organ failure assessment score ($r^2 = 0.815$), lung injury score ($r^2 = 0.361$), and PaO_2/FiO_2 ($r^2 = 0.472$). Significantly different LUSs were found between the non-survivor and survivor groups ($F = 77.64$, $P < 0.01$) by repeated-measures analysis of variance. There were no significant differences between the two groups on different days. The areas under the receiver operating characteristic curves of LUS and EVLW measured by PiCCO were 0.846 ($P < 0.01$) and 0.918 ($P < 0.01$), respectively. The cut-off of LUS for prognosis prediction was 16.5.

Conclusions: Lung ultrasonography is a non-invasive, economic, simple, user-friendly, and radiation-free bedside method for predicting the prognosis of ARDS patients. Early measurement of LUS is a better prognostic indicator in patients with ARDS.

Background

Acute respiratory distress syndrome (ARDS) is a common complication in critically ill patients. In the intensive care unit (ICU), 19 % of patients with mechanical ventilation are diagnosed with ARDS, which is characterized by increased extravascular lung water (EVLW) and refractory hypoxemia, with mortality rates as high as 32–65 % [1]. Diagnostic methods, such as physical examination, bedside X-ray chest film, and computed tomography (CT), provide a basic clinical evaluation of EVLW in severe cases, and they are useful for assessing lung involvement in ARDS. However, the accuracy of the former two methods is less than optimal [2]. CT scans increase safety risks because they require patient transport. Pulse index continuous cardiac output (PiCCO) technology is a highly accurate quantitative method for determination of EVLW, but it is invasive and may cause

* Correspondence: jiangli@sina.com
[1]Intensive Care Unit, Fuxing Hospital affiliated with Capital Medical University, Beijing 100038, China
Full list of author information is available at the end of the article

catheter-related infections [3]. Lung ultrasound is used to detect pulmonary edema in the early period, and 'B-lines' indicate loss of lung aeration, which may be caused by an increase in EVLW [4]. However, some researchers have introduced LUS, according to the different pulmonary ultrasonography of ARDS patients, to determine EVLW semi-quantitatively [5].

In the present study, the correlation between lung ultrasound and PiCCO monitoring was investigated to determine EVLW and evaluate the value of these two examinations in predicting ICU prognosis of ARDS patients. This economic and noninvasive bedside examination is expected to be used in the prognostic evaluation of ARDS patients.

Methods

Patients

Criteria for inclusion: (1) ARDS patients admitted to the ICU of Fu Xing Hospital affiliated with the Capital University of Medical Sciences from June 2012 to May 2013; (2) Patients meeting the diagnostic criteria of ARDS [6].

Criteria for exclusion:(1) Patients who spent ≤ 24 h in the ICU; (2) Patients whose mechanical ventilation time was ≤ 24 h; (3) Patients with severe hemodynamic instability who were unable to safely change body positions; (4) Patients with severely deformed chest cage or subcutaneous emphysema who were unfit for lung ultrasound; (5) Patients who agreed to limit or withdraw life support treatment during hospitalization;(6) Patients whose family did not sign the informed consent.

Data collection

All patients were confirmed to have ARDS by chest CT on the first day of admission to the hospital. Patients were studied on the first, second, and third day after diagnosis of ARDS by lung ultrasound, bedside X-ray film, and PiCCO monitoring. Lung ultrasound was performed immediately after PiCCO monitoring.

Epidemiological data were collected, including sex, age, height, ideal weight, ARDS etiology, incidence period, and ICU outcome. The sequential organ failure assessment (SOFA) scores and lung injury score (LIS) scores of the patients were recorded every day. Parameters of mechanical ventilation were also collected every day, including tidal volume index, positive end-expiratory pressure (PEEP), static respiratory system compliance (Crs), and PaO_2/FiO_2 (P/F).

The study was approved by the Ethics Committee of Beijing Fuxing Hospital, Capital Medical University and met all ethical requirements. All participants in both groups voluntarily joined this study and provided written informed consent.

EVLW assessment

Lung ultrasound

Lung ultrasound was performed to diagnose ARDS. A Philips C5 ultrasound system (frequency 5Hz; Philips Medical Systems, Suresnes, France) with an ordinary convex probe was used. Chest ultrasound was performed using the 12 regions method. All intercostal spaces of the upper and lower parts of the anterior, lateral, and posterior regions of the left and right chest walls were examined. Each region of interest was extensively examined. The worst ultrasound abnormality detected was considered to characterize the region being examined. Four ultrasound aeration patterns as shown in Fig. 1 were defined [5]: a. normal aeration (N): line sliding sign associated with respiratory movement or less than 3 B lines; b. moderate loss of lung aeration: a clear number of multiple visible B-lines with horizontal spacing between adjacent B lines ≤ 7 mm (B1 lines); c. severe loss of lung aeration: multiple B lines fused together that were difficult to count with horizontal spacing between adjacent B lines ≤ 3 mm, including'white lung' (B2 lines); and d. pulmonary consolidation (C), hyperechoic lung tissue, accompanied by dynamic air bronchogram.

LUS was determined based on four lung ultrasonographs: N = 0, B1 = 1, B2 = 2, and C = 3. All patients underwent a lung ultrasound, and each of the 12 lung areas was examined. The final LUS of the patient was the sum of each regional ultrasound score (ranging from 0 to 36).

All lung ultrasound images were examined by two ultrasound doctors. Both doctors were blind to the clinical data of the patients and to the other doctor's ultrasound diagnosis.

PiCCO monitoring

EVLW was measured using a PiCCO system (Pulsiocath PV8115; Pulsion Medical Systems, Feldkirchen, Germany). For each patient, after 15 ml of 0 °C 0.9 % saline bolus was injected into the central vein, artery temperature was detected using a temperature sensor in a femoral artery catheter, and EVLW was calculated. The final EVLW was the average of three consecutive injections [7]. Extravascular lung water index (EVLWI) was the surface distribution of extra-vascular lung water in a predicted body weight (PBW). Male: PBW(kg) = 0.91(height (cm) – 152.4) +50; female: PBW(kg) = 0.91 (height (cm) –152.4) +45.5 [8].

Statistical analysis

With ICU mortality as the end point, all patients were divided into a survivor group and a non-survivor group. Normally distributed continuous quantitative data were described as means ± standard deviation (mean ± standard deviation (SD)). Normal continuous variables were compared using the t test, and non-normal continuous data were compared using the Mann-Whitney U test. One-way analysis of variance was used to compare more than two independent variables. To access ICU outcome, a linear regression model was built that included LUS and other ARDS prognostic indices. Additionally, scatter grams (GraphPad Prism5) and receiver operating characteristic (ROC) analyses were performed.

Results

Twenty-nine ARDS patients were selected from June 2012 to March 2013. Eight of these patients matched the exclusion criteria, including three patients who died within 24 h, two patients who were unable to complete the lung ultrasound, and three patients who signed restrictions or asked for withdrawal from life support. The clinical characteristics of 21 patients with ARDS are shown in Table 1. The average age of all patients was 78 ± 6 years, their average height was 169 ± 8 cm, and their average weight was 66 ± 7 kg. ARDS was caused by pneumonia in 13 patients (62 %), aspiration in three patients (14 %), cardiopulmonary resuscitation in another three patients (14 %), and trauma in one patient (5 %). Fifteen patients (72 %) in the ICU were diagnosed with ARDS within 48 h. Thirteen patients (62 %) died in the ICU.

Table 1 Clinical characteristics of 21 patients with acute respiratory distress syndrome

Variable	Mean ± SD
Age (years)	78 ± 6
Gender	
Male	14 (67 %)
Female	7 (33 %)
Height (cm)	169 ± 8
PBW (kg)	66 ± 7
CRX quadrants	
3	9 (43 %)
4	12 (57 %)
Etiology of ARDS	
Pneumonia	13 (62 %)
Aspiration	3 (14 %)
Sepsis	3 (14 %)
CPR	1 (5 %)
Trauma	1 (5 %)
Onset	
<48 h	15 (72 %)
>48 h	6 (28 %)
ICU mortality	
Survival	13 (62 %)
Non-survival	8 (38 %)

PBW predicted body weight, *CRX* chest X-ray, *CPR* cardio pulmonary resuscitation

As shown in Table 2, the LUS of ARDS patients in the non-survivor group was significantly higher than that in the survivor group (20 ± 5*vs.* 15 ± 5, $P = 0.022$). EVLWI (16.8 ± 4.4 mL/kg), SOFA (15 ± 2), LIS (3 ± 0.3), and Crs (39 ± 8) in the non-survivor group were significantly higher than in the survivor group on the first day, while age, height, PBW, and tidal volume were not significantly different between the two groups. Moreover, Crs and P/F in the non-survivor group were significantly lower (34 ± 8 mL/cmH_2O, 160 ± 42 mmHg) than those in the survivor group. LUS of the non-survivor group was markedly higher than in the survivor group in the first 3 days following diagnosis of acute respiratory distress syndrome, and the other examined indicators (EVLWI, SOFA, LIS, Crs, P/F) exhibited the same tendencies with the degree of disease (Fig. 2). The average LUS and the EVLWI, SOFA, P/F, and LIS on the third day were significantly correlated (r^2 = 0.906,0.815,0.472,0.361, $P < 0.01$) (Fig. 3).

Significant differences in LUS and EVLWI overall for 3 days were found between the non-survivor group and the survivor group ($F = 11.82$, 22.08, $P < 0.01$). The non-survivor group had significantly higher LUS and EVLWI values than the survivor group. The ROC curves of the average LUS and EVLWI values on the third day were valuable for evaluating clinical prognosis. There were no significant differences between the two groups in LUS or EVLWI on different days. The areas under the ROC curves of LUS and EVLW as determined by PiCCO were 0.846($P < 0.01$) and 0.918($P < 0.01$), respectively. The cut-off of LUS for prognosis prediction was 16.5 (Fig. 4).

Table 2 The characteristics of patients on day 1

	All	Survivors	Non-survivors	p
	(n = 21)	(n = 8)	(n = 13)	
Age (years)	78 ± 6	76 ± 3	80 ± 2	0.228
Male (n (%))	14 (67)	5 (63)	9 (69)	<0.01
Height (cm)	169 ± 8	170 ± 9	169 ± 8	0.866
PBW (kg)	66 ± 7	66 ± 8	65 ± 7	0.866
SOFA	13 ± 2.6	10 ± 2	15 ± 2	<0.01
PEEP (cm H_2O)	10 ± 3	8 ± 2	11 ± 3	0.036
Crs (mL/cm H_2O)	34 ± 8	39 ± 8	31 ± 6	0.013
P/F (mmHg)	160 ± 42	184 ± 23	145 ± 45	0.019
VT (ml/kg PBW)	6.6 ± 0.5	6.4 ± 0.5	6.7 ± 0.5	0.109
LIS	2.8 ± 0.4	2.4 ± 0.3	3 ± 0.3	0.001
LUS	18.1 ± 5.3	15 ± 5	20 ± 5	0.022
EVLWI	16.8 ± 4.4	13 ± 3.6	19 ± 3	<0.01

PBW predicted body weight, *SOFA* sequential organ failure assessment score, *PEEP* positive end expiratory pressure, *Crs* static respiratory system compliance, *P/F* PaO2/FiO2, *VT* tidal volume, *LIS* lung injury score, *LUS* lung ultrasound score, *EVLWI* extra-vascular lung water indexed to PBW

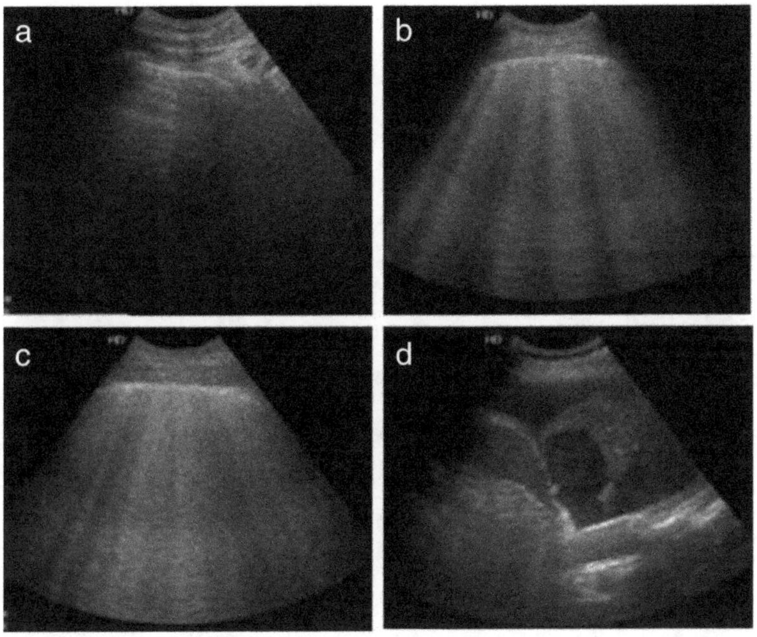

Fig. 1 Four ultrasound patterns according to lung aeration. **a** normal aeration (N): presence of lung sliding with A lines or fewer than two isolated B lines; **b** moderate loss of lung aeration: multiple, well-defined B lines (B1 lines); **c** severe loss of lung aeration: multiple coalescent B lines (B2 lines); and **d** lung consolidation (C), the presence of a tissue pattern. For a given region of interest, points were allocated according to the worst ultrasound pattern observed: N = 0, B1 lines = 1, B2 lines = 2, C = 3

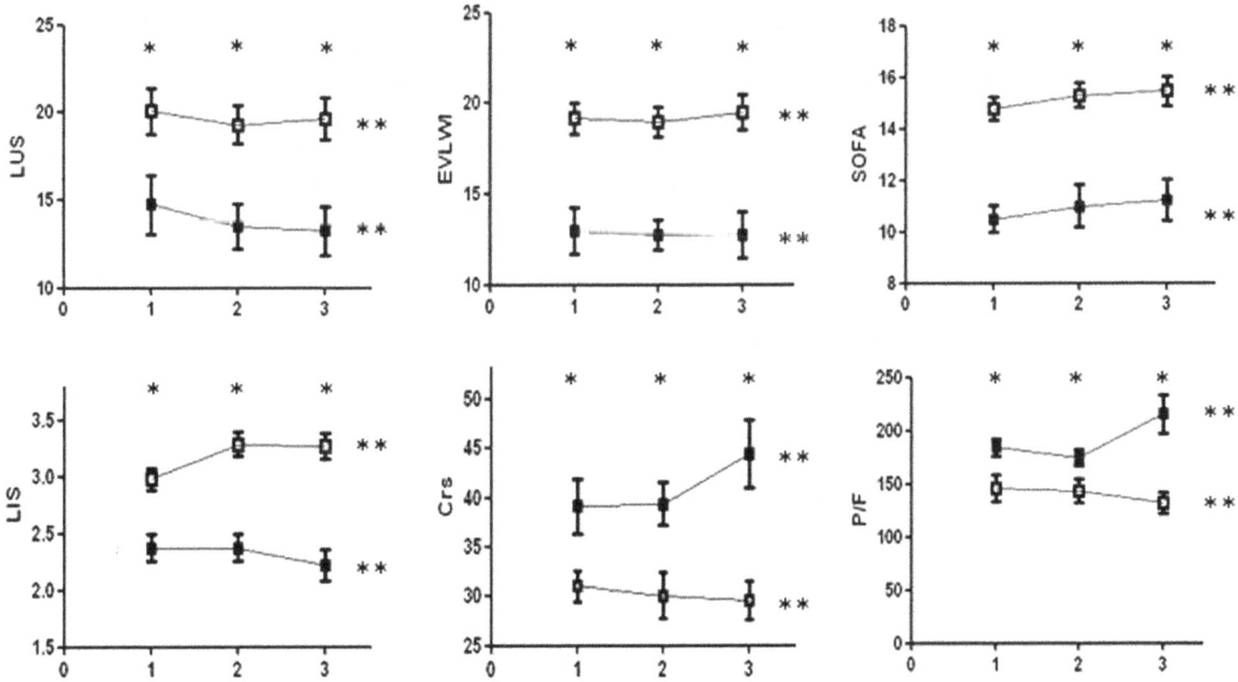

Fig. 2 Lung dysfunction in the first 3 days following diagnosis of acute respiratory distress syndrome. Non-survivors are represented by unfilled squares and survivors are represented by filled ones. Plots show the means of values of 3 days vs. time for the following: lung ultrasound score (LUS); EVLWI: extra-vascular lung water indexed to predicted body weight (EVLWI) measured by pulse index continuous cardiac output (PiCCO); sequential organ failure assessment (SOFA); lung injury score (LIS); static respiratory system compliance (Crs); PaO_2/FiO_2(P/F). *: $P < 0.05$, significant differences were found between the non-survivor and survivor groups. **: $P > 0.05$, no significant differences were found between the two groups on different days

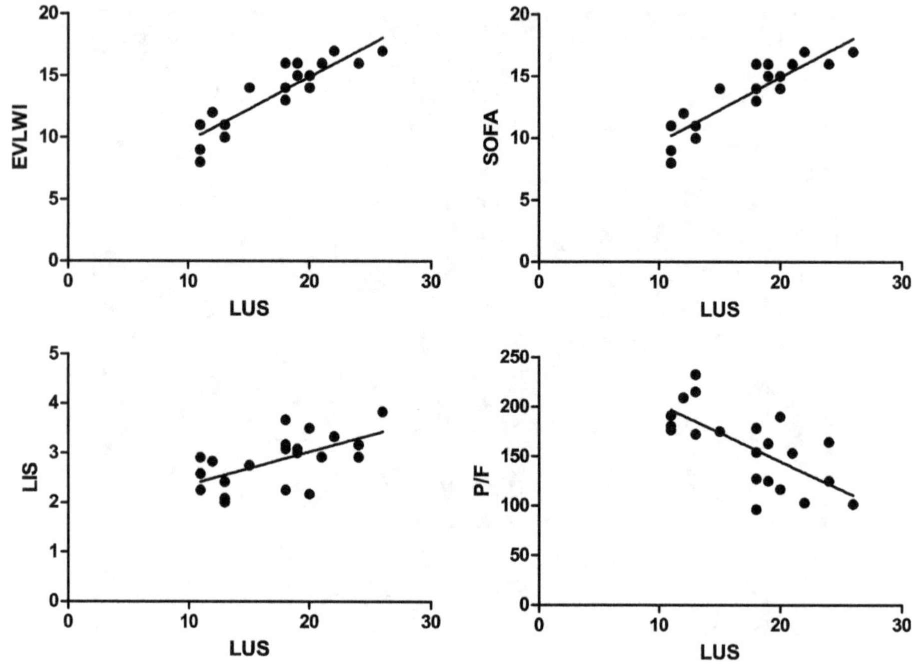

Fig. 3 Scatterplots demonstrating the correlation between lung ultrasound score (LUS) and lung dysfunction. The graphs show pooled average data for all 3 days for survivors and non-survivors. EVLWI, extravascular lung water indexed to predicted body weight; P/F PaO_2/FiO_2; SOFA, sequential organ failure assessment score; LIS, lung injury score. Significant positive linear correlations were found between LUS and EVLWI, SOFA, LIS, P/F (r^2 = 0.906, 0.815, 0.361, 0.472, $P < 0.01$)

Discussion

Increased EVLW is the most important pathophysiological sign of ARDS. Additionally, the severity of pulmonary edema is closely related to the prognosis of ARDS patients. Several quantitative methods are clinically used to assess EVLW [9]. Bedside chest X-ray film is the simplest method but it is difficult to immediately detect changes in EVLW using this method. Although semi-quantitative determinations of EVLW have been made, the scores obtained were found to have a large respective divergence and to be inaccurate [10, 11]. CT is the gold standard for assessing EVLW. Changes in CT images in regard to pleural effusion, pulmonary interstitial syndrome, and pulmonary consolidation clearly confirm the diagnosis of ARDS. Moreover, chest CT software has been developed to accurately measure EVLW. However, to perform a CT scan, the patient has to be moved to the CT room. This movement is particularly dangerous, especially for patients with severe unstable hemodynamics, and it may even threaten the patient's life [12, 13]. Recently, PiCCO technology has become widely used in clinics [14]. Kuzkovet al. found a positive linear correlation between EVLW and acute lung injury severity index (Crs, P/F, and LIS), and this

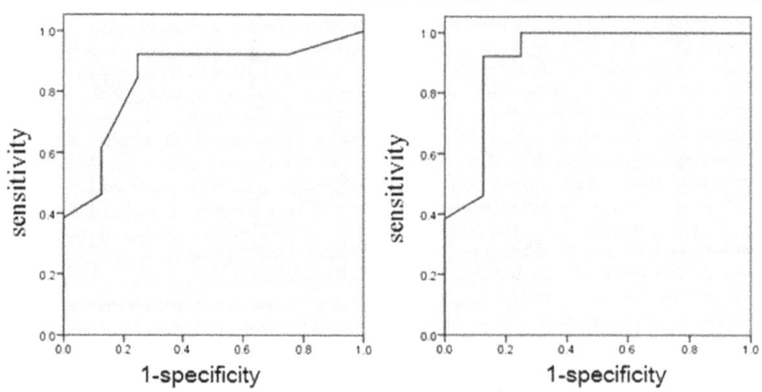

Fig. 4 Receiver operating characteristic curves of lung ultrasound score (LUS) and extra-vascular lung water (EVLW) for mortality. The area under the curve (95 % confidence interval [CI]) was 0.846 ± 0.91 and 0.918 ± 0.72 for LUS and EVLW, respectively

correlation can help doctors to effectively characterize the clinical prognosis of patients [15]. PiCCO technology can provide a quantitative determination of EVLW, and EVLWI has emerged as a widely used method to evaluate the severity of pulmonary edema. However, PiCCO technology is expensive, and the procedure is invasive, therefore it puts patients at risk of infection because of the use of a catheter, and this limits its clinical application.

Lung ultrasonography has been widely used to assess EVLW clinically in recent years. Jambrik et al. determined the relationship between lung ultrasound and chest X-ray using PiCCO technology to assess EVLW [16]. To date, lung ultrasound has been applied in differential diagnosis of the acute respiratory failure etiology [17], in the EVLW assessment of hemodialysis (HD) patients [18, 19], even more in the extravascular lung water assessment of heart failure patients [20, 21], concluding that lung ultrasound is a relatively new method which has gained a growing acceptance as a bedside diagnostic tool to assess pulmonary interstitial fluid and alveolar oedema [22]. Also, lung ultrasound has been applied in the selection of the best PEEP of ARDS patients [23]. PEEP > 5cmH_2O might aid in the prevention of alveolar collapse, improve the oxygenation state, and reduce ventilator-induced lung injury [24]. The strategy of low tidal volume and high PEEP ventilation could significantly reduce 28-day mortality in ARDS patients [25], increase the number of days of weaning success, and reduce the incidence of organ failure [26, 27]. However, the strategies of high PEEP ventilation and low PEEP ventilation did not show significant differences in regard to the prognosis of ARDS patients [28–30]. A meta-analysis showed that a high PEEP level could reduce the mortality of patients with moderate or severe ARDS (P/F ≤ 200 mmHg) but had no effect on the mortality of patients with mild ARDS [31].

Lung ultrasonography is rarely used in prognostic evaluation of ARDS patients. Frassi et al. divided patients with chest pain and dyspnea into mild, moderate, and severe groups based on the number of lung ultrasound comet tails (ULCs) and found a direct correlation between the number of ULCs and mortality rate [32]. Acute Physiology and Chronic Health Evaluation II and SOFA scores are good predictors of death risk in ARDS patients, while LIS and P/F have lower prognostic abilities [33–35]. Recently, EVLWI measured using PiCCO technology is being used with increasing frequency to assess ARDS prognosis. EVLWI is directly correlated with LIS, Crs, and, obviously, P/F [36–38]. Additionally, EVLWI of pediatric patients with acute respiratory distress could predict survival prognosis and mechanical ventilation duration [39]. A meta-analysis covering 670 patients in 11 studies of 9 countries showed that EVLWI was a better predictor of the mortality of severe patients [40].

In this study, LUS was closely related to several ARDS prognostic indices (EVLWI, LIS, Crs, and P/F) and was able to predict death risk and served as a diagnostic marker of ARDS. Early measurement of LUS is a better diagnostic indicator of acute lung injury than late measurement. Compared with other examinations, lung ultrasound is a non-invasive, economic, repeatable, simple, user-friendly, radiation-free bedside method for the prognosis of ARDS patients and for determination of the best treatment plan.

Conclusions

In summary, significant positive correlations were found between LUS and EVLWI measured by PiCCO. Both were effective clinical examination tools for the evaluation of ICU outcome in ARDS patients. Lung ultrasound diagnosis is simple, quick, non-invasive, economic, and rather accurate and is recommended for clinical use.

Abbreviations

ARDS: Acute respiratory distress syndrome; PiCCO: Pulse index continuous cardiac output; LUS: Lung ultrasound score; PBW: Predicted body weight; EVLW: Extra-vascular lung water; EVLWI: Extra-vascular lung water indexed to PBW; SOFA: Sequential organ failure assessment score; LIS: Lung injury score; P/F: PaO_2/FiO_2; ICU: Intensive care unit; PEEP: Positive end expiratory pressure; Crs: Static respiratory system compliance.

Competing interests

The authors declare that they have no competing interests.

Authors' contributions

LJ and ZZ conceived and planned the program. XMX participated in the design of the study and performed the statistical analysis. ZZ drafted the manuscript and revised it critically for important intellectual content. BZ and QJ recorded the patients' information. ZZ and MPW collected, analyzed, and interpreted the data. JX and DZ helped with lung ultrasound training. All authors read and approved the final manuscript.

Acknowledgments

The authors sincerely thank Dr. Bin Du (Division of Intensive Care Unit, Peking Union Medical College Hospital, China) for kindly contributing suggestions for the conception and design of this study. The authors also sincerely thank Dr. Xiaoxia Peng (School of Public Health, Capital Medical University, China) for her advice on the statistical analysis of the data. The study was undertaken with funding support from Beijing Municipal Science & Technology Commission No.Z121107001012125.

Author details

[1]Intensive Care Unit, Fuxing Hospital affiliated with Capital Medical University, Beijing 100038, China. [2]Department of Ultrasonography, Fuxing Hospital affiliated with Capital Medical University, Beijing 100038, China.

References

1. Irish Critical Care Trials Group. Acute lung injury and the acute respiratory distress syndrome in Ireland: a prospective audit of epidemiology and management. Critical Care. 2008;12:R30.
2. Rubenfeld G, Caldwell E, Granton J, Hudson LD, Matthay MA. Interobserver variability in applying a radiographic definition for ARDS. Chest. 1999;116:1347–53.
3. Rossi P, Rudehill A, Konrad D, Weitzberq E, Oldner A. Comparison of a single indicator and gravimetric technique for estimation of extravascular lung water in endotoxemic pigs. Crit Care Med. 2006;34:1437–43.
4. Volpicelli G. Lung sonography. J Ultrasound Med. 2013;32:165–17.

5. Volpicelli G, Skurzak S, Boero E, Carpinteri G, Tengattini M, Stefanone V, et al. Lung ultrasound predicts well extravascular lung water but is of limited usefulness in the prediction of wedge pressure. Anesthesiology. 2014;121:320–7.
6. ARDS Definition Task Force, Rubenfeld GD, Thompson BT, Ferguson ND, Galdwell E, Fan E, et al. Acute respiratory distress syndrome: the Berlin Definition. JAMA. 2012;307.
7. Katzenelson R, Perel A, Berkenstadt H, Preiman S, Kogan S, Sternik L, et al. Accuracy of transpulmonary thermodilution versus gravimetric measurement of extravascular lung water. Crit Care Med. 2004;32:1550–4.
8. Devine B. Gentamicin therapy. Drug Intell Clin Pharm. 1974;8:650–5.
9. Halperin BD, Feeley TW, Mihm FG, Chiles C, Guthaner DF, Blank NE. Evaluation of the portable chest roentgenogram for quantitating extravascular lung water in critically ill adults. Chest. 1985;88:649–52.
10. Giuntini C, Pistoles M, Miniati M, Fazio F. Theoretical and practical considerations of measuring extravascular lung water. J Thorac Imaging. 1988;3:36–43.
11. Pistolesi M, Giuntini C. Assessment of extravascular lung water. Radiol Clin North Am. 1978;16:551–74.
12. Malbouisson LM, Preteux F, Puybasset L, Grenier P, Coriat P, Rouby JJ. Validation of a software designed for computed tomographic (CT) measurement of lung water. Intensive Care Med. 2001;27:602–8.
13. Rouby JJ, Puybasset L, Nieszkowska A, Lu Q. Acute respiratory distress syndrome: lessons from computed tomography of the whole lung. Crit Care Med. 2003;31:S285–295.
14. Effros RM, Pornsuriyasak P, Porszasz J, Casaburi R. Indicator dilution measurements of extravascular lung water: basic assumptions and observations. Am J Physiol Lung Cell Mol Physiol. 2008;294:L1023–1031.
15. Kuzkov VV, Kirov MY, Sovershaev MA, Kuklin VN, Suborov EV, Waerhaug K, et al. Extravascular lung water determined with single transpulmonary thermodilution correlates with the severity of sepsis-induced acute lung injury. Crit Care Med. 2006;34:1647–53.
16. Jambrik Z, Monti S, Coppola V, Agricola E, Mottola G, Miniati M. Usefulness of ultrasound lung comets as a nonradiologic sign of extravascular lung water. Am J cardiol. 2004;93:1265–70.
17. Lichtenstein DA, Meziere GA. Relevance of lung ultrasound in the diagnosis of acute respiratory failure: the BLUE protocol. Chest. 2008;134:117–25.
18. Noble VE, Murray AF, Capp R, Syivia-reardon MH, Steele DJ, Liteplo A. Ultrasound assessment for extravascular lung water in patients undergoing hemodialysis. Time course for resolution. Chest. 2009;135:1433–9.
19. Mallamaci F, Benedetto FA, Tripepi R, Rastelli S, Castellino P, Tripepi G, et al. Detection of pulmonary congestion by chest ultrasound in dialysis patients. JACC Cardiovasc Imaging. 2010;3:586–94.
20. Agricola E, Bove T, Oppizzi M, Marino G, Zangriuo A, Margonato A, et al. "Ultrasound comet-tail images": a marker of pulmonary edema: a comparative study with wedge pressure and extravascular lung water. Chest. 2005;127:1690–5.
21. Agricola E, Picano E, Oppizzi M, Pisani M, Meris A, Fragasso G, et al. Assessment of stress-induced pulmonary interstitial edema by chest ultrasound during exercise echocardiography and its correlation with left ventricular function. J Am Soc Echocardiogr. 2006;19:457–63.
22. Volpicelli G, Melniker LA, Cardinale L, Lamorte A, Frascisco MF. Lung ultrasound in diagnosing and monitoring pulmonary interstitial fluid. Radiol Med. 2013;118:196–205.
23. Bouhemad B, Brisson H, Le-Guen M, Arbelot C, Lu Q, Rouby JJ. Bedside ultrasound assessment of positive end-expiratory pressure-induced lung recruitment. Am J Respir Crit Care Med. 2011;183:341–7.
24. Gattinoni L, Caironi P, Cressoni M, Chiumello D, Ranieri VM, Quintel M, et al. Lung recruitment in patients with the acute respiratory distress syndrome. N Engl J Med. 2006;354:1775–86.
25. The Acute Respiratory Distress Syndrome Network. Ventilation with lower tidal volumes as compared with traditional tidal volumes for acute lung injury and the acute respiratory distress syndrome. N Engl J Med. 2000;342:1301–8.
26. Amato MB, Barbas CS, Medeiros DM, Magaldi RB, Schetlino GP, Lorenzi-Filho G, et al. Effect of a protective-ventilation strategy on mortality in the acute respiratory distress syndrome. N Engl J Med. 1998;338:347–54.
27. Villar J, Kacmarek RM, Perez-Mendez L, Aguirre-Jaime AA. A high positive end-expiratory pressure, low tidal volume ventilatory strategy improves outcome in persistent acute respiratory distress syndrome: a randomized, controlled trial. Crit Care Med. 2006;34:1311–8.
28. Mercat A, Richard JC, Vielle B, Jaber S, Osman D, Diehl JL, et al. Positive end-expiratory pressure setting in adults with acute lung injury and acute respiratory distress syndrome: a randomized controlled trial. JAMA. 2008;299:646–55.
29. Meade MO, Cook DJ, Guyatt GH, Slutsky AS, Arabi YM, Cooper DJ, et al. Ventilation strategy using low tidal volumes, recruitment maneuvers, and high positive end-expiratory pressure for acute lung injury and acute respiratory distress syndrome: a randomized controlled trial. JAMA. 2008;299:637–45.
30. Brower RG, Lanken PN, MacIntyre N, Matthay MA, Morris A, Ancukiewicz M, et al. Higher versus lower positive end-expiratory pressures in patients with the acute respiratory distress syndrome. N Engl J Med. 2004;351:327–36.
31. Briel M, Meade M, Mercat A, Brower RG, Talmor D, Walter SD, et al. Higher vs lower positive end-expiratory pressure in patients with acute lung injury and acute respiratory distress syndrome: systematic review and meta-analysis. JAMA. 2010;303:865–73.
32. Frassi F, Gargani L, Tesorio P, Raciti M, Mottola G, Picano E. Prognostic value of extravascular lung water assessed with ultrasound lung comets by chest sonography in patients with dyspnea and/or chest pain. J Card Fail. 2007;13:830–5.
33. Luecke T, Muench E, Roth H, Friess U, Paul T, Kleinhuber K, et al. Predictors of mortality in ARDS patients referred to a tertiary care centre: a pilot study. Eur J Anaesthesiol. 2006;23:403–10.
34. Agarwal R, Aggarwal AN, Gupta D, Behera D, Jindal SK. Etiology and outcomes of pulmonary and extrapulmonary acute lung injury/ARDS in a respiratory ICU in North India. Chest. 2006;130:724–9.
35. Monchi M, Bellenfant F, Cariou A, Joly LM, Thebert D, Laurent I, et al. Early predictive factors of survival in the acute respiratory distress syndrome. A multivariate analysis. Am J Respir Crit Care Med. 1998;158:1076–81.
36. Berkowitz DM, Danai PA, Eaton S, Moss M, Martin GS. Accurate characterization of extravascular lung water in acute respiratory distress syndrome. Crit Care Med. 2008;36:1803–9.
37. Phillips CR, Chesnutt MS, Smith SM. Extravascular lung water in sepsis-associated acute respiratory distress syndrome: indexing with predicted body weight improves correlation with severity of illness and survival. Crit Care Med. 2008;36:69–73.
38. Craig TR, Duffy MJ, Shyamsundar M, McDowell C, McLaughlin B, Elborn JS, et al. Extravascular lung water indexed to predicted body weight is a novel predictor of intensive care unit mortality in patients with acute lung injury. Crit Care Med. 2010;38:114–20.
39. Lubrano R, Cecchetti C, Elli M, Tomasello C, Guido G, Di Nardo M, et al. Prognostic value of extravascular lung water index in critically ill children with acute respiratory failure. Intensive Care Med. 2011;37:124–31.
40. Zhang Z, Lu B, Ni H. Prognostic value of extravascular lung water index in critically ill patients: a systematic review of the literature. J Crit Care. 2012;27:420.e1–8.

3

Clinical course and complications following diagnostic bronchoalveolar lavage in critically ill mechanically ventilated patients

R M Schnabel[1*], K van der Velden[1], A Osinski[1], G Rohde[2], P M H J Roekaerts[1] and D C J J Bergmans[1]

Abstract

Background: Flexible, fibreoptic bronchoscopy (FFB) and bronchoalveolar lavage (BAL) have been used for diagnostic purposes in critically ill ventilated patients. The additional diagnostic value compared to tracheal aspirations in ventilator-associated pneumonia (VAP) has been questioned. Nevertheless, BAL can provide extra information for the differential diagnosis of respiratory disease and good antibiotic stewardship. These benefits should outweigh potential hazards caused by the invasiveness of this diagnostic technique. The focus of the present study was on the clinical course and complications of patients following BAL procedures up to 24 h.

Methods: Hundred sixty-four FFB guided BAL procedures for suspected pneumonia were analysed in an observational study. The clinical course of patients was monitored by respiratory and haemodynamic data before BAL, 1 and 24 h after BAL. Complications were defined and registered. Factors associated with complications were analysed by logistic regression.

Results: Clinical course: a decrease in average pO_2/FiO_2 ratio 1 h after BAL from 29 kPa (218 mmHg) to 25 kPa (189 mmHg) ($p < 0.05$) was observed which fully recovered within 24 h. Respiratory complications: the incidence of procedure related hypo-oxygenation ($SaO_2 \leq 88$ %) and/or bronchospasm was 9 %; a decrease of >25 % PaO_2/FiO_2 ratio 1 h after BAL was found in 29 % of patients; no bleeding or pneumothorax were registered. Haemodynamic complications: there were no cases of hypertension and cardiac rhythm disturbances; haemodynamic instability within the first 24 h after BAL was recorded in 22 %; this was correlated with a cardiovascular diagnosis at admission (OR 2.9; 95 % CI 1.2 - 6.7) and the presence of cardiovascular co-morbidity (OR 3.5; 95 % CI 1.5 – 8.3). The incidence of bacteraemia was 7 %. There was no case of procedure related death.

Discussion: Frequently occurring haemodynamic and respiratory instability but no cases of cardiac rhythm disturbances, bleeding, pneumothorax or procedure related death were attributable to diagnostic FFB and BAL. The procedures should be conducted under careful supervision by experienced physicians. Only a randomized controlled trial that compares diagnostic FFB and BAL with a non-invasive strategy could ultimately establish the safety profile and clinical utility of these procedures in critically ill ventilated patients.

Keywords: Bronchoalveolar lavage, Pneumonia, Safety, Complications, Critical care

* Correspondence: r.schnabel@mumc.nl
Summary at a glance: Benefits of bronchoalveolar lavage should outweigh potential hazards caused by the invasiveness of this diagnostic technique. The present study is the largest investigation on periprocedural complications and clinical course.
[1]Department of Intensive Care Medicine, Maastricht University Medical Centre+, P. Debyelaan 25, PO Box 5800, 6202 AZ Maastricht, The Netherlands
Full list of author information is available at the end of the article

Background

Flexible, fibreoptic bronchoscopy (FFB) and bronchoalveolar lavage (BAL) have been established for diagnostic purposes in critically ill ventilated patients in intensive care units (ICUs). The technique is applicable at the bedside and therefore makes potentially hazardous patient transfers outside the ICU unnecessary. With regard to the diagnosis of ventilator-associated pneumonia (VAP) there is no consensus in the literature and between clinicians. Bronchoscopic BAL from the presumed site of infection with cytological analysis and quantitative microbiological culture of the lavage fluid is thought by many to be a specific diagnostic approach to identify patients with a true infection of the lungs and to enable tailored antibiotic therapy. The most cited benefit of BAL is the prevention of incorrect use of antibiotics. The administration of unnecessary antibiotics is associated with risks of toxicity and development of multiresistance [1–3]. Others question the use of BAL because several investigations have shown similar outcome and overall use of antibiotics when clinical diagnostic criteria added by non-quantitative culture results from tracheal aspirations were used in the diagnosis of VAP [4, 5]. However, there are other benefits associated with the performance of BALs. Direct visualisation of the airway by FFB delivers additional clinical information and guides the selection of lung areas where specimens are taken [6, 7]. Moreover, the information provided by BAL analysis is more comprehensive than from tracheal aspirates as it not only can benefit the diagnosis of bacterial VAP [8] but can also support the diagnosis of alternative infectious causes [9] or other respiratory diseases [10].

In order to evaluate FFB and BAL as a diagnostic tool in ICU patients, it is necessary to balance benefits with potential hazards caused by the invasiveness of the technique. The focus of the present study is on the clinical tolerance of FFB and BAL. The clinical course and complications of critically ill mechanically ventilated patients after a diagnostic FFB and BAL were investigated. Clinical data were collected before BAL, 1 and 24 h after BAL. The frequency of haemodynamic, respiratory and procedure related complications were registered. This information can contribute to the discussion whether or not utility and benefits of the more invasive diagnostic approach outweigh its potential risks.

Methods

The study was conducted in the Maastricht University Medical Centre+, a tertiary-care, university hospital in the Netherlands with 1,700 ICU admissions per year. Adult critically ill, mechanically ventilated patients with a clinical suspicion of infectious pneumonia who underwent a diagnostic FFB and BAL were included in the analysis. Exclusion criteria for the procedure were thrombocytopenia (<40,000/μL) and other coagulation abnormalities. Only clinical data were used in the study. The data were collected retrospectively in 43 cases and prospectively in 121 cases in the period from 2011 to 2014. Patients consented to the use of clinical data for scientific analysis according to the admission regulations of the hospital if they did not opt out. This is approved by the local ethics commission (Medisch Ethische Toetsingscommissie azM).

Senior registrars or consultant pulmonologists conducted all BAL procedures. The fraction of inspired oxygen (FiO_2) was increased to 1.0 for 5 to 15 min prior to and during FFB and BAL procedures. Patients were *anaesthetised* by an experienced intensive care physician, present during the whole procedure, with either propofol or midazolam and fentanyl continuous infusion and as required rocuronium for muscle relaxation. Patients had tracheal tubes with an inner diameter varying from 7.5 to 8.5 mm or a Portex® tracheal cannula with an inner diameter of 8 mm in place. A flexible, fibreoptic bronchoscope (Pentax® FB-15H/FB-15X, Pentax Medicals, Tokyo, Japan) with a calibre of 4.9 mm was introduced and 'wedged' into the affected segmental or subsegmental bronchus. Before performing BAL, a quick inspection of all the major airways in both lungs was carried out. Sterile saline (0.9 % sodium chloride at room temperature) was instilled. An initial aliquot of 20 mL and subsequent four aliquots of 50 mL were immediately aspirated and recovered. After completing the BAL, the bronchoscope was removed, and the patient was monitored closely by continuous pulse oximetry and arterial blood gases while the FiO_2 was then gradually decreased. BAL samples were transported to the laboratory within 15 min after collection and processed immediately upon arrival. Information about the quality of BAL sampling was collected. The BAL fluid was regarded non-representative if the volume of recovery was <20 mL, the total cell count was < 60.000/mL, the presence of squamous epithelial cells was >1 %, the presence of bronchial epithelial cells was >5 % or in the presence of extensive amounts of debris and damaged cells. Further BAL workup in the laboratory included: a differential cell count, microscopic investigation of a Gram-stained preparation, quantitative bacterial and fungal culture. BAL fluid analysis was considered to support the diagnosis of VAP when Memphis Consensus Conference criteria were met. These criteria include: ≥2 % BAL fluid cells containing intracellular organisms, and/or identification of a bacterial micro-organism in the BAL fluid in a concentration of $\geq 10^4$ colony forming units/ml (cfu/mL) [11, 12]. Demographic characteristics and Acute Physiology and Chronic Health Evaluation (APACHE-II) scores were recorded on admission. All diagnoses apart from the principal reason for admission to the ICU were regarded as co-morbidities: 1. cardiovascular: severe ischemic heart disease, NYHA IV heart failure, disabling peripheral vascular disease; 2. respiratory: disabling chronic pulmonary disease, COPD Gold III and IV, continuous additional oxygen therapy; 3. chronic renal failure: chronic dialysis, serum creatinine level chronically > 177 µmol/L; 4. immunocompromised: disease and drug effects, prednisone equivalent > 7.5 mg/day; 5. active malignancy; 6. neurologic impairment: cerebral haemorrhage, meningitis, encephalitis, severe paresis; 7. chronic coagulation disorder; 8. chronic hepatic failure: hepatic encephalopathy, Child C cirrhosis, portal hypertension. Patients were classified as "severe sepsis" following the Surviving Sepsis Campaign criteria [13]. Clinical parameters were collected at baseline, at 1 h and 24 h after the BAL procedure. Blood cultures were obtained before and 24 h after the procedure, chest X-rays were performed within 24 h after BAL and sputum cultures were taken prior to the procedure. In general, the results of Gram staining, differential cell count and percentage of intracellular organisms of samples obtained by BAL were available within 2 h after bronchoscopy, preliminary culture results after 1 day, and definite culture results after 4 days. When BAL fluid analysis rejected the diagnosis of bacterial pneumonia, additional steps followed to determine an alternative diagnosis. Empirical antibiotic therapy was directed towards pathogens isolated from clinical and surveillance cultures of sputum cultures, and patients with VAP were treated with antibiotics for 8 to 14 days according to causative microorganisms. In case of clinical suspicion of pneumonia, antibiotic therapy was initiated after BAL had been performed. When a patient was receiving antibiotics for more than 48 h for another unrelated infection or for prophylaxis on the day that the criteria for a clinical suspicion of pneumonia were met, antibiotics were not changed until the BAL procedure.

The clinical course of the patients was monitored for 24 h after diagnostic FFB and BAL. PaO_2/FiO_2 ratios, positive end-expiratory pressure (PEEP) levels, fractions of oxygen (FiO_2), ph, $PaCo_2$, mean arterial pressure (MAP), heart rate and dosages of norepinephrine and dobutamine were assessed. Clinical complications of BAL were defined as complications occurring during the BAL procedure and up to 24 h after BAL. *1. Respiratory complications:* hypooxygenation ($SaO_2 \leq 88$ %) during BAL and/or bronchospasm; a decrease in PaO_2/FiO_2 ratio >25 % compared to baseline; bleeding defined as haemoptysis requiring medical intervention and/or interruption of the procedure; pneumothorax. *2. Haemodynamic complications:* hypertension defined as an increase of MAP >25 % baseline; cardiac rhythm disturbances defined as newly developed pathologic rhythm (atrial fibrillation, ventricular tachycardia, ventricular fibrillation, asystole) or bradycardia or rapid atrial fibrillation with decrease in MAP; haemodynamic instability defined as a decrease of MAP < 55 mmHg at any time and/or necessity to initiate norepinephrine > 0.15 µg/kg/min or dubutamine >5 µg/kg/min and/or the necessity to more than double the dose of norepinephrine or dobutamine. *3. Bacteraemia:* positive blood cultures following BAL. *4. Death:* procedure related death within 24 h. Possible correlations of demographic and clinical items (age, gender, APACHE II, SOFA, diagnosis at admission, severe sepsis, comorbidities) with a respiratory and hemodynamic complication following BAL were analysed by multiple logistic regression. Odds ratios with 95 % confidence interval were calculated.

Data were analysed using the SPSS version 20 statistical package for MS Windows. Quantitative variables were expressed as means with standard deviations (SD). Qualitative variables were reported with the percentage distribution of each of the categories. Fisher's Exact Test and Chi Square Test were used for the analyses of categorical variables and ANOVA analysis and Kruskal-Wallis test for numerical variables. Linear mixed models analysis was performed in all patients, excluding consecutive BALs in the same patients who underwent more than one BAL.

Results

A total of 164 datasets of FFB and BAL procedures were recorded during the study period.

Patient demographics are shown in Table 1. In 68 patients (41 %) analysis of BAL fluid supported the diagnosis bacterial pneumonia. The most frequently acquired micro-organisms were *Pseudomonas aeruginosa* (12), *Staphylococcus aureus* (5) and *Escherichia coli* (5). In retrospection 92 % of all BAL positive patients received adequate empiric antibiotic treatment. Ninety-six BAL fluid analyses were classified as negative. However, in 68 % of these an alternative diagnosis could be established in the following diagnostic process [Table 2]. In 26 patients there was a significant presence of viruses in the BAL fluid. In seven patients *Pneumocystis jiroveci* could be detected. Further diagnostic workup including computed tomography, lung biopsy, ultrasound examinations and advanced laboratory tests revealed a broad spectrum of alternative diagnoses in the putative ventilator-associated pneumonia patient not meeting lavage-based diagnostic criteria.

The clinical course of patients following diagnostic FFB and BAL is illustrated in Table 3. Baseline data before BAL were compared with data after 1 h and 24 h. The average PaO_2/FiO_2 ratio declined from 29 kPa (218 mmHg) to 25 kPa (189 mmHg) ($p < 0.05$) after 1 h but had reached baseline again after 24 h. The average PEEP level of 9.4 cmH_2O was not significantly increased after 1 h and kept constant after 24 h. After 1 h, PEEP level was increased in 7 % of patients and in

Table 1 Patient demographics

Age (years)		61	±14
Gender	male	116	71 %
	female	48	29 %
APACHE II		21	±9
SOFA (at time of BAL)		7	±4
Parameters (at time of BAL)	pH <7.25	10	6 %
	$PaCO_2 \geq$ 7.5kPa (56 mmHg)	9	5 %
	$PaO_2 \leq$ 8kPa (60 mmHg)	10	6 %
	PaO2/FiO2 ratio ≤ 13kPa (100 mmHg)	12	7 %
Diagnosis upon admission	respiratory	64	38 %
	cardiovascular	37	22 %
	haematological	19	11 %
	gastrointestinal	16	10 %
	trauma/orthopaedic	10	6 %
	neurological	12	7 %
	urogenital	3	2 %
	other	7	4 %
Severe Sepsis at admission		52	32 %
Co-morbidity	none	53	33 %
	one item	72	44 %
	two items	35	21 %
	≥ three items	4	2 %
Co-morbidity	cardiovascular	34	21 %
	respiratory	12	7 %
	chronic renal failure	8	5 %
	immunocompromised	47	29 %
	active malignancy	32	20 %
	neurologic impairment	17	10 %
	coagulation disorder	3	2 %
	chronic hepatic failure	2	1 %
BAL positive		68	41 %
ICU mortality		80	49 %
In-hospital mortality		90	55 %
Cause of death	cardiovascular	13	15 %
	persistent respiratory failure	24	27 %
	neurological impairment	9	10 %
	multi organ failure	10	11 %
	active malignancy	28	31 %
	other	4	4 %
	unknown	2	2 %

Results are given either as number, percentages or mean ± standard deviation

Table 2 Alternative diagnosis in patients with negative bacterial growth BAL result

BAL negative ($n = 96$)	
Viral	26
Pneumocystis jirovecii	7
Fungal	6
Heart failure	4
Bronchiolitis obliterans organizing pneumonia	3
Usual interstitial pneumonia	1
All trans retinoic acid (ATRA) syndrome	1
Pulmonary embolism; obstructive shock	2
Endocarditis	1
Abdominal sepsis with ARDS	4
Necrotizing pancreatitis	2
Abdominal ischaemia	1
Urinary tract sepsis with ARDS	2
Ovarian cancer with pulmonary metastases	1
Systemic lupus erythematosus	1
Toxic epidermal necrolysis	1
Postanoxic encephalopathy with multiple infarction	1
Myasthenia gravis	1
None established	31

15 % after 24 h. The average FiO_2 level of 52 % was not significantly altered after 1 h and had decreased to 43 % ($p < 0.0001$) 24 h after BAL. One hour after BAL, 27 % of patients had an increased FiO_2 of ≥ 10 % compared to baseline; after 24 h 8 % of patients had an increased FiO_2 of ≥ 10 % compared to baseline. The pH and $paCO_2$ were unchanged after 1 and 24 h compared to baseline. The averages of haemodynamic parameters (MAP, heart rate, number of patients receiving norepinephrine and/or dobutamine and dose) were not significantly different after 1 and 24 h from baseline.

The following complications of diagnostic FFB and BAL were registered. *1. Respiratory complications*: hypo-oxygenation ($SaO_2 \leq 88$ %) during BAL and/or bronchospasm was documented in 9 % of patients; a decrease of >25 % PaO_2/FiO_2 ratio compared to baseline was registered in 29 % of patients 1 h after BAL; in half of these patients a persisting decrease of >25 % PaO_2/FiO_2 ratio was found 24 h after BAL; no cases of clinically significant bleeding requiring interruption of the procedure or treatment were reported. Further analysis could not establish a significant correlation of respiratory complications with demographic or clinic items [Fig. 1]. *2. Haemodynamic complications:* no patients had hypertension or cardiac rhythm disturbances during the FFB and BAL procedure; hemodynamic instability (as defined in the methods section) was found

Table 3 Results - clinical course 1 h and 24 h after BAL procedure

	Before BAL	1 h after BAL	24 h after BAL
PaO_2/FiO_2 [kPa]	29 (CI 25–32)	25 (CI 23–29) $p < 0.05$	31 (CI 27–33)
PaO_2/FiO_2 [mmHg]	218 (CI 188–240)	189 (CI 173–218)	233 (CI 203–248)
PaO_2/FiO_2 decreased >25 % baseline [% of patients]		29 %	14 %
PEEP mean [cmH_2O]	9.4 (CI 9.1–9.8)	9.6 (CI 9.2–9.9)	9.6 (CI 9.2–10)
PEEP increased		7 %	15 %
FiO_2 mean [%]	52 (CI 49–55)	54 (CI 51–57)	43 (CI 41–46) $p < 0.0001$
FiO_2 increased ≥ 10 % baseline [% of patients]		27 %	8 %
pH mean	7.41 (CI 7.40–7.42)	7.40 (CI 7.39–7.41)	7.41 (CI 7.40–7.42)
pCO_2 mean [kPa]	5.2 (CI 5.0–5.4)	5.4 (CI 5.2–5.6)	5.2 (CI 5.0–5.4)
pCO_2 mean [mmHg]	39 (CI 38–41)	41 (CI 39–42)	39 (CI 38–41)
MAP mean [mmHg]	84 (CI 81–86)	79 (CI 76–81)	83 (CI 81–86)
Heart rate mean [beats/min]	96 (CI 93–100)	94 (CI 93–99)	91 (CI 88–94)
Norepinephrine [% of patients]	58 %	57 %	62 %
Norepinephrine median	0.125	0.109	0.125
1. quartile/3. Quartile [μg/kg/min]	0.050/0.201	0.075/0.202	0.068/0.219
Dobutamine [% of patients]	3 %	3 %	3 %
Dobutamine median	5	5	3
1. quartile/3. Quartile [μg/kg/min]	3/5	2/5	3/5
Hemodynamic instability[a] [% of patients]		5 %	7 %
Hemodynamic instability[a] at any time within 24 h [% of patients]			22 %

CI 95 % confidence interval, *MAP* mean arterial pressure, *PEEP* positive end-expiratory pressure, *FiO_2* fraction of inspired oxygen, *PaO_2* arterial partial oxygen pressure, *SOFA* sequential organ failure assessment
[a]decrease of mean arterial pressure (MAP) < 55 mmHg and/or necessity to initiate norepinephrine > 0.15 μg/kg/min / dubutamine >5 μg/kg/min and/or the necessity to more than double the dose of norepinephrine or dobutamine

in 5 % of patients 1 h after BAL and 7 % of patients 24 h after BAL. However, 22 % of patients had hemodynamic instability at any time during the first 24 h after BAL. This was correlated with a cardiovascular diagnosis at admission (OR 2.9; 95 % CI 1.2 - 6.7) and the presence of cardiovascular co-morbidity (OR 3.5; 95 % CI 1.5 - 8.3) [Fig. 2]. Multiple logistic regression revealed that the correlation was independent from age and gender (OR 2.3; 95 % CI 1 – 5.6 / OR 2.8; 95 % CI 1.1 – 6.7) and the APACHE II score at admission (OR 3.5; 95 % CI 1.5 – 8.5 / OR 3.5; 95 % CI 1.4 – 8.6) 3. *Bacteraemia:* newly positive blood cultures were observed in 7 % of patients. 4. *Death:* no case of procedure related death was reported.

Discussion

The present observational study monitored the 24 h clinical course and complications following diagnostic FFB and BAL in critically ill ventilated patients. Patients' characteristics illustrate the severity of illness before BAL procedures. The high percentage of patients with active malignancy, immunosuppression and neurologic impairment can be explained by the function of the hospital as referral centre for haematology, oncology, immunologic diseases and neurosurgery.

Following diagnostic FFB and BAL there were no cases of cardiac rhythm disturbances, bleeding, pneumothorax or procedure related death during this study. Nevertheless, haemodynamic (22 %) and respiratory (29 %) instability

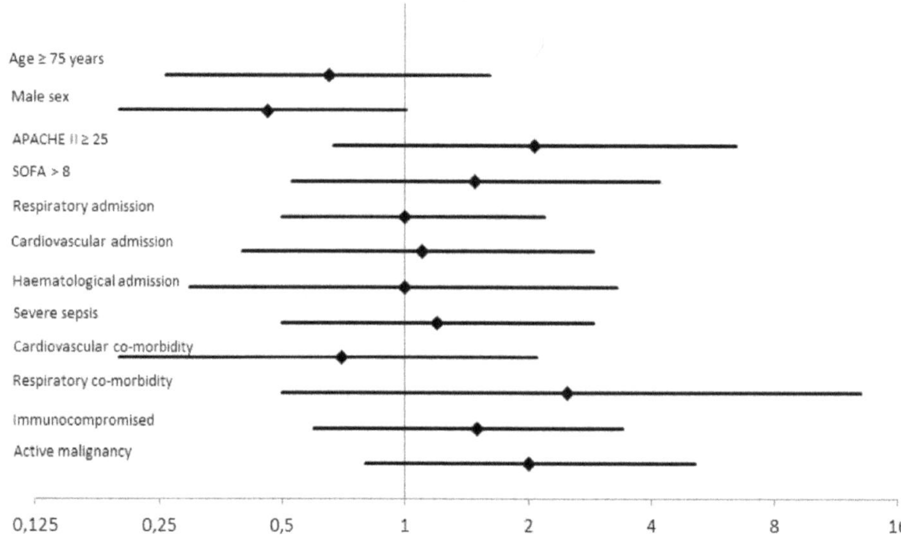

Fig. 1 Results – Odds ratios and 95 % confidence interval for respiratory complications[1] of BAL. [1] Decrease of the $PaO_2/FiO_2 > 25$ % compared to baseline within 1 h after BAL

according to the applied definitions were frequently recorded. Due to the complexity of human nature, physiology and pathophysiologic mechanisms of diseases, there might be no simple and consistent definition of respiratory and haemodynamic instability. It has been notoriously difficult to define cut-off variables with regard to vital parameters in clinical trials and practice [14–16]. A single vital parameter or even a set of absolute values of vital parameters will rarely suffice. For example in patients with preserved or abolished

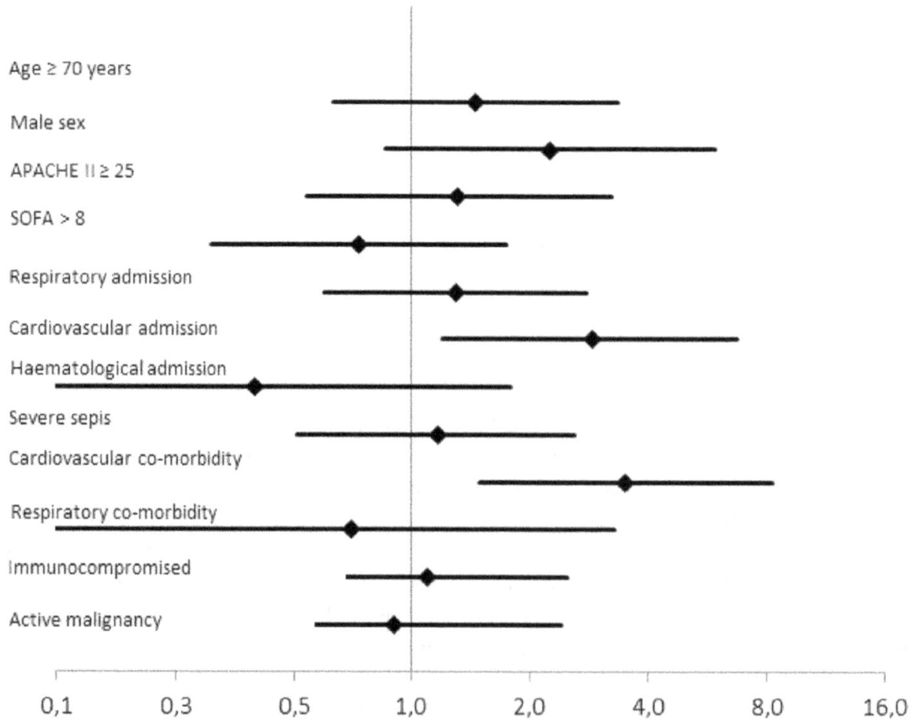

Fig. 2 Results – Odds ratios with 95 % confidence interval for hemodynamic complications [1] of BAL. A cardiovascular diagnosis upon admission and cardiovascular co-morbidity are associated with significantly more hemodynamic complications. [1]Decrease of mean arterial pressure (MAP) < 55 mmHg at any time and/or necessity to initiate norepinephrine > 0.15 μg/kg/min / dubutamine >5 μg/kg/min and/or the necessity to more than double the dose of norepinephrine or dobutamine

autoregulation the same absolute value of MAP can have different effects on the blood flow and vital functions. Hemodynamic and respiratory variables in critical care and ventilated patients markedly interact. MAP and heart rate should be related to dosages of inotropic and vasoactive medication; partial pressure of oxygen should always be correlated with the applied fraction of oxygen and PEEP level. Relative changes of vital parameters with regard to baseline might provide a better assessment of the impact of invasive diagnostic techniques. The definitions for respiratory and hemodynamic complications in the present study were eventually based on pathophysiologic reasoning, earlier publications of bronchoscopy associated complications [17, 18] and literature [19]. Haemodynamic instability in the study population was associated with a cardiovascular diagnosis at admission or presence of cardiovascular co-morbidity reflecting an expected causal relationship. Interestingly these two risk factors were independent from age, gender and APACHE II score. Haemodynamic changes could have been influenced by cardiovascular effects of the applied anaesthetic drugs to facilitate the procedure, as judged by the supervising physician. Hypo-oxygenation ($SaO_2 \leq 88$ %) during BAL and/or bronchospasm occurred in 9 % of patients and was always manageable and did not necessitate terminating the procedure. Nevertheless, 1 h after BAL there was a significant decrease in the average PaO_2/FiO_2 ratio which fully recovered to baseline after 24 h. Average PEEP and FiO_2 levels remained constant. After 24 h more patients had PEEP adjustment than 1 h after BAL explaining the decrease of the average FiO_2 from 52 to 43 %.

Altogether, haemodynamic and respiratory instability could be attributed to FFB and BAL in a substantial number of patients. This is in line with previous studies concerning the safety of bronchoscopic diagnostic techniques in critical care patients. Table 4 provides an overview of the literature [17, 18, 20–25]. The studies differ in patient population, setting, applied diagnostic technique and length of observation. All authors described a certain impact of diagnostic FFB on respiratory mechanics, respiratory and hemodynamic parameters.

To warrant a high procedural safety level of FFB and BAL in ICU patients, a structured approach is mandatory [6]. An experienced bronchoscopist should concentrate on the procedure while another physician surveys the patient, regulates analgosedation and adjusts the support of vital functions as necessary. The benefits of a BAL should be weighed against the potential additional harm for the patient secondary to the invasiveness of the procedure and the additional costs as compared to less invasive diagnostic measures. There is ongoing discussion on the pros and cons of BAL in the diagnosis of VAP. In this study, the majority of patients had a substantial benefit from the BAL. In 41 % of patients the diagnosis of bacterial pneumonia was confirmed by BAL fluid analysis. In a further 24 % of patients a viral or fungal infection or *Pneumocystis jiroveci* pneumonia could be diagnosed. When no infectious cause in the BAL fluid analysis was detected, the medical team was urged to look for non-infectious diagnoses without any delay and to adjust the therapy. This practice could beneficially affect the patients' outcome and at the same time reduce unnecessary antibiotic use. The

Table 4 Results of studies with regard to bronchoscopically guided diagnostic techniques in ICU patients

Reference	Year	Patients	Setting	Results
Trouillet et al. [20]	1990	$N = 107$	acutely ill ventilated patients; bronchial brush	26 % of patients ($p < 0.01$) with a drop in PaO_2; modest alterations in mean systolic blood pressure related to sedation; six patients developed arrhythmias during the procedure
Montravers et al. [21]	1993	$N = 30$	mechanically ventilated patients; BAL	mild haemodynamic variations but a marked decrease in PaO_2 during bronchoscopy with a maximum at the end of the procedure that not fully recovered up to 2 h thereafter
Steinberg et al. [17]	1993	$N = 110$	ARDS patients; BAL	21 patients with a moderate to severe drop in PaO_2/FiO_2; four patients with a decrease of mean arterial pressure < 60 mmHg; six patients developed arrhythmias during the procedure; one pneumothorax; two cases of bacteraemia within 24 h
Turner et al. [25]	1994	$N = 107$	intensive care patients; bronchial brush	study describes therapeutic and diagnostic fiberoptic bronchoscopies; 23 bronchial brush procedures included; low rate of complications (4.1 %); none with long-term sequelae
Bauer et al. [22]	2001	$N = 37$	mechanically ventilated patients; BAL	patients showed a lower PaO_2/FiO_2 ratio and higher MAP after BAL up to 24 h
Chou et al. [23]	2009	$N = 56$	mechanically ventilated patients; BAL	alterations in respiratory mechanics more pronounced by BAL in patients with intrinsic positive end-expiratory pressure before the procedure was started
Estella [24]	2010	$N = 50$	Mechanically ventilated patients; BAL	respiratory mechanics during BAL procedures showed significant decrease in lung compliance and increase in resistance that only reached baseline after 90 min to 3 h
Estella [18]	2012	$N = 148$	ICU patients; BAL	desaturations <90 % (7 %), supraventricular tachycardia (4 %) and slight bronchial bleeding (2 %)

latter becomes increasingly important with the rapid emergence and dissemination of multi-drug resistant microorganisms particularly in the ICU environment worldwide [26]. Antibiotic stewardship programs (ASPs) were developed to address the problem and ensure a responsible use of antimicrobial drugs [27, 28]. The diagnostic BAL can be implemented in an ASP and deliver important information to confirm an infectious disease, to optimize antimicrobial treatment (e.g. in the presence of *Pneumocystis jiroveci*), to de-escalate and narrow antibiotic therapy once the responsible pathogen is known and to stop antibiotic therapy in patients unlikely to have infections [27, 29].

Limitations of the study are its observational design of FFB and BAL as standard of care in a single centre without a randomized control group. Part of the included cases were retrospectively collected. In the assessment of a long term clinical course it might be difficult to differentiate the natural course of the underlying disease from the impact of the bronchoscopic intervention. Evidently, FFB and BAL procedures should not be performed in patients in a deplorable clinical condition. Unfortunately, the present study does not allow to define clear-cut clinical criteria for withholding FFB and BAL because the limited number of patients with severe acidosis (pH < 7.25; n = 10), hypercapnia (PaCo2 ≥ 7.5kPa/56 mmHg; n = 9) and hypoxia (PaO2 ≤ 8kPa/60 mmHg; n = 10 or PaO2/FiO2 ratio ≤13kPa/100 mmHg; n = 12). Further limitation is the lack of the measurement of respiratory mechanics before, during and after FFB.

Conclusion

Frequently occurring haemodynamic and respiratory instability could be attributable to diagnostic FFB and BAL but no cases of cardiac rhythm disturbances, bleeding, pneumothorax or procedure related death were observed in the present study. The procedures should be conducted under careful supervision by experienced physicians. Only a randomized controlled trial that compares diagnostic FFB and BAL with a non-invasive strategy could ultimately establish the safety profile and clinical utility of these procedures in critically ill ventilated patients.

Competing interests

The authors declare that they have no competing interests.

Authors' contributions

RS, DB and PR participated in the design of the study. RS, KvdV and AO collected the data and participated in the statistical analysis. GR gave advise with regard to bronchoalveolar lavage procedures. RS and KvdV drafted the manuscript. All authors read and approved the final manuscript.

Authors' information

Not applicable.

Acknowledgments

The authors acknowledge Bjorn Winkens for advise and support with regard to the statistical analysis.

Funding

There was no funding or financial support of this study.

Author details

[1]Department of Intensive Care Medicine, Maastricht University Medical Centre+, P. Debyelaan 25, PO Box 5800, 6202 AZ Maastricht, The Netherlands. [2]Department of Respiratory Medicine, Maastricht University Medical Centre+, Maastricht, The Netherlands.

References

1. Fagon JY, Chastre J, Wolff M, Gervais C, Parer-Aubas S, Stephan F, et al. Invasive and noninvasive strategies for management of suspected ventilator-associated pneumonia. A randomized trial. Ann Intern Med. 2000;132:621–30.
2. Shorr AF, Sherner JH, Jackson WL, Kollef MH. Invasive approaches to the diagnosis of ventilator-associated pneumonia: a meta-analysis. Crit Care Med. 2005;33:46–53.
3. Fagon JY. Diagnosis and treatment of ventilator-associated pneumonia: fiberoptic bronchoscopy with bronchoalveolar lavage is essential. Semin Respir Crit Care Med. 2006;27:34–44. doi:10.1055/s-2006-933672.
4. Canadian Critical Care Trials, G. A randomized trial of diagnostic techniques for ventilator-associated pneumonia. N Engl J Med. 2006;355:2619–30. doi:10.1056/NEJMoa052904.
5. Berton DC, Kalil AC, Teixeira PJ. Quantitative versus qualitative cultures of respiratory secretions for clinical outcomes in patients with ventilator-associated pneumonia. Cochrane Database Syst Rev. 2014;10:CD006482. doi:10.1002/14651858.CD006482.pub4.
6. Meduri GU, Chastre J. The standardization of bronchoscopic techniques for ventilator-associated pneumonia. Chest. 1992;102:557S–64.
7. Timsit JF, Misset B, Azoulay E, Renaud B, Garrouste-Orgeas M, Carlet J. Usefulness of airway visualization in the diagnosis of nosocomial pneumonia in ventilated patients. Chest. 1996;110:172–9.
8. Kirtland SH, Corley DE, Winterbauer RH, Springmeyer SC, Casey KR, Hampson NB, et al. The diagnosis of ventilator-associated pneumonia: a comparison of histologic, microbiologic, and clinical criteria. Chest. 1997;112:445–57.
9. Linssen CF, Jacobs JA, Stelma FF, van Mook WN, Terporten P, Vink C, et al. Herpes simplex virus load in bronchoalveolar lavage fluid is related to poor outcome in critically ill patients. Intensive Care Med. 2008;34:2202–9. doi:10.1007/s00134-008-1231-4.
10. Linssen KC, Jacobs JA, Poletti VE, van Mook W, Cornelissen EI, Drent M. Reactive type II pneumocytes in bronchoalveolar lavage fluid. Acta Cytol. 2004;48:497–504.
11. Linssen CF, Jacobs JA, Schouten JS, van Mook WN, Ramsay G, Drent M. Influence of antibiotic therapy on the cytological diagnosis of ventilator-associated pneumonia. Intensive Care Med. 2008;34:865–72. doi:10.1007/s00134-008-1015-x.
12. Bonten MJ, Bergmans DC, Stobberingh EE, van der Geest S, De Leeuw PW, van Tiel FH, et al. Implementation of bronchoscopic techniques in the diagnosis of ventilator-associated pneumonia to reduce antibiotic use. Am J Respir Crit Care Med. 1997;156:1820–4. doi:10.1164/ajrccm.156.6.9610117.
13. Dellinger RP, Levy MM, Rhodes A, Annane D, Gerlach H, Opal SM, et al. Surviving Sepsis Campaign: international guidelines for management of severe sepsis and septic shock, 2012. Intensive Care Med. 2013;39:165–228. doi:10.1007/s00134-012-2769-8.
14. Bijker JB, van Klei WA, Kappen TH, van Wolfswinkel L, Moons KG, Kalkman CJ. Incidence of intraoperative hypotension as a function of the chosen definition: literature definitions applied to a retrospective cohort using automated data collection. Anesthesiology. 2007;107:213–20. doi:10.1097/01.anes.0000270724.40897.8e.
15. Lonjaret L, Lairez O, Minville V, Geeraerts T. Optimal perioperative management of arterial blood pressure. Integr blood press control. 2014;7:49–59. doi:10.2147/IBPC.S45292.
16. Sevransky JE, Nour S, Susla GM, Needham DM, Hollenberg S, Pronovost P. Hemodynamic goals in randomized clinical trials in patients with sepsis: a systematic review of the literature. Crit Care. 2007;11:R67. doi:10.1186/cc5948.

17. Steinberg KP, Mitchell DR, Maunder RJ, Milberg JA, Whitcomb ME, Hudson LD. Safety of bronchoalveolar lavage in patients with adult respiratory distress syndrome. Am Rev Respir Dis. 1993;148:556–61. doi:10.1164/ajrccm/148.3.556.
18. Estella A. Analysis of 208 flexible bronchoscopies performed in an intensive care unit. Med Intensiva. 2012;36:396–401. doi:10.1016/j.medin.2011.11.005.
19. Walsh M, Devereaux PJ, Garg AX, Kurz A, Turan A, Rodseth RN, et al. Relationship between intraoperative mean arterial pressure and clinical outcomes after noncardiac surgery: toward an empirical definition of hypotension. Anesthesiology. 2013;119:507–15. doi:10.1097/ALN.0b013e3182a10e26.
20. Trouillet JL, Guiguet M, Gibert C, Fagon JY, Dreyfuss D, Blanchet F, et al. Fiberoptic bronchoscopy in ventilated patients. Evaluation of cardiopulmonary risk under midazolam sedation. Chest. 1990;97:927–33.
21. Montravers P, Gauzit R, Dombret MC, Blanchet F, Desmonts JM. Cardiopulmonary effects of bronchoalveolar lavage in critically ill patients. Chest. 1993;104:1541–7.
22. Bauer TT, Torres A, Ewig S, Hernandez C, Sanchez-Nieto JM, Xaubet A, et al. Effects of bronchoalveolar lavage volume on arterial oxygenation in mechanically ventilated patients with pneumonia. Intensive Care Med. 2001;27:384–93.
23. Chou MY, Ou CY, Chen CW. Alterations in respiratory mechanics in mechanically ventilated patients following bronchoalveolar lavage. J Formos Med Assoc. 2009;108:704–12. doi:10.1016/S0929-6646(09)60393-4.
24. Estella A. Effects on respiratory mechanics of bronchoalveolar lavage in mechanically ventilated patients. J bronchology & interv pulmonol. 2010;17:228–31. doi:10.1097/LBR.0b013e3181e846ee.
25. Turner JS, Willcox PA, Hayhurst MD, Potgieter PD. Fiberoptic bronchoscopy in the intensive care unit–a prospective study of 147 procedures in 107 patients. Crit Care Med. 1994;22:259–64.
26. Laxminarayan R, Duse A, Wattal C, Zaidi AK, Wertheim HF, Sumpradit N, et al. Antibiotic resistance-the need for global solutions. Lancet Infect Dis. 2013;13:1057–98. doi:10.1016/S1473-3099(13)70318-9.
27. Arnold HM, Micek ST, Skrupky LP, Kollef MH. Antibiotic stewardship in the intensive care unit. Semin Respir Crit Care Med. 2011;32:215–27. doi:10.1055/s-0031-1275534.
28. Goff DA. Antimicrobial stewardship: bridging the gap between quality care and cost. Curr Opin Infect Dis. 2011;24 Suppl 1:S11–20. doi:10.1097/01.qco.0000393484.17894.05.
29. Luyt CE, Brechot N, Trouillet JL, Chastre J. Antibiotic stewardship in the intensive care unit. Crit Care. 2014;18:480. doi:10.1186/s13054-014-0480-6.

4

Diagnostic accuracy of nasal nitric oxide for establishing diagnosis of primary ciliary dyskinesia

Panayiotis Kouis[1*], Stefania I. Papatheodorou[1] and Panayiotis K. Yiallouros[1,2]

Abstract

Background: To date, diagnosis of Primary Ciliary Dyskinesia (PCD) remains difficult and challenging. We systematically evaluated the diagnostic performance of nasal Nitric Oxide (nNO) measurement for the detection of PCD, using either velum-closure (VC) or non-velum-closure (non-VC) techniques.

Methods: All major electronic databases were searched from inception until March 2015 using appropriate terms. The sensitivity and specificity of nNO measurement was calculated in PCD patients diagnosed by transmission electron microscopy, high speed video-microscopy or genetic testing. Summary receiver operating characteristic (HSROC) curves were drawn using the parameters of the fitted models.

Results: Twelve studies provided data for 13 different populations, including nine case–control ($n = 793$) and four prospective cohorts ($n = 392$). The overall sensitivity of nNO measured by VC techniques was 0.95 (95 % CI 0.91–0.97), while specificity was 0.94 (95 % CI 0.88–0.97). The positive likelihood ratio (LR+) of the test was 15.8 (95 % CI 8.1–30.6), whereas the negative likelihood ratio (LR-) was 0.06 (95 % CI 0.04–0.09). For non-VC techniques, the overall sensitivity of nNO measurement was 0.93 (95 % CI 0.89–0.96) whereas specificity was 0.95 (95 % CI 0.82–0.99). The LR+ of the test was 18.5 (95 % CI 4.6–73.8) whereas the LR- was 0.07 (95 % CI 0.04–0.12).

Conclusions: Diagnostic accuracy of nNO measurement both with VC and non-VC maneuvers is high and can be effectively employed in the clinical setting to detect PCD even in young children, thus potentiating early diagnosis. Measurement of nNO merits to be part of a revised diagnostic algorithm with the most efficacious combination of tests to achieve PCD diagnosis.

Keywords: Primary Ciliary Dyskinesia, Nitric oxide, Kartagener syndrome, Diagnosis

Background

Primary ciliary dyskinesia (PCD) is a rare, hereditary disorder characterized by impaired mucociliary clearance [1]. Apart from situs inversus in ~50 % of the cases, the main manifestations of the disease are not specific. Nevertheless, the associated recurrent sinopulmonary infections eventually lead to severe chronic lung disease and development of bronchiectasis [2, 3].

While some centers began using targeted genetic testing [4], the diagnosis of PCD in the majority of centers currently relies on an array of different sophisticated tests namely the High Speed Video Microscopy (HSVM) for ciliary motility assessment [5], Transmission Electron Microscopy (TEM) for the examination of cilia ultrastructure [6] and nasal nitric oxide (nNO) measurement [7]. The diversity of the employed diagnostic tests reflects the lack of a golden diagnostic standard and the weaknesses and inaccuracies that characterize each of these tests. In particular, TEM examination of ciliary axonemes exhibits normal ultrastructure in confirmed patients with biallelic mutations in certain disease-causing genes such as DNAH11 [8], while the motility patterns observed by HSVM vary widely depending on the implicated genetic variant [9, 10].

Nasal nitric oxide (nNO) is abnormally low in PCD patients [11] and it has been part of the diagnostic work-up

* Correspondence: panagiotis.kouis@cut.ac.cy
[1]Cyprus International Institute for Environmental & Public Health in Association with Harvard School of Public Health, Cyprus University of Technology, 95 Irenes Street, 3041 Limassol, Cyprus
Full list of author information is available at the end of the article

in many PCD centers [12]. Current American Thoracic Society/European Respiratory Society (ATS/ERS) guidelines for nNO measurements recommend air aspiration via a nasal probe while the subject exhales through the mouth against resistance in order to maintain velum closure. Alternative techniques to maintain velum closure such as breath hold or pursed- lip breathing via the mouth are also acceptable [13]. However, velum closure requires cooperation and this precludes the performance of these techniques in young children. Few reports have investigated the discriminative ability of nNO measurements with the velum open as in the case of tidal breathing [3, 14] with encouraging findings for the usefulness of this technique in screening for PCD in younger children and adults unable to perform velum closure.

In view of the above specific restrictions and weaknesses, for the clinicians and the patients it remains of key importance to appraise the potential diagnostic value of each of the available diagnostic tests for PCD, in order to find its place in the armamentarium for elicitation of the diagnosis of the disease. A recent systematic review and meta-analysis summarized the published evidence on the measurement of nNO in PCD and reported on the mean difference of nNO production values obtained during velum closure techniques in PCD patients versus healthy controls (231 nL/min, 95 % CI: 193.3–268.9) and cystic fibrosis patients (114.1 nL/min, 95 % CI: 101.5–126.8) [15]. However, that report did not perform a meta-analysis on the diagnostic accuracy of nNO measurements in order to provide synthesized data on the potential diagnostic value this test may have in future algorithms for PCD diagnosis, which would be particularly informative in clinical decision making. The aim of this study was to systematically evaluate the diagnostic performance of nNO measurement as obtained either with a velum-closure or a non-velum-closure technique in screening for PCD so as to provide appropriate summary estimates of diagnostic accuracy with each breathing technique and demonstrate the summary trade-off between sensitivity and specificity across the included studies.

Methods

Search strategy and selection criteria

The electronic databases PubMed, SCOPUS, Cochrane Database of Systematic Reviews and Google Scholar were searched from inception until March 2015 using the keywords: 'nasal nitric oxide', "nNO", "nasal NO", "Primary Ciliary Dyskinesia", "PCD", "lung", "pulmonary", "pulm*", "cilia" either in the title or the abstract or using MeSH terms. The references of eligible studies were further examined for possible missing articles. We included studies which were identified after two reviewers (PK, SIP) independently screened the title and abstract of the obtained search results. Final selection was based on full text evaluation. Any disagreements were resolved by discussion and in case of discrepancy, by a third researcher (PKY). As this study is based on a systematic review of the previously published literature, an ethical approval was not obtained, since there is no potential of participant identification and ethical approval and consent was already obtained at the individual study level. The guidelines of the Preferred Reporting Items for Systematic Reviews and Meta-Analyses (PRISMA) were followed.

The validity of each primary study was assessed using the Quality Assessment of Diagnostic Accuracy Studies -2 (QUADAS-2) tool [16], that evaluates the risk of bias and applicability of diagnostic accuracy studies. It consists of four key domains: patient selection, index test, reference standard, flow and timing. Each is assessed in terms of risk of bias and the first three in terms of issues regarding applicability.

Studies were considered eligible if they provided data on the sensitivity and specificity of nNO for the diagnosis of PCD in order to construct a 2 × 2 table for each study calculating true positives (TP), false negatives (FN), false positives (FP) and true negatives (FN) for the presence or not of PCD according to nNO values set as a cut-off in each study. In some studies, the numbers were not provided per se but it was possible to extract them from other manuscript data sources. In case of incomplete information, we contacted the authors of the primary studies. Studies that reported only mean values of nNO were not included in our analyses as they did not provide data for computing summary diagnostic accuracy estimates (sensitivity, specificity, positive and negative likelihood ratio). Disease status in each selected study was required to have been confirmed by TEM and/or HSVM or genetic testing. Additional information on NO analyzer type, flow rate and breathing maneuver was also collected and used in data synthesis. Studies that did not report the equipment and flow rate used were not considered eligible as well as studies that may have used flow rate outside of the ATS/ERS recommended range (0.25–3 L/min) [13]. Cut-off values for the nNO test, were usually reported in parts per billion (ppb) and were transformed to NO production rate units (nl/min), using the conversion formula concentration (ppb) × sampling rate (L/min) as used previously [7], in order to account for the used different flow rates. Breathing maneuvers such as breath hold (BH) and exhalation against resistance (ER) were categorized as velum closure (VC) techniques and in case of both maneuvers performed by the study subjects; only results for the ER maneuver were included as the most validated technique according to ATS/ERS guidelines [13]. For studies employing the non-velum closure (non-VC) technique, only results of nNO measurements that were performed during tidal breathing (TB) with mouth open were included in the meta-analysis.

Data extraction

The name of author, study design, publication year, country of origin, study population sample size, age distribution of study population subgroups, nNO cut-off levels, information on the measurement method and the test(s) used for the diagnosis of PCD were recorded for each study. Data on the values of TP, TN, FP, FN were extracted independently by two reviewers (PK, SIP). A third investigator (PKY) settled any discrepancies and consensus was reached for all data.

Analysis

A bivariate model was used to calculate estimates of overall sensitivity and overall specificity. We fitted a two-level mixed logistic regression model conditional on the sensitivity and the specificity of each study and a bivariate normal model for the sensitivity and specificity between studies [17]. This method combines information from multiple thresholds and the output is expressed as a hierarchical summary receiver operator curve (HSROC). The HSROC describes the relationship between sensitivity and specificity derived from the individual receiver operator curves (ROC) of each study. Following this method, it describes the 'average' relationship between a continuous cut-off value and discriminatory ability in the 'average' population. This maximizes the amount of information used in the evidence synthesis and better represents the available data. The advantage of this method is that it allows clinicians to estimate how changing thresholds will alter the diagnostic utility of the test under study. All calculations are performed using STATA (Version 12, StataCorp, College Station, Texas) with the commands metandi and metandi plots for analyses of four studies and above [18].

We also reported the summary likelihood ratios across all studies. These measures also combine in their calculation both sensitivity and specificity. Positive likelihood ratio (LR+) is the ratio of sensitivity/(1-specificity), whereas negative likelihood ratio (LR-) is defined as the ratio of (1-sensitivity)/specificity. When there is absolutely no discriminating ability for a diagnostic test, both ratios are equal to 1. The discriminating ability is better with higher LR+ and lower LR-. A good diagnostic test has typically LR+ greater than 5.0 and LR- less than 0.2 [19].

VC and non-VC measurements were analyzed separately and this allowed us to arrive at estimates on overall sensitivity, specificity and likelihood ratios for nNO depending on VC status. We also performed a sensitivity analysis including only studies in which PCD status was defined by TEM and at least one more diagnostic test, with the rationale to examine whether the diagnostic accuracy of nNO measurement differs with the inclusion of a more representative spectrum of PCD population. Measurements of nNO were compared to PCD diagnosis obtained through a combination of tests which included TEM and HSVM or DNA testing.

Results

Eligible studies

Of the 1940 items retrieved through online search, 1866 were excluded based on the title and abstract and the remaining 74 were downloaded for detailed, full text assessment. Two additional studies were identified through references screening and were also evaluated. Studies with overlapping populations were cross-checked and final selection was based on the largest number of participating PCD patients. In summary, 26 studies did not provide data on sensitivity and specificity, 13 items involved overlapping populations, 15 items were review papers while the remaining items that were excluded were case reports (2), editorials (3) and guidelines papers (2) (Fig. 1). Of the total 76 studies assessed in detail, 15 provided enough data for the construction of a 2×2 table. Among these, two studies did not report type of NO analyzer and flow rate and despite our effort to obtain this information after contacting the authors, this was not feasible and they were excluded from the analysis [20, 21]. Finally, quantitative synthesis included data on 13 different populations from 12 studies (Marthin et al. included data on more than one population) and two separate analyses were carried out, based on the employed breathing maneuver.

Study characteristics

Descriptive characteristics of the included studies are presented in Table 1. From 12 studies, 325 PCD patients and 711 non-PCD subjects were included in the meta-analysis for the diagnostic performance of VC nNO testing. In the case of non-VC nNO testing, 210 PCD patients and 471 non-PCD subjects from seven studies were included. The majority of the studies were performed in Western Europe and only two in North America. Four studies evaluated the diagnostic efficacy of nNO in cohorts of referred suspect patients for PCD testing [7, 22–24] whereas the rest of the studies had a case–control design. Controls were non-PCD subjects, either healthy subjects only [22, 25–28] or healthy subjects and patients with other respiratory diseases [14, 29–31].

The number of PCD patients (range: 9–59) and controls (range: 14–188) per case–control study varied widely. All case–control studies confirmed PCD status by TEM findings while in 55 % of them HSVM was also performed. Of the four prospective studies, Beydon et al. used a combination of TEM, HSVM and genetic testing to confirm PCD diagnosis [24] while Marthin et al. used TEM and HSVM in their cohort of consecutive referrals [22]. Leigh et al. confirmed PCD via a combination of ultrastructure assessment and genetic testing [7] while the smallest cohort study confirmed PCD only via ultrastructural assessment

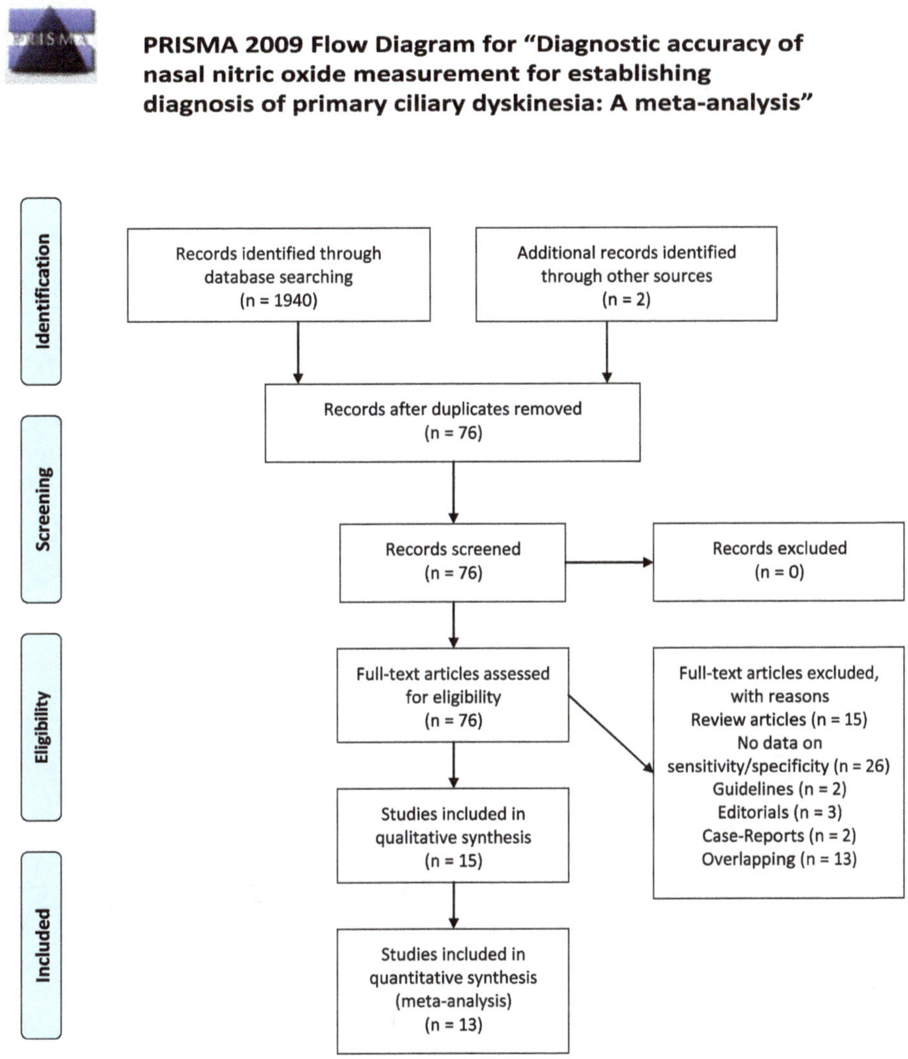

Fig. 1 PRISMA diagram. PRISMA diagram for the search strategy and selected studies. *From*: Moher D, Liberati A, Tetzlaff J, Altman DG, The PRISMA Group (2009). Preferred Reporting Items for Systematic Reviews and Meta-Analyses: The PRISMA Statement.

[23]. The sensitivity and specificity of each included study with VC and non-VC technique are shown in Fig. 2.

Quality assessment

Reporting of the meta-analysis is based on PRISMA guidelines [32]. Based on the QUADAS-2 tool, the quality assessment of the primary studies is shown in Table 2. In general, the analyzed studies had overall reasonably good methodology and this offers relative reassurance that results have not been substantially influenced from bias.

Data synthesis

The overall sensitivity of abnormal (low) nNO measured by VC techniques for all the included studies was 0.95 (95 % CI 0.91–0.97), while the specificity was 0.94 (95 % CI 0.88–0.97). The LR+ of the test was 15.8 (95 % CI 8.1–30.6), whereas the LR- was 0.06 (95 % CI 0.04–0.09). The HSROC curve is shown in Fig. 3.

For the non-VC techniques the overall sensitivity of nNO to detect PCD was 0.93 (95 % CI 0.89–0.96) whereas the specificity was 0.95 (95 % CI 0.82–0.99). The LR+ of the test was 18.5 (95 % CI 4.6–73.8) whereas the LR- was 0.07 (95 % CI 0.04–0.12). The HSROC curve is shown in Fig. 3.

When we performed a sensitivity analysis, to calculate the nNO diagnostic accuracy in studies that only included PCD populations diagnosed by more than one test (combination of TEM and HSVM or genetic testing) [7, 14, 22, 24, 26, 27, 30], the results did not change significantly. Similarly, after performing a post hoc

Table 1 Characteristics of the included studies

#	Author/Study	Country	Study Design	Study Population[a]	Age range (yrs) (Mean, range/SD)	Analyzer	Flow rate (L/min)	Measurement Method[b]	Cut – off (nL/min)	Inclusion criteria/ Diagnosis
1	Narang I (2002) [26]	United Kingdom	Case - Control	31 PCD 53 HC	PCD: 11.0 (5.5–17.3) HC: 10.7 (5.5–19.0)	LR 2000	0.25	BH	62.5	HSVM and TEM
2	Corbelli R (2004) [23]	Switzerland	Prospective Cohort	17 PCD 17 non PCD (BE,B)	All: 11.4 (1.2)	CLD88sp	1.20	BH	126	TEM
3	Piacentini G (2008) [25]	Italy	Case - Control	10 PCD 27 HC	PCD: 17 (–) HC: 7 (–)	NIOX Flex	0.30	BH	21.3	TEM
4	Mateos Coral D (2011) [31]	Canada	Case – Control (with longitudinal follow-up in a subsample)	20 PCD 65 non PCD (CF,BE,HC)	PCD: 11.4 (3.5) HC: 11.0 (3.7) CF: 11.0 (3.4) BE: 10.9(3.3)	CLD88sp	0.33	ER & TB	ER: 58.5 TB: 37.1	TEM
5	Marthin JK (2011) [22] Substudy 3	Denmark	Prospective Cohort	20 PCD 97 non PCD	All: 6.9 (0.0–62.4)[c]	NIOX Flex	0.30	BH & TB	BH: 52.5 TB: 47.4	HSVM and TEM
6	Marthin JK (2011) [22] Substudy 2	Denmark	Case - Control	59 PCD 57 HC	PCD: 17.4 (3.6–65.8)[c] Non PCD:29.5 (3.1–63.6)[c]	NIOX Flex	0.30	BH & TB	BH: 52.5 TB: 47.4	HSVM and/or TEM
7	Leigh M (2013) [7]	United States	Prospective Cohort	71 PCD 84 non-PCD	PCD: 23.3(18) Non PCD: 31.8 (22.3)	Sievers 280i CLD88sp NIOX Flex	0.50 0.33 0.30	ER	76.9	TEM and DNA
8	Boon M (2014) [30]	Belgium	Case - Control	38 PCD 188 non PCD (HC, CF, Asthma, HID)	PCD: 14.3 (8.8–18.1)[c] HC: 14.9 (10.8–20.4)[c] CF: 14.0 (9.2–17.9)[c] Asthma: 12.1 (9.8–16.5)[c] HID: 10.7 (8.2–15.6)[c]	CLD88sp	0.30	ER & TB	ER: 90 TB: 60	HSVM and TEM (and culture)
9	Harris A (2014) [14]	United Kingdom	Case - Control	13 PCD 37 non PCD (HC,CF, CSLD)	PCD: 23 (5–71) HC: 31 (8–65) CF: 15(6–29) CSLD: 36 (8–79)	NIOX Flex NIOX MINO	0.30	BH & TB	BH: 38 TB: 30	HSVM and TEM (and culture for some)
10	Montella S (2012) [27]	Italy	Case - Control	23 PCD 23 HC	PCD: 15.8 (4.6–32.8)[c] HC: 15.7 (4.3–32.1)[c]	NIOX MINO	0.30	TB	17.4	HSVM and TEM
11	Santamaria F (2008) [28]	Italy	Case - Control	14 PCD 14 HC	PCD: 15 (7–27) HC:16 (7–27)	NIOX Flex	0.28	BH	7.2	TEM
12	Moreno Caldo A (2010) [29]	Spain	Case Control	9 PCD 112 non PCD (HC, CF, Asthma,BE)	PCD: – (7–14) HC: – (–) CF: – (6–14) Asthma: (6–17) BE: – (6–14)	LR2000	0.25	BH	28	TEM
13	Beydon M 2015 [24]	France	Prospective Cohort	49 PCD 37 non-PCD	PCD: 11.4 (7,13.9)[d] Non PCD: 7.9 (4.9,11.6)[d]	NIOX Flex Endono 8000	0.30	BH/ER TB	BH/ER: 82.2 TB: 39.9	HSVM, TEM and/or DNA

PCD: Primary Ciliary Dyskinesia, HC: Healthy Controls, B: Bronchitis, CF: Cystic Fibrosis, BE: non CF non PCD Bronchiectasis, CSLD: Chronic Suppurative Lung Disease, HID: Humoral Immunodeficiency Disorders, TEM: Transmission Electron Microscopy, HSVM: High Speed Video Microscopy, DNA: Genetic testing

[a]Study population refers to subgroups that comparisons (sensitivity, specificity, PPV, NPV) were reported for in the original articles

[b]Measurements methods taken into account for the meta-analysis, BH: Breath Hold, ER: Exhalation against Resistance, TB: Tidal Breathing

[c]Median (range)

[d]Median (IQR)

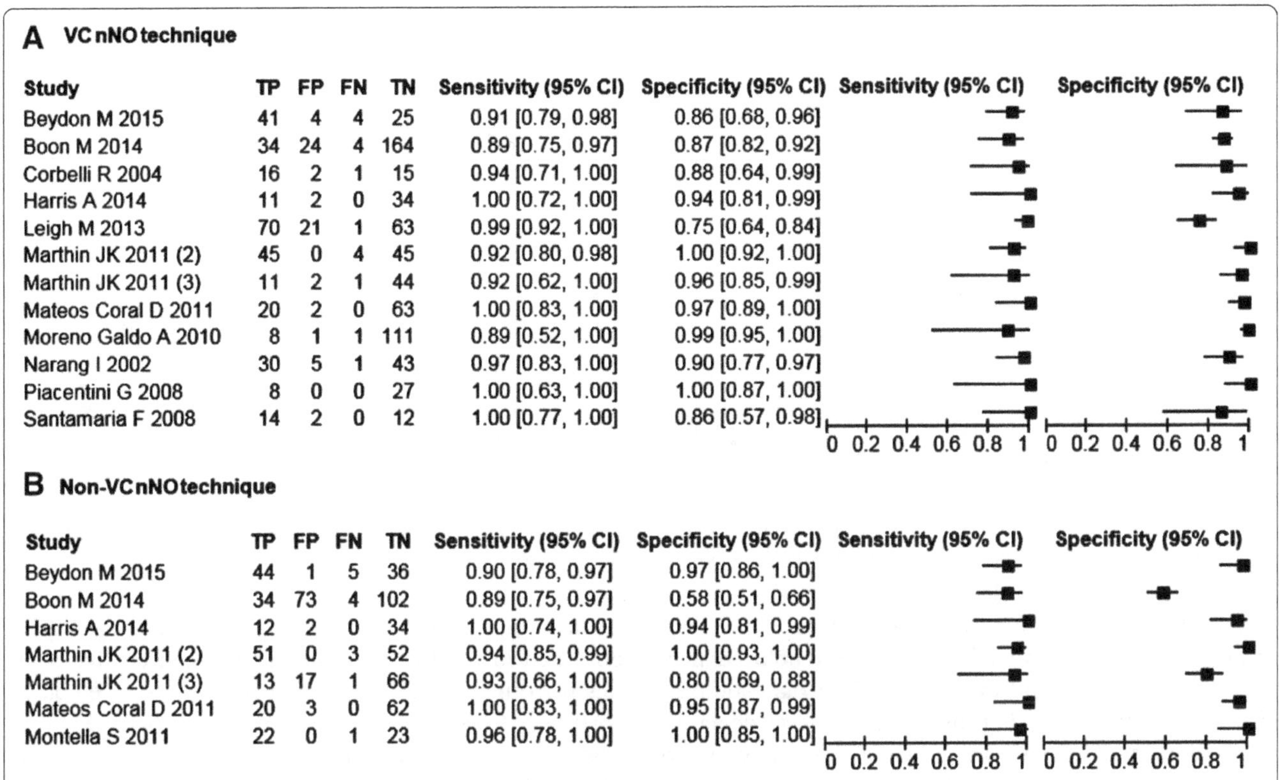

Fig. 2 Forest plots for sensitivity and specificity. Forest plot of sensitivity and specificity of nNO for detecting PCD with the 95 % CI for each population of the included studies. **a** Forest plot for studies employing a VC breathing technique and **b** Forest plot for studies employing a non-VC breathing technique

sensitivity analysis, with the exclusion of studies that used the electrochemical devise NIOX MINO [14, 27], the resulting estimates of overall sensitivity and overall specificity for the non-VC maneuver do not significantly differ from the estimates of the main analysis.

Discussion

In this meta-analysis we demonstrated that nNO measurement with VC techniques has overall sensitivity of 95 % and a specificity of 94 % whereas nNO measurement with the non-VC technique has comparable and

Table 2 QUADAS-2 Quality Assessment results

Study	Risk of bias				Applicability concerns		
	Patient selection	Index test	Reference Standard	Flow and timing	Patient selection	Index test	Reference standard
Boon 2014 [30]	L	U	L	L	L	L	L
Mateos Coral 2011 [31]	U	L	L	L	U	L	L
Piacentini 2008 [25]	U	L	L	L	U	L	L
Santamaria 2008 [28]	L	U	L	L	L	L	L
Montela 2012 [27]	U	L	U	L	L	L	L
Corbelli 2004 [23]	L	U	L	L	L	L	L
Narang 2002 [26]	L	L	L	L	L	L	L
Harris 2014 [14]	L	U	L	L	L	L	L
Leigh 2013 [7]	L	L	L	L	L	L	L
Marthin 2011 [22]	L	U	L	L	L	L	L
Moreno Galdo 2010 [29]	U	U	L	L	U	L	L
Beydon M 2015 [25]	L	L	L	U	L	L	L

QUADAS 2 consists of four key domains covering patient selection, index test, reference standard and flow of patients through the study and timing of the index test and reference standard ("flow and timing"). Each domain is assessed in terms of the risk of bias and the first three are also assessed in terms of concerns regarding applicability

U: Unknown, L: Low, H: High

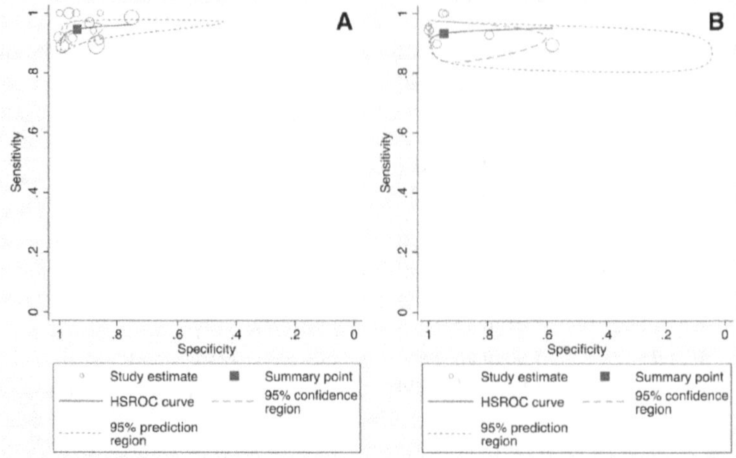

Fig. 3 VC and non-VC HSROC curves. HSROC curves for the included studies. **a** HSROC curve for studies employing a VC breathing technique and **b** HSROC curve for studies employing a non-VC breathing technique

very similar sensitivity (93 %) and specificity (95 %). We applied a different approach to the one employed in a previous report [15] and evaluated nNO diagnostic performance metrics by using all the available evidence in the literature. These summary estimates allow us to make comparisons between the various proposed and established diagnostic tests for PCD, which are essential for clinical decision making. We also provide a graphical representation of our results using the hierarchical summary receiver operating characteristic (HSROC) curve incorporating the different cut-offs between primary studies. The clinical utility of nNO measurement is underlined by the high LR+ (VC: 15.8, non-VC: 18.5) and low LR- (VC: 0.06, non-VC: 0.07), meaning that an abnormal (low) nNO leads to a steep increase in the post-test probability of PCD, compared to the pretest probability, while in the case of a normal nNO measurement the opposite is also true [19]. However, since the sensitivity and specificity of the test are not 100 %, in the presence of strong clinical suspicion for PCD [33], even in the case of a negative nNO test, a more detailed diagnostic work-up (HSVM, TEM, genetics) is indicated.

Current ATS/ERS recommendations for nNO include only VC maneuvers although recent evidence [14, 30, 31], that is supported by the results of this meta-analysis, highlights the discriminative ability of nNO during TB. TB is the only method available to obtain nNO measurements in young children (<5 years), which is particularly important as disease manifestations appear very early in life. Of course, the validity of nNO measurements in infants (<6 months) has been questioned, as nNO output in infancy is reduced due to the partial development of paranasal sinuses [25] where the majority of NO is produced [11] whereas the number of patients under 5 years which were evaluated in these studies [14, 22, 24, 27, 30, 31] is very small . The usefulness of nNO during TB has been demonstrated in the Danish cohort of 117 consecutive referrals with median age 6.9 years, where 83 % were able to perform TB versus 50 % for BH and 31 % for ER [22]. There is evidence that patients that have earlier diagnosis of this disease might have better clinical and functional outcomes [34, 35] and the application of this promising screening method in preschool children could not only lead to diagnosis at an earlier age but could also contribute towards the reduction of unnecessary cilia biopsies. Nevertheless, our results for the non-VC techniques should be interpreted with caution. Their low 95 % CI limit for specificity is at 82 % which suggests that a significant number of suspect PCD referrals is possible to give a falsely low nNO and prompt further diagnostic testing, thus increasing costs both to the healthcare system and the patient. Only seven studies were eligible for inclusion in the meta-analysis of non-VC maneuver, as opposed to 12 studies for the VC maneuver, and the low 95 % CI limit of the former may be due to the limited sample size. Furthermore, two of the non-VC studies used the NIOX MINO portable device which uses electrochemical analysis of NO as opposed to the better validated chemiluminescence method of the stationary devices (NIOX FLEX, Ecomedics CLD88). Nevertheless, we performed a post hoc analysis with the exclusion of these studies which did not influence the diagnostic accuracy of the non-VC maneuver and the quantitative synthesis includes data from all seven non-VC studies.

NIOX MINO is a simpler and cheaper tool for measuring nNO, and validation studies have already been published [14, 36, 37]. However, as NIOX MINO was designed for exhaled NO measurement in asthmatic individuals, issues relating to its accuracy [37] and repeatability [14] have been reported when used for nNO measurement in subjects referred for PCD evaluation. In addition, while the manufacturer recommends measurements of nNO with BH for at least 45 s, this is usually not possible by many patients and instead NIOX MINO is frequently used with the alternative TB maneuver regardless of patient's age [14, 37]. These limitations question the suitability of NIOX MINO as a stand-alone diagnostic test and additional studies on the diagnostic accuracy of NIOX MINO measurements during TB are needed to confirm the validity of this method. However, the low cost and simple use potentiate the consideration of NIOX MINO as a promising first line screening test in a future diagnostic algorithm for PCD.

Currently, there is no universally accepted cutoff for abnormally low nNO. The included studies in this meta-analysis proposed a variety of cutoffs for nNO production by VC (7.2–126 nl/min) and non-VC (17.4–60 nl/min) techniques. This variability demonstrates the need for standardization of nNO measurements and agreement on cutoffs for the different breathing maneuvers. A recent, large, multicenter study has proposed a cutoff equal to 77 nl/min for VC [7], whereas the meta-analysis by Collins et al. reported that a cutoff of 75.2 nl/min would include 99.85 % of PCD patients performing VC maneuvers [15]. Regarding the non-VC maneuver however, no cutoff value has been proposed by a large enough study, thus additional studies are needed for the establishment of such cutoffs and further standardization of the technique.

Our study has some limitations. The main limitation is the heterogeneity and the weaknesses of the diagnostic standard that the published studies are employing for the definition of PCD status. As a result, the captured spectrum of the disease might not be totally representative of the true PCD population. TEM, which is the most commonly used test for PCD status definition in published studies, misses approximately 30 % of patients with PCD [38] and this should be taken into account in the assessment of the diagnostic efficacy of nNO. However, in the sensitivity analysis, when we included the studies that had employed more than one (in addition to TEM) diagnostic test to establish PCD diagnosis, our results did not change substantially thus providing relative certainty to the accuracy of nNO as a diagnostic test. There is considerable variation between individual studies in the number of cases, total sample size and cut-off values. However, the bivariate meta-analysis and HSROC curve analyses take explicitly this diversity into account and can accommodate studies with populations of different risks and different definition thresholds. Another issue for the synthesis of the data is that the majority of the included studies were diagnostic case–control studies. Empirical evidence has shown that case–control studies, as opposed to cohort studies, may overestimate the diagnostics Odds Ratio (DOR) [39]. Nevertheless, we think that the possibility of overestimation is limited, as the case–control studies included here were diagnostic studies designed to assess the test accuracy and not to provide evidence on associations between a risk factor and the disease [40]. Additionally, given the rarity of PCD, it is expected that the majority of studies will have a case–control design. Due to the same reason, both case–control and prospective cohort studies included relatively small numbers of subjects. However the synthesis of the included studies led to the inclusion of data for several hundreds of PCD and non-PCD subjects and allowed the use of the appropriate statistical models and provided the estimates we report. It should be underlined of course that these estimates apply provided that the ATS/ERS guidelines are followed for the performance of the test and the obtained values are compared to the normal values obtained from samples of healthy subjects in the respective populations.

Conclusions

In summary, measurement of nNO, both with VC and non-VC maneuvers, has high overall diagnostic accuracy and provides a clinically significant diagnostic tool for large uninvestigated populations of suspect cases worldwide where access to TEM and HSVM is not easy. Furthermore, the high overall diagnostic accuracy of nNO calls for re-evaluation of the diagnostic accuracy of each of the available diagnostic tests for PCD (nNO, TEM and HSVM) with the aim to develop an algorithm with the most efficacious combination of tests to achieve PCD diagnosis.

Abbreviations

ATS/ERS: American Thoracic Society/European Respiratory Society; BH: Breath hold; ER: Exhalation against resistance; FN: False negatives; FP: False positives; HSVM: High Speed Video Microscopy; nNO: nasal Nitric Oxide; PCD: Primary Ciliary Dyskinesia; ppb: parts per billion; TB: Tidal breathing; TEM: Transmission Electron Microscopy; TP: True positives; TN: True negatives; VC: Velum closure.

Competing interests

The authors wish to declare that they have no competing interests.

Authors' contributions

PK performed the search and extraction of information from the papers, organized the material and prepared the first draft of the manuscript. SIP provided advice on the methodology of the search and selection of the papers, contributed to the interpretation of the findings, critically revised the manuscript and contributed towards the final version of the manuscript. PKY conceived the hypothesis of the manuscript, coordinated the whole work, contributed to the interpretation of the findings and contributed intellectually towards the final version of the manuscript. All authors read and approved the final manuscript.

Authors' information

S.I.P. is the main advisor of P.K for his doctoral studies. PK was supported by the European Union's Seventh Framework Program EC-GA No. 305404 BESTCILIA. The sponsors had no role or involvement in study design; in the collection, analysis and interpretation of data; in the writing of the report; and in the decision to submit the article for publication.

Acknowledgements
This work was performed at the Cyprus International Institute for Environmental and Public Health in association with Harvard School of Public Health, Cyprus University of Technology, Limassol, Cyprus.

Author details
[1]Cyprus International Institute for Environmental & Public Health in Association with Harvard School of Public Health, Cyprus University of Technology, 95 Irenes Street, 3041 Limassol, Cyprus. [2]Department of Pediatrics, Hospital "Archbishop Makarios III", Nicosia, Cyprus.

References

1. Leigh MW, Pittman JE, Carson JL, Ferkol TW, Dell SD, Davis SD, et al. Clinical and genetic aspects of primary ciliary dyskinesia/Kartagener syndrome. Genet Med. 2009;11(7):473–87.
2. Noone PG, Leigh MW, Sannuti A, Minnix SL, Carson JL, Hazucha M, et al. Primary ciliary dyskinesia: diagnostic and phenotypic features. Am J Respir Crit Care Med. 2004;169(4):459–67.
3. Boon M, Jorissen M, Proesmans M, De Boeck K. Primary ciliary dyskinesia, an orphan disease. Eur J Pediatr. 2013;172(2):151–62.
4. Kim RH, A Hall D, Cutz E, Knowles MR, Nelligan KA, Nykamp K, et al. The Role of Molecular Genetic Analysis in the Diagnosis of Primary Ciliary Dyskinesia. Ann Am Thorac Soc. 2014;11(3):351–9.
5. Stannard WA, Chilvers MA, Rutman AR, Williams CD, O'Callaghan C. Diagnostic testing of patients suspected of primary ciliary dyskinesia. Am J Respir Crit Care Med. 2010;181(4):307–14.
6. Papon JF, Coste A, Roudot-Thoraval F, Boucherat M, Roger G, Tamalet A, et al. A 20-year experience of electron microscopy in the diagnosis of primary ciliary dyskinesia. Eur Respir J. 2010;35(5):1057–63.
7. Leigh MW, Hazucha MJ, Chawla KK, Baker BR, Shapiro AJ, Brown DE, et al. Standardizing nasal nitric oxide measurement as a test for primary ciliary dyskinesia. Ann Am Thorac Soc. 2013;10(6):574–81.
8. Schwabe GC, Hoffmann K, Loges NT, Birker D, Rossier C, De Santi MM, et al. Primary ciliary dyskinesia associated with normal axoneme ultrastructure is caused by DNAH11 mutations. Hum Mutat. 2008;29(2):289–98.
9. Lucas JS, Adam EC, Goggin PM, Jackson CL, Powles-Glover N, Patel SH, et al. Static respiratory cilia associated with mutations in Dnahc11/DNAH11: a mouse model of PCD. Hum Mutat. 2012;33(3):495–503.
10. Raidt J, Wallmeier J, Hjeij R, Onnebrink JG, Pennekamp P, Loges NT, et al. Ciliary beat pattern and frequency in genetic variants of primary ciliary dyskinesia. Eur Respir J. 2014
11. Lundberg J, Farkas-Szallasi T, Weitzberg E, Rinder J, Lidholm J, Änggåard A, et al. High nitric oxide production in human paranasal sinuses. Nat Med. 1995;1(4):370–3.
12. Strippoli MP, Frischer T, Barbato A, Snijders D, Maurer E, Lucas JS, et al. ERS Task Force onPrimary Ciliary Dyskinesia in Children: Management of primary ciliary dyskinesia in European children: recommendations and clinical practice. Eur Respir J. 2012;39(6):1482–91.
13. American Thoracic Society, European Respiratory Society. ATS/ERS recommendations for standardized procedures for the online and offline measurement of exhaled lower respiratory nitric oxide and nasal nitric oxide, 2005. Am J Respir Crit Care Med. 2005;171(8):912–30.
14. Harris A, Bhullar E, Gove K, Joslin R, Pelling J, Evans HJ, et al. Validation of a portable nitric oxide analyzer for screening in primary ciliary dyskinesias. BMC Pulm Med. 2014;14(1):18.
15. Collins SA, Gove K, Walker W, Lucas JS. Nasal nitric oxide screening for primary ciliary dyskinesia: systematic review and meta-analysis. Eur Respir J. 2014;44(6):1589–99.
16. Whiting PF, Rutjes AW, Westwood ME, Mallett S, Deeks JJ, Reitsma JB, et al. QUADAS-2: a revised tool for the quality assessment of diagnostic accuracy studies. Ann Intern Med. 2011;155(8):529–36.
17. Chu H, Cole SR. Bivariate meta-analysis of sensitivity and specificity with sparse data: a generalized linear mixed model approach. J Clin Epidemiol. 2006;59(12):1331–2.
18. Harbord R. METANDI: Stata module to perform meta-analysis of diagnostic accuracy. In: Statistical Software Components S456932, Boston College Department of Economics, 2008. https://ideas.repec.org/c/boc/bocode/s456932.html. Assessed 15 May 2015.
19. Deeks JJ, Altman DG. Diagnostic tests 4: likelihood ratios. BMJ. 2004; 329(7458):168–9.
20. Pifferi M, Bush A, Maggi F, Michelucci A, Ricci V, Conidi ME, et al. Nasal nitric oxide and nitric oxide synthase expression in primary ciliary dyskinesia. Eur Respir J. 2011;37(3):572–7.
21. Morgan L, Buddle L, Rogers P, Seccombe L, MacKenney K, Hughes L. Nasal nitric oxide is useful in an Australian Primary Ciliary Dyskinesia clinic. Cilia. 2012;1 Suppl 1:7.
22. Marthin JK, Nielsen KG. Choice of nasal nitric oxide technique as first-line test for primary ciliary dyskinesia. Eur Respir J. 2011;37(3):559–65.
23. Corbelli R, Bringolf-Isler B, Amacher A, Sasse B, Spycher M, Hammer J. Nasal nitric oxide measurements to screen children for primary ciliary dyskinesia. CHEST J. 2004;126(4):1054–9.
24. Beydon N, Chambellan A, Alberti C, de Blic J, Clément A, Escudier E, et al. Technical and practical issues for tidal breathing measurements of nasal nitric oxide in children. Pediatr Pulmonol. 2015; :n/a-n/a.
25. Piacentini GL, Bodini A, Peroni D, Rigotti E, Pigozzi R, Pradal U, et al. Nasal nitric oxide for early diagnosis of primary ciliary dyskinesia: practical issues in children. Respir Med. 2008;102(4):541–7.
26. Narang I, Ersu R, Wilson NM, Bush A. Nitric oxide in chronic airway inflammation in children: diagnostic use and pathophysiological significance. Thorax. 2002;57(7):586–9.
27. Montella S, Alving K, De Stefano S, Di Micco LL, Di Giorgio A, Santamaria F. Nasal nitric oxide measurement using continuous aspiration by hand-held device discriminates patients with primary ciliary dyskinesia from healthy subjects. Eur Respir J. 2012;40 Suppl 56:3338.
28. Santamaria F, De Stefano S, Montella S, Barbarano F, Iacotucci P, Ciccarelli R, et al. Nasal nitric oxide assessment in primary ciliary dyskinesia using aspiration, exhalation, and humming. Med Sci Monit. 2008;14(2):CR80–5.
29. Moreno Galdo A, Vizmanos Lamotte G, Reverte Bover C, Gartner S, Cobos Barroso N, Rovira Amigo S, et al. Value of nasal nitric oxide in the diagnosis of primary ciliary dyskinesia. An Pediatr (Barc). 2010;73(2):88–93.
30. Boon M, Meyts I, Proesmans M, Vermeulen FL, Jorissen M, De Boeck K. Diagnostic accuracy of nitric oxide measurements to detect primary ciliary dyskinesia. Eur J Clin Invest. 2014;44(5):477–85.
31. Mateos-Corral D, Coombs R, Grasemann H, Ratjen F, Dell SD. Diagnostic value of nasal nitric oxide measured with non-velum closure techniques for children with primary ciliary dyskinesia. J Pediatr. 2011;159(3):420–4.
32. Moher D, Liberati A, Tetzlaff J, Altman DG. Preferred reporting items for systematic reviews and meta-analyses: the PRISMA statement. Ann Intern Med. 2009;151(4):264–9.
33. Barbato A, Frischer T, Kuehni CE, Snijders D, Azevedo I, Baktai G, et al. Primary ciliary dyskinesia: a consensus statement on diagnostic and treatment approaches in children. Eur Respir J. 2009;34(6):1264–76.
34. Yiallouros PK, Kouis P, Middleton N, Nearchou M, Adamidi T, Georgiou A, et al. Clinical features of primary ciliary dyskinesia in Cyprus with emphasis on lobectomized patients. Respir Med. 2015;109(3):347–56.
35. Coren M, Meeks M, Morrison I, Buchdahl R, Bush A. Primary ciliary dyskinesia: age at diagnosis and symptom history. Acta Paediatr. 2002;91(6):667–9.
36. Maniscalco M, Laurentiis G, Weitzberg E, Lundberg J, Sofia M. Validation study of nasal nitric oxide measurements using a hand-held electrochemical analyser. Eur J Clin Invest. 2008;38(3):197–200.
37. Marthin JK, Nielsen KG. Hand-held tidal breathing nasal nitric oxide measurement–a promising targeted case-finding tool for the diagnosis of primary ciliary dyskinesia. PLoS One. 2013;8(2):e57262.
38. Knowles MR, Leigh MW, Carson JL, Davis SD, Dell SD, Ferkol TW, et al. Genetic Disorders of Mucociliary Clearance Consortium: Mutations of DNAH11 in patients with primary ciliary dyskinesia with normal ciliary ultrastructure. Thorax. 2012;67(5):433–41.
39. Lijmer JG, Mol BW, Heisterkamp S, Bonsel GJ, Prins MH, van der Meulen JH, et al. Empirical evidence of design-related bias in studies of diagnostic tests. JAMA. 1999;282(11):1061–6.
40. Rutjes AW, Reitsma JB, Vandenbroucke JP, Glas AS, Bossuyt PM. Case–control and two-gate designs in diagnostic accuracy studies. Clin Chem. 2005;51(8):1335–41.

5

Radial endobronchial ultrasound with a guide sheath for diagnosis of peripheral cavitary lung lesions

Manabu Hayama[1*], Norio Okamoto[1], Hidekazu Suzuki[1], Motohiro Tamiya[1], Takayuki Shiroyama[1], Ayako Tanaka[1], Takuji Nishida[1], Takashi Nishihara[1], Nobuko Uehara[1], Naoko Morishita[1], Kunimitsu Kawahara[2] and Tomonori Hirashima[1]

Abstract

Background: Radial endobronchial ultrasound with a guide sheath (EBUS-GS) has improved the diagnostic outcomes of peripheral lung lesions. However, to our knowledge, reports on the use of EBUS-GS for diagnosis of cavitary lesions are unavailable. Therefore, this study aimed to assess the effectiveness and safety of EBUS-GS for diagnosis of peripheral cavitary lung lesions (PCLLs).

Methods: This study was a single-institution retrospective review of PCLLs examined by using EBUS-GS between July 2013 and October 2015. The diagnostic results of different EBUS-GS samples, including cytologic, histopathologic, and microbiologic samples, were analysed separately.

Results: Of 696 radial EBUS procedures performed during the study period, 50 were performed for examination of PCLLs. The overall diagnostic yield for EBUS-GS was 80 % (40/50). Regarding 27 malignant lesions, the diagnostic yields for cytologic and histopathologic samples were 63.0 % (17/27) and 74.1 % (20/27), respectively. Regarding 23 benign lesions, the diagnostic yields for histopathologic and microbiologic samples were 69.6 % (16/23) and 47.8 % (11/23), respectively. Uni- and multivariate analyses indicated that the EBUS probe being within the lesion was the only factor significantly associated with increased diagnostic yield (odds ratio, 7.04; $P = 0.03$). Although pulmonary infection occurred after the procedure in 1 patient (2.0 %), no other complications, including pneumothorax or significant haemorrhage, were reported.

Conclusion: EBUS-GS was found to be an effective and safe procedure for diagnosis of PCLLs.

Keywords: Radial endobronchial ultrasound, Endobronchial ultrasound with a guide sheath, Lung cancer, Cavity, peripheral lung lesion, Transbronchial biopsy, Bronchoscopy

Background

A pulmonary cavity is defined as a gas-filled area within a pulmonary consolidation, mass, or nodule that may or may not contain a fluid level and is surrounded by a wall, usually of varied thickness [1]. Various malignant and benign diseases can present as cavitary lung lesions. Because findings on chest radiography and computed tomography (CT) often overlap between malignant and benign cavitary lesions, minimally invasive specimen collection is often necessary for accurate diagnosis [2]. However, sufficient diagnostic biopsy samples may not be obtained due to the limited target area of the cavity wall and the surrounding reactive normal tissue [3].

According to the guidelines of the American College of Chest Physicians, the sensitivity of transbronchial biopsy (TBB) for diagnosis of peripheral lung lesions is 63 % for lesions >20 mm, and only 34 % for lesions <20 mm [4]. On the other hand, the pooled sensitivity of transthoracic needle aspiration (TTNA) for diagnosis of peripheral lung cancer is 90 %, making it the preferred method for preoperative diagnosis [4]. However, TTNA carries a high

* Correspondence: manabuhayama@gmail.com
[1]Department of Thoracic Malignancy, Osaka Prefectural Medical Center for Respiratory and Allergic Diseases, 3-7-1, Habikino, Habikino City, Osaka 583-8588, Japan
Full list of author information is available at the end of the article

risk of complications, such as pneumothorax, air embolism, and tumour seeding [5, 6]. With regard to bronchoscopy for diagnosis of peripheral lung lesions, a recent meta-analysis reported a diagnostic yield of 70 % with use of electromagnetic navigation bronchoscopy, radial endobronchial ultrasound (R-EBUS) with or without a guide sheath, virtual bronchoscopic navigation (VBN), and ultrathin bronchoscopes; among these, the pooled diagnostic yield was highest with use of a guide sheath [7]. Therefore, because of its safety profile and sufficient diagnostic yield, R-EBUS with a guide sheath (EBUS-GS) is now becoming a common procedure for examination of peripheral lung lesions [8].

However, reports on the use of R-EBUS for diagnosis of cavitary lung lesions with a relatively high probability of infectious disease are limited [9]. Because it is unknown whether a lung lesion is malignant or benign before diagnostic bronchoscopy, malignant and benign lesions usually are examined by using the same procedure [10]. The aim of this study was to assess the effectiveness and safety of EBUS-GS for diagnosis of peripheral cavitary lung lesions (PCLLs).

Methods

Study approval

This study was a retrospective review of a prospectively maintained database and medical records at our institution. The Institutional Review Board of Osaka Prefectural Medical Center for Respiratory and Allergic Diseases approved this study without the need to obtain informed consent. Written informed consent for bronchoscopy was obtained from all eligible patients.

Patient selection

Patient information (age, sex, type of procedure) and lesion characteristics were collected prospectively in the database before diagnostic bronchoscopy. Lesion characteristics, including type (solid, part-solid, pure ground-glass opacity [GGO], cavitary, or other [i.e., atelectasis, diffuse or lobar consolidation]), maximum diameter, target bronchus, and presence of bronchus sign, were evaluated on thin-section chest CT images during regular team discussions that included board-certified bronchoscopists, pulmonologists, and medical oncologists. VBN (LungPoint, Bronchus Ltd.) was used when the target bronchus was small and difficult to trace [11].

PCLLs examined by using EBUS-GS at our institution between July 2013 and October 2015 were included in this study. Cases in which ultrathin bronchoscopes (BF-XP260, Olympus Ltd.) were additionally used were excluded. A PCLL was defined as a bronchoscopically invisible lung lesion that had an internal gas-filled area and was surrounded by pulmonary parenchyma [1, 8]. Maximum cavity wall thickness and minimum distance from the costal pleura were additionally assessed on chest CT transverse images.

EBUS-GS procedure

All EBUS-GS procedures were performed by expert bronchoscopists or trainees with sufficient experience with conventional bronchoscopy and EBUS-GS assistance. During all the procedures, the trainees were supervised by the experts.

EBUS-GS procedures were carried out by using one of the following bronchoscopes (Olympus Ltd.): BF-1T260, BF-P260, BF-F260, or BF-Y0053, a new middle-range bronchoscope with a 5.1-mm outer diameter and a 2.6-mm working channel [12]. A guide sheath kit (K-202 or K-204, Olympus Ltd.) was used in combination with an R-EBUS probe (UM-S20-17S, Olympus Ltd.). All bronchoscopies were performed via an oral route under local anaesthesia with intravenous midazolam for mild sedation.

Upon insertion of the scope to reach the target bronchus, the guide sheath together with the R-EBUS probe was inserted through the working channel and advanced under fluoroscopic guidance. EBUS images before transbronchial sampling were categorized into 3 patterns: 'within' (the probe was located in a bronchus that was inside the lesion), 'adjacent to' (the probe was located in a bronchus that ran alongside the lesion), or 'invisible' (the probe was not able to reach the lesion) [8]. After locating the lesion, the probe was removed while the guide sheath was kept in place for subsequent sampling, also under fluoroscopic guidance. Transbronchial needle aspiration (TBNA) with or without a guide sheath was additionally performed when the operator deemed that the sample amount was insufficient [11, 13].

Brush and needle smears and tissue stumps on glass slides were sent for cytologic examination. Tissue samples obtained by using forceps were sent for histopathologic examination. After each sampling, the brush, needles, and forceps were rinsed with 5 mL normal saline (device wash) [14]. After all the samplings, the guide sheath was removed and the lumen was flushed with the device wash liquid. Then, the device wash sample was divided into 2 test tubes, which were sent for cytologic and microbiologic examinations, respectively (Fig. 1). Routine microbiologic examination comprised Gram stain, acid-fast bacilli smear, polymerase chain reaction of *Mycobacterium tuberculosis* (TB), and cultures including TB. Although additional bronchial wash was performed in 2 patients, those results were not assessed in this study.

Diagnostic criteria

Final diagnosis was determined based on either one or a combination of the results of EBUS-GS, EBUS-TBNA,

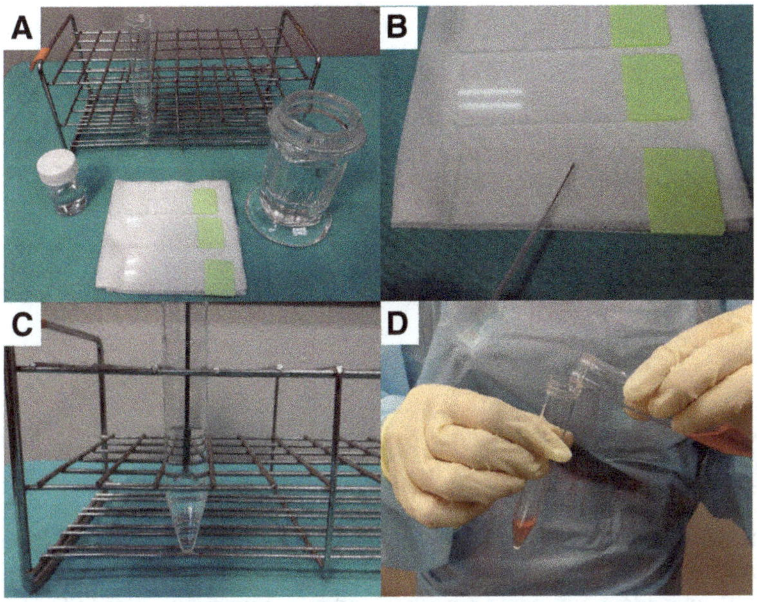

Fig. 1 Specimen collection set for endobronchial ultrasound with a guide sheath (EBUS-GS). (**a**) A specimen collection set for EBUS-GS routinely consists of 10 % formalin (*lower left*), glass slides (*lower centre*), 95 % alcohol (*lower right*), and 5 mL normal saline (*upper*). (**b**) Brush and needle smears and tissue stumps on glass slides are sent for cytologic examination. (**c**) After each sampling, the brush, needles, and forceps are rinsed with 5 mL normal saline (device wash). (**d**) The device wash sample is divided into 2 test tubes, which are sent for cytologic and microbiologic examinations, respectively

surgery, or clinical follow-up for at least 3 months. A lesion was designated as inflammation if it showed no significant pathologic or clinical findings, and it decreased in size on follow-up CT.

For malignant lesions, class IV/V results on cytology or specific malignant findings on histopathology were considered as diagnostic. For benign lesions, specific benign findings on histopathology (e.g. necrotizing epithelioid granuloma, acute-angle branching hyphae, or inflammation) or positive cultures on microbiology were considered as diagnostic. Histopathologic results were reviewed by 2 investigators (MH and KK). Overall, EBUS-GS was considered as diagnostic when at least 1 of the cytologic, histopathologic, or microbiologic results was diagnostic.

Complications of EBUS-GS

All bronchoscopies were performed in inpatient settings. After every procedure, chest radiography was performed and oral antibiotics (cefcapene pivoxil 300 mg/day for 3 days) were administered. A major complication was defined as an event that necessitated premature termination of the procedure or a symptomatic postprocedure sequela, including pneumothorax, haemorrhage, infection, air embolism, or other untoward life-threatening outcome [8].

Statistical analysis

Descriptive statistics are presented as frequency, percentage, and median (range). Univariate analyses were performed by using Fisher's exact test for categorical data. Multivariate logistic regression analysis was performed to determine the factors associated with increased diagnostic yield. Variables for the multivariate analysis model were chosen from the results of the univariate analyses and experimentally predicted factors, such as lesion size and bronchus sign. A 2-tailed P value of <0.05 was considered to indicate statistical significance. All statistical analyses were performed by using EZR (Saitama Medical Center, Jichi Medical University, Saitama, Japan), a graphical user interface for R (The R foundation for Statistical Computing, Vienna, Austria) [15].

Results

Among 696 R-EBUS procedures performed between July 2013 and October 2015 at our institution, 50 PCLLs examined by using EBUS-GS were included in this study (Fig. 2). A summary of the baseline characteristics of the 50 patients is shown in Table 1. The study population had a median age of 67 years and mostly consisted of male patients. Median lesion size, cavity wall thickness, and distance from the costal pleura were 33.5, 11 , and 0 mm, respectively. Most lesions were located in the lower lobe (54 %), and bronchus sign was positive in the majority of cases (82 %). VBN was used for route planning in 27 patients (54 %).

Details of the final diagnoses are shown in Table 2. Among 27 malignant lesions, 21 were successfully

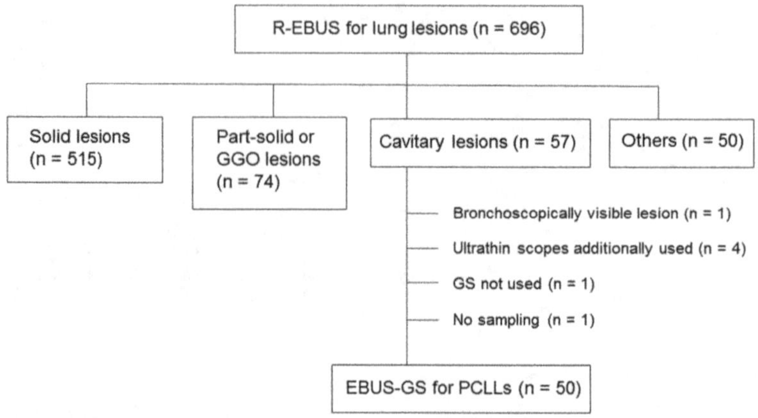

Fig. 2 Study diagram. *Abbreviations*: *EBUS-GS* endobronchial ultrasound with a guide sheath, *GGO* ground-glass opacity, *GS* guide sheath, *PCLL* peripheral cavitary lung lesion, *R-EBUS* radial endobronchial ultrasound

diagnosed by using EBUS-GS (diagnostic yield, 77.8 %), 4 were diagnosed according to other examinations after EBUS-GS (EBUS-TBNA in 1 lung adenocarcinoma, surgery in 2 lung adenocarcinomas and 1 lung squamous carcinoma), and the remaining 2 were clinically diagnosed as lung cancer according to more than 6 months of CT follow-up and multidisciplinary team discussions. Among 23 benign lesions, 19 were successfully diagnosed by using EBUS-GS (diagnostic yield, 82.6 %), 3 were diagnosed according to other examinations after EBUS-GS (surgery in 1 nontuberculous mycobacteria [NTM], sputum culture in 2 NTMs), and the remaining 1 was clinically diagnosed as rheumatoid nodule based on its marked decrease in size by immunosuppressive therapy for rheumatoid arthritis. Overall, sensitivity, specificity, positive predictive value and negative predictive value for diagnosing malignancy were 77.8, 100, 100 and 79.3 %, respectively.

Table 1 Baseline characteristics of patients with peripheral cavitary lung lesions

Variable	All (n = 50)
Age, median (range), year	67 (45–86)
Sex, *n* (%)	
Male	32 (64)
Female	18 (36)
Lesion size, median (range), mm	33.5 (16–100)
Cavity wall thickness, median (range), mm	11 (3–64)
Distance from costal pleura, median (range), mm	0 (0–22)
Lobar location, *n* (%)	
Upper	21 (42)
Middle	2 (4)
Lower	27 (54)
Bronchus sign, *n* (%)	
Positive	41 (82)
Negative	9 (18)
VBN, *n* (%)	
Yes	27 (54)
No	23 (46)
EBUS, *n* (%)	
Within	26 (52)
Adjacent to	18 (36)
Invisible	6 (12)

Abbreviations: *EBUS* endobronchial ultrasound, *VBN* virtual bronchoscopic navigation

The diagnostic yields for cytologic, histopathologic and microbiologic samples also are shown in Table 2. For 27 malignant lesions, 17 (63.0 %) cytologic and 20 (74.1 %) histopathologic samples were diagnostic. With respect to histologic type of lung cancer, squamous cell carcinoma was more diagnosable by histopathology than adenocarcinoma (86.7 vs 70 %). For 23 benign lesions, 16 (69.6 %) histopathologic and 11 (47.8 %) microbiologic samples were diagnostic. For 15 lesions with mycobacterial infection (TB in 3, NTM in 12), the sensitivity of EBUS-GS was 80 % (12/15), and 9 (60 %) and 11 (73.3 %) lesions were successfully diagnosed by using histopathologic and microbiologic samples, respectively. All of the other infectious diseases, including 4 lung abscesses and 1 Aspergillosis, were successfully diagnosed by histopathologic samples only.

The overall diagnostic yield for EBUS-GS was 80 % (40/50). Univariate analyses indicated that PCLLs in which the EBUS probe could be placed within the lesion had a significantly higher diagnostic yield compared with when the EBUS probe was adjacent to the lesion or invisible (92.3 vs. 66.7 %, $P = 0.03$). Multivariate logistic regression analyses using the possible cofounders of lesion size, bronchus sign and EBUS probe 'within' also revealed that the only significant factor affecting diagnostic yield was EBUS probe 'within' (odds ratio, 7.04; $P = 0.03$) (Table 3). Among the 50 procedures, pulmonary

Table 2 Final diagnoses and diagnostic yields according to sample category

Final diagnosis	All ($n = 50$)	Diagnosed by EBUS-GS, n (%)	Diagnosed by cytologic sample, n (%)	Diagnosed by histologic sample, n (%)	Diagnosed by microbiologic sample, n (%)
Lung cancer	27	21 (77.8)	17 (63.0)	20 (74.1)	0 (0)
Adenocarcinoma	10	7 (70)	6 (60)	7 (70)	0 (0)
Squamous cell carcinoma	15	14 (93.3)	11 (73.3)	13 (86.7)	0 (0)
Clinically diagnosed	2	0 (0)	0 (0)	0 (0)	0 (0)
Benign	23	19 (82.6)	0 (0)	16 (69.6)	11 (47.8)
TB	3	3 (100)	0 (0)	3 (100)	3 (100)
NTM	12	9 (75)	0 (0)	6 (50)	8 (66.7)
Lung abscess	4	4 (100)	0 (0)	4 (100)	0 (0)
Aspergillosis	1	1 (100)	0 (0)	1 (100)	0 (0)
Rheumatoid nodule	1	0 (0)	0 (0)	0 (0)	0 (0)
Inflammation	2	2 (100)	0 (0)	2 (100)	0 (0)

Abbreviations: *EBUS-GS* endobronchial ultrasound with a guide sheath, *NTM* nontuberculous mycobacteria, *TB Mycobacterium tuberculosis*

infection occurred in 1 patient (2.0 %). In this case, although fever and increased inflammatory reaction occurred after EBUS-GS, such symptoms were resolved by intravenous antibiotic therapy. No other major complications, including pneumothorax or significant haemorrhage that necessitated premature termination of the procedure, were reported.

A representative case is shown in Fig. 3. The EBUS image before sampling was 'adjacent to' the lesion, which showed the thin wall of the lesion. With the guide sheath located just before the cavity wall, samples were obtained by using a brush and forceps. Cytologic and histologic specimens showed adenocarcinoma.

Discussion

Although EBUS-GS has improved the diagnostic yield for peripheral lung lesions, reports on the use of EBUS-GS specifically for cavitary lesions are unavailable. To the best of our knowledge, this is the first report on the efficacy and safety of EBUS-GS for diagnosis of PCLLs. In addition, the utility of the practical sampling method of EBUS-GS for malignant and benign PCLLs was carefully evaluated in this study. Two important clinical observations were made. First, EBUS-GS had a high diagnostic yield (80 %) for PCLLs with a low risk of significant complications (2.0 %). Second, the EBUS-GS sampling method combined with cytologic, histopathologic, and microbiologic samples was effective for diagnosis of both benign and malignant PCLLs.

A cavity is the result of such pathologic processes as necrosis, cystic dilation of pulmonary structures, and displacement of lung tissue by cystic structures [16]. In addition, malignant lesions can become hollowed out due to treatment-related necrosis, internal cyst formation, or internal desquamation of tumour cells [17]. Active infectious and malignant diseases require a prompt and accurate diagnosis to minimize adverse outcomes and apply appropriate management. Although thin-section chest CT findings, such as cavity wall thickness, are helpful for diagnosis of cavitary lesions, sufficient pathologic or microbiologic samples are often necessary to ensure correct diagnosis [16]. TTNA is a useful nonsurgical method for examination of peripheral lung lesions, but its risk of complication is generally higher than TBB, and thus, it may have concerns about safety for cavitary lesions because of internal necrosis and inflammatory reactions [18, 19]. Actually, Zhuang et al. reported that although TTNA had an accuracy of 96.1 % for diagnosis of 102 cavitary lung lesions, complications included pneumothorax (8.8 %), alveolar haemorrhage (13.7 %), and hemoptysis (1 %) [20].

Currently, EBUS-GS is becoming a standard procedure for diagnosis of peripheral lung lesions based on its useful and safe profile. Therefore, confirmation of its diagnostic utility for PCLLs is also demanded in clinical practice. In the present study, we first reported a high diagnostic yield (80 %) for EBUS-GS for PCLLs. This result is comparable to the diagnostic yield for R-EBUS for peripheral lung lesions reported in recent studies. Therefore, EBUS-GS can be considered as a standard procedure for diagnosis of peripheral lung lesions and PCLLs [9, 21–23]. Moreover, we demonstrated that the diagnostic yield was better when the R-EBUS probe was within the lesion, which has been similarly shown in previous studies [24–26]. However, in the present study, no other important factors, such as bronchus sign, lesion size, or cavity wall thickness, were found to be associated with increased diagnostic yield, despite the small sample size. Especially in larger lesions, the inflammatory reaction

Table 3 Factors affecting diagnostic yield of EBUS-GS for peripheral cavitary lung lesions

Variable	Univariate analysis		Multivariate analysis	
	Diagnostic yield, (%)	*P* value	OR (95 % CI)	*P* value
Age, year				
≥ 70	17/20 (85)	0.72	–	
< 70	23/30 (76.7)			
Sex				
Male	26/32 (81.3)	1	–	
Female	14/18 (77.8)			
Lesion size, mm				
> 30	25/31 (80.6)	1	1.19 (0.24–5.95)	0.83
≤ 30	15/19 (78.9)			
Cavity wall thickness, mm				
> 10	22/27 (81.5)	1	–	
≤ 10	18/23 (78.3)			
Distance from costal pleura, mm				
> 10	10/11 (90.9)	0.42	–	
≤ 10	30/39 (76.9)			
Lobar location				
Lower	21/27 (77.8)	0.74	–	
Upper/middle	19/23 (82.6)			
Bronchus sign				
Positive	32/41 (78.0)	0.67	0.26 (0.02–2.90)	0.27
Negative	8/9 (88.9)			
VBN				
Yes	22/27 (81.5)	1	–	
No	18/23 (78.3)			
EBUS image				
Within	24/26 (92.3)	0.03	7.04 (1.27–38.90)	0.03
Adjacent to/invisible	16/24 (66.7)			

Abbreviations: *CI* confidence interval, *EBUS* endobronchial ultrasound, *EBUS-GS* endobronchial ultrasound with a guide sheath, *OR* odds ratio, *VBN* virtual bronchoscopic navigation

around the cavity wall might interfere with obtaining diagnostic samples even if bronchus sign is positive. A previous study on the use of TTNA for diagnosis of cavitary lung lesions reported that more nondiagnostic samples were obtained from lesions with thin walls [20]. Repeated biopsies at precise locations might contribute to accurate diagnosis even for PCLLs with thin walls, as shown in the representative case.

The complication rate in the present study was 2.0 % (pulmonary infection), which is lower than that reported in previous studies on the use of TTNA for diagnosis of cavitary lung lesions [3, 20]. There was no case of pneumothorax or significant haemorrhage, which are major complications of TBB for peripheral lung lesions. Precise localisation by R-EBUS and the tamponade effect of the guide sheath might reduce the risk of complications, even for PCLLs. Although TBB using R-EBUS has been reported as a safe procedure for diagnosis of peripheral lung lesions, a previous study showed that among 965 peripheral lung lesions examined by using EBUS-GS, pulmonary infection occurred in 5 patients (0.5 %), 2 of which had PCLLs [8]. Therefore, although EBUS-GS was found to be safe for diagnosis of PCLLs in the present study, we should be mindful of the risk of pulmonary infection.

This study also demonstrated that the EBUS-GS sampling method combined with cytologic, histopathologic, and microbiologic samples was effective for diagnosis of both benign and malignant PCLLs. In the present study, diagnostic tissue samples were obtained by using TBB for 74.1 % of malignant lesions and 69.6 % of benign lesions. Recently, histopathologic diagnosis of lung cancer is becoming important for definitive treatment including chemotherapy and tyrosine kinase inhibitors [27].

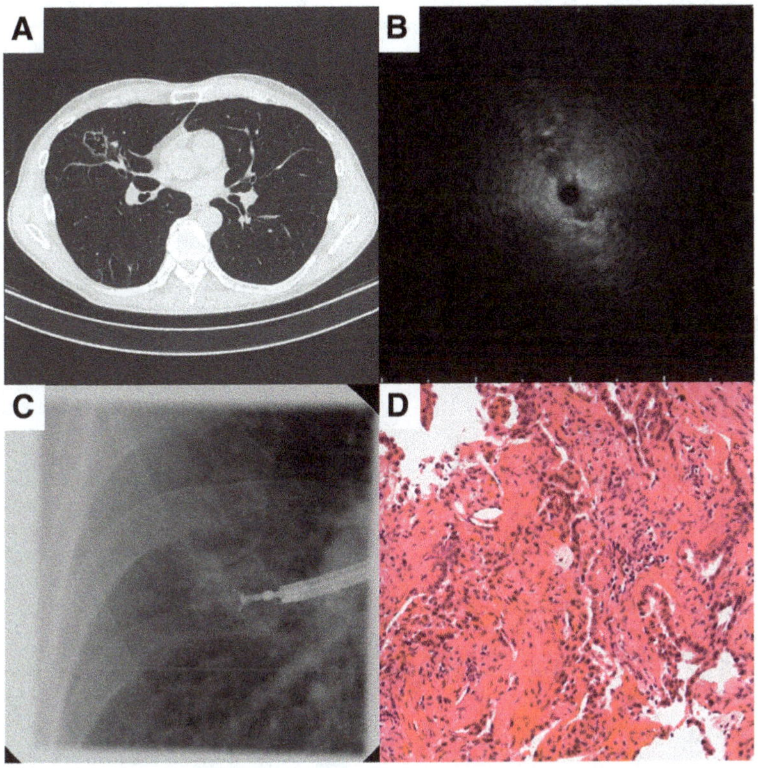

Fig. 3 Case of a 64-year-old man with an abnormal shadow in the right middle lobe. (**a**) Computed tomography scan, showing a 32-mm peripheral cavitary lung lesion with a thin wall (3 mm). (**b**) Endobronchial ultrasound image is 'adjacent to' the lesion. (**c**) Fluoroscopic image during transbronchial biopsy through a guide sheath. (**d**) Histologic specimen obtained by using forceps, showing adenocarcinoma (hematoxylin and eosin stain, magnification ×200)

Moreover, because cavitary lung cancer has a worse prognosis than non-cavitary lung cancer, successful histopathologic diagnosis using a safe technique is demanded [28]. This should also be applied to benign cavitary lesions. Chan et al. recently reported that necrotizing granulomatous inflammation was demonstrated by using EBUS-GS in 10 of 22 patients with pulmonary TB, and that histopathologic diagnosis of TB might contribute to prompt treatment [9]. Certainly, histopathologic diagnosis is necessary for appropriate treatment not only for malignant lesions but also for benign lesions. Even for PCLLs, EBUS-GS has the advantages of locating lesions accurately, controlling bleeding, and obtaining adequate tissue samples.

In the present study, microbiologic samples demonstrated a diagnostic yield of 47.8 % for benign diseases; the diagnostic yield was particularly high for mycobacterium infection, which is the main cause of a cavitary lung lesion (100 % in TB, 66.7 % in NTM). Microbiology results were negative for infectious cases with lung abscess or Aspergillosis, though anaerobic or *Aspergillus* culture was not performed routinely. Because the culture sensitivities of these diseases using bronchoscopy samples are not satisfactory [29, 30], routine bronchial wash or bronchoalveolar lavage after removing the guide sheath may not be necessary. Instead, obtaining adequate tissue samples can contribute to definitive treatment. Although the guide sheath has to be introduced into the lesion for adequate tissue sampling, the R-EBUS probe was located within the lesion in only 26 patients (52 %) in the present study, despite a positive bronchus sign in the majority of cases (82 %). Although this may be due to a lack of skills in the trainees, additional TBNA may be important for improved diagnosis of PCLLs, especially when they are not located by using R-EBUS [13, 31–33].

The present study has several limitations. First, this was a retrospective, nonrandomised, single-institution study with a small sample size. Second, the procedures were not performed by the same operator. Thus, it remains unclear whether the results can be generalized to other institutions.

Conclusions

In conclusion, we presented the first report on EBUS-GS for PCLLs based on our clinical experience. Our results indicate that EBUS-GS is a safe and effective procedure for diagnosis of PCLLs. Sufficient cytologic, histopathologic, and microbiologic samples can be obtained for both benign and malignant PCLLs. Further multicenter prospective studies are recommended in the future.

Abbreviations

CT: computed tomography; EBUS: endobronchial ultrasound; EBUS-GS: endobronchial ultrasound with a guide sheath; GGO: ground-glass opacity; NTM: nontuberculous mycobacteria; PCLL: peripheral cavitary lung lesion; R-EBUS: radial endobronchial ultrasound; TB: *Mycobacterium tuberculosis*; TBB: transbronchial biopsy; TBNA: transbronchial needle aspiration; TTNA: transthoracic needle aspiration; VBN: virtual bronchoscopic navigation.

Competing interests

The authors declare that they have no competing interests.

Authors' contributions

MH designed the overall study and performed the statistical analysis. All authors substantially contributed to the acquisition, interpretation, and consolidation of data. All authors wrote the manuscript and approved the final version.

Acknowledgments

We thank the staff members of the Department of Thoracic Malignancy at Osaka Prefectural Medical Center for Respiratory and Allergic Diseases for their efforts in data collection.

Funding

None.

Author details

[1]Department of Thoracic Malignancy, Osaka Prefectural Medical Center for Respiratory and Allergic Diseases, 3-7-1, Habikino, Habikino City, Osaka 583-8588, Japan. [2]Department of Pathology, Osaka Prefectural Medical Center for Respiratory and Allergic Diseases, Osaka, Japan.

References

1. Tuddenham WJ. Glossary of terms for thoracic radiology: recommendations of the Nomenclature Committee of the Fleischner Society. AJR Am J Roentgenol. 1984;143:509–17.
2. Honda O, Tsubamoto M, Inoue A, Johkoh T, Tomiyama N, Hamada S, et al. Pulmonary cavitary nodules on computed tomography: differentiation of malignancy and benignancy. J Comput Assist Tomogr. 2007;31:943–9.
3. Belet U, Findik S, Ozmen Z, Atici AG, Akan H. Percutaneous cavitary lavage in the diagnosis of pulmonary cavities. J Thorac Dis. 2013;5:440–5.
4. Rivera MP, Mehta AC, Wahidi MM. Establishing the diagnosis of lung cancer: diagnosis and management of lung cancer, 3rd ed: American College of Chest Physicians evidence-based clinical practice guidelines. Chest. 2013; 143(5 Suppl):e142S–65.
5. Tomiyama N, Yasuhara Y, Nakajima Y, Adachi S, Arai Y, Kusumoto M, et al. CT-guided needle biopsy of lung lesions: a survey of severe complication based on 9783 biopsies in Japan. Eur J Radiol. 2006;59:60–4.
6. Wiener RS, Schwartz LM, Woloshin S, Welch HG. Population-based risk for complications after transthoracic needle lung biopsy of a pulmonary nodule: an analysis of discharge records. Ann Intern Med. 2011;155:137–44.
7. Wang Memoli JS, Nietert PJ, Silvestri GA. Meta-analysis of guided bronchoscopy for the evaluation of the pulmonary nodule. Chest. 2012;142:385–93.
8. Hayama M, Izumo T, Matsumoto Y, Chavez C, Tsuchida T, Sasada S. Complications with endobronchial ultrasound with a guide sheath for the diagnosis of peripheral pulmonary lesions. Respiration. 2015;90:129–35.
9. Chan A, Devanand A, Low SY, Koh MS. Radial endobronchial ultrasound in diagnosing peripheral lung lesions in a high tuberculosis setting. BMC Pulm Med. 2015;15:90.
10. Shinagawa N, Nakano K, Asahina H, Kikuchi E, Ito T, Matsuno Y, et al. Endobronchial ultrasonography with a guide sheath in the diagnosis of benign peripheral diseases. Ann Thorac Surg. 2012;93:951–7.
11. Tamiya M, Okamoto N, Sasada S, Shiroyama T, Morishita N, Suzuki H, et al. Diagnostic yield of combined bronchoscopy and endobronchial ultrasonography, under LungPoint guidance for small peripheral pulmonary lesions. Respirology. 2013;18:834–9.
12. Sasada S, Izumo T, Chavez C, Matsumoto Y, Tsuchida T. A new middle-range diameter bronchoscope with large channel for transbronchial sampling of peripheral pulmonary lesions. Jpn J Clin Oncol. 2014;44:826–34.
13. Hayama M, Izumo T, Chavez C, Matsumoto Y, Tsuchida T, Sasada S. Additional transbronchial needle aspiration through a guide sheath (GS-TBNA) for peripheral pulmonary lesions that cannot be detected by radial EBUS. Clin Respir J. 2015 Nov 25. [Epub ahead of print]
14. Izumo T, Sasada S, Chavez C, Matsumoto Y, Hayama M, Tsuchida T. The diagnostic value of histology and cytology samples during endobronchial ultrasound with a guide sheath. Jpn J Clin Oncol. 2015;45:362–6.
15. Kanda Y. Investigation of the freely available easy-to-use software 'EZR' for medical statistics. Bone Marrow Transplant. 2013;48:452–8.
16. Gadkowski LB, Stout JE. Cavitary pulmonary disease. Clin Microbiol Rev. 2008;21:305–33.
17. Miura H, Taira O, Hiraguri S, Hagiwara M, Kato H. Cavitating adenocarcinoma of the lung. Ann Thorac Cardiovasc Surg. 1998;4:154–8.
18. Seo H, Cha SI, Shin KM, Lim J, Yoo SS, Lee J, et al. Focal necrotizing pneumonia is a distinct entity from lung abscess. Respirology. 2013;18: 1095–100.
19. Kim NR, Han J. Pathologic review of cystic and cavitary lung diseases. Korean J Pathol. 2012;46:407–14.
20. Zhuang YP, Wang HY, Zhang J, Feng Y, Zhang L. Diagnostic accuracy and safety of CT-guided fine needle aspiration biopsy in cavitary pulmonary lesions. Eur J Radiol. 2013;82:182–6.
21. Oki M, Saka H, Ando M, Asano F, Kurimoto N, Morita K, et al. Ultrathin bronchoscopy with multimodal devices for peripheral pulmonary lesions. A randomized trial. Am J Respir Crit Care Med. 2015;192:468–76.
22. Steinfort DP, Bonney A, See K, Irving LB. Sequential multimodality bronchoscopic investigation of peripheral pulmonary lesions. Eur Respir J. 2016;47:607–14.
23. Matsumoto Y, Izumo T, Sasada S, Tsuchida T, Ohe Y. Diagnostic utility of endobronchial ultrasound with a guide sheath under the computed tomography workstation (ziostation) for small peripheral pulmonary lesions. Clin Respir J. 2015 June 15. [Epub ahead of print]
24. Chavez C, Sasada S, Izumo T, Watanabe J, Katsurada M, Matsumoto Y, et al. Endobronchial ultrasound with a guide sheath for small malignant pulmonary nodules: a retrospective comparison between central and peripheral locations. J Thorac Dis. 2015;7:596–602.
25. Tay JH, Irving L, Antippa P, Steinfort DP. Radial probe endobronchial ultrasound: factors influencing visualization yield of peripheral pulmonary lesions. Respirology. 2013;18:185–90.
26. Yamada N, Yamazaki K, Kurimoto N, Asahina H, Kikuchi E, Shinagawa N, et al. Factors related to diagnostic yield of transbronchial biopsy using endobronchial ultrasonography with a guide sheath in small peripheral pulmonary lesions. Chest. 2007;132:603–8.
27. Hirashima T, Suzuki H, Okamoto N, Morishita N, Yamadori T, Tamiya M, et al. Important factors for achieving survival of five years or more in non-small cell lung cancer patients with distant metastasis. Oncol Lett. 2014;8:327–34.
28. Watanabe Y, Kusumoto M, Yoshida A, Suzuki K, Asamura H, Tsuta K. Surgically resected solitary cavitary lung adenocarcinoma: association between clinical, pathologic, and radiologic findings and prognosis. Ann Thorac Surg. 2015;99:968–74.

29. Ascioglu S, Rex JH, de Pauw B, Bennett JE, Bille J, Crokaert F, et al. Defining opportunistic invasive fungal infections in immunocompromised patients with cancer and hematopoietic stem cell transplants: an international consensus. Clin Infect Dis. 2002;34:7–14.
30. Hammond JM, Potgieter PD, Hanslo D, Scott H, Roditi D. The etiology and antimicrobial susceptibility patterns of microorganisms in acute community-acquired lung abscess. Chest. 1995;108:937–41.
31. Chao TY, Chien MT, Lie CH, Chung YH, Wang JL, Lin MC. Endobronchial ultrasonography-guided transbronchial needle aspiration increases the diagnostic yield of peripheral pulmonary lesions: a randomized trial. Chest. 2009;136:229–36.
32. Ost DE, Ernst A, Lei X, Kovitz KL, Benzaquen S, Diaz-Mendoza J, et al. Diagnostic yield and complications of bronchoscopy for peripheral lung lesions. Results of the AQuIRE registry. Am J Respir Crit Care Med. 2016;193: 68–77.
33. Bellinger CR, Chatterjee AB, Adair N, Houle T, Khan I, Haponik E. Training in and experience with endobronchial ultrasound. Respiration. 2014;88:478–83.

6

From "traction bronchiectasis" to honeycombing in idiopathic pulmonary fibrosis: A spectrum of bronchiolar remodeling also in radiology?

Sara Piciucchi[1*], Sara Tomassetti[2], Claudia Ravaglia[2], Christian Gurioli[2], Carlo Gurioli[2], Alessandra Dubini[3], Angelo Carloni[4], Marco Chilosi[5], Thomas V Colby[6] and Venerino Poletti[2,7]

Abstract

Background: The diagnostic and prognostic impact of traction bronchiectasis on high resolution CT scan (HRCT) in patients suspected to have idiopathic pulmonary fibrosis (IPF) is increasing significantly.

Main body: Recent data demonstrated that cysts in honeycombing areas are covered by epithelium expressing bronchiolar markers. In IPF bronchiolization is the final consequence of a variety of pathogenic events starting from alveolar stem cell exhaustion, and ending in a abnormal/dysplastic proliferation of bronchiolar epithelium. CT scan features of traction bronchiectasis and honeycombing should be interpreted under the light of these new pathogenetic and morphologic considerations.

Short conclusion: We suggest that in IPF subjects traction bronchiectasis and honeycombing -now defined as distinct entities on HRCT scan- are actually diverse aspects of a continuous spectrum of lung remodeling.

Keywords: Traction bronchiectasis, Honeycombing, Fibroblastic Foci, Bronchiolar dysplastic proliferation

Background

Histologically, Usual Interstitial Pneumonia (UIP) is characterized by a combination of "patchy fibrosis" and fibroblastic foci displaying a "patchwork pattern". Disease progression is characterized by the appearance of airspaces lined by plump cuboidal or even ciliated columnar cells showing a immunohistochemical and molecular bronchiolar phenotype [1–3].

In the recent years, the role of bronchiolar epithelium in the development of UIP pattern (in IPF subjects) has been widely emphasized [4–8].

Factors leading to lung remodeling include senescence, alveolar stem cell exhaustion and consequently aberrant activation of the wnt-β-catenin and hedgehog pathways that normally regulate branching morphogenesis in the lungs [6, 9].

Mechanical stress may contribute to the subpleural and usually basilar localization of UIP changes [10, 11].

The final stage of this "bronchiolization" process corresponds radiologically to honeycombing, typically seen first in the subpleural regions of the lower lobes [2, 3].

Main text

By CT, a "definite" usual interstitial pneumonia (UIP) pattern, as seen in IPF, is characterized by the presence of reticulation, traction bronchiectasis and honeycombing in a basal and peripheral predominant distribution. The presence of honeycombing and traction bronchiectasis, besides reticulation, is crucial [12–19].

However if we reconsider morphological aspects in light of the pathogenic events discussed above, we identify some interesting key points in the interpretation of CT findings.

First, the sites in which mechanical stress and remodeling are highest, correspond to the areas in which traction bronchiectasis and honeycombing appear.

* Correspondence: piciucchi.sara@gmail.com
[1]Department of Radiology, Azienda USL Romagna, Ospedale GB Morgagni, Via C. Forlanini, Forlì FC 34-47121, Italy
Full list of author information is available at the end of the article

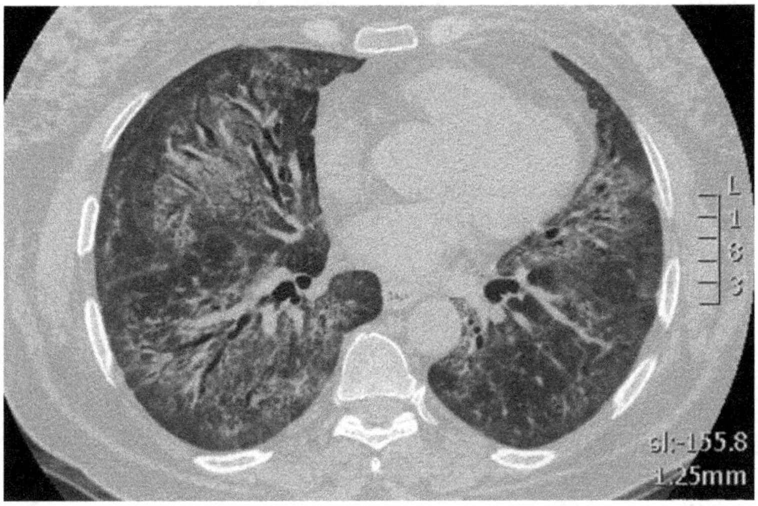

Fig. 1 CT scan of a 52 years old lady, affected by idiopathic NSIP. Bilateral, peribronchovascular ground glass attenuation, due to intralobular fibrotic changes. Traction bronchiectasis are present bilaterally surrounded by ground glass,"fibrotic" attenuation, mainly in the right middle lobe and in both lower lobes. No honeycombing is present. A relative subpleural sparing is also visible

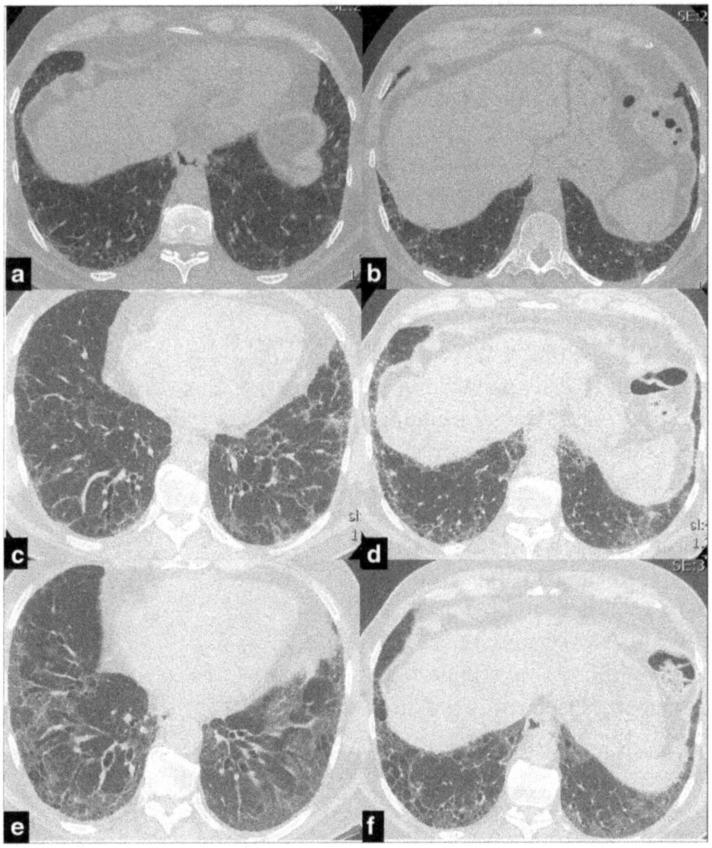

Fig. 2 Serial CT images of a 63 years old male affected by IPF. UIP pattern has been diagnosed through surgical lung biopsy at diagnosis. CT shows the progressive worsening of the coarseness. In 2007 (**a**, **b**) a moderate peripheral fibrotic reticulation is present. In the following years it progressively gets worse, particularly in the right lower lobe, with increase of the extension of traction bronchiectasis in 2010 (**c**, **d**) and with honeycombing and traction bronchiectasis in 2014 (**e**, **f**)

Second, most of the "scarred" tissue is in the region distal to the traction bronchiectasis, beneath the pleura, and does not concentrically surround the dilated bronchi. Conversely in nonspecific Interstitial Pneumonia (NSIP), traction bronchiectasis is completely surrounded by the fibrotic tissue (Fig. 1).

Furthermore as the fibrosis progresses, dilatation of the airways increases in severity from the periphery to the inner third of the lungs, passing from a score 1 (more peripheral) to 3 (from periphery to the inner third of the parenchyma) [score proposed by Edey et al. [20]] (Fig.2).

In CT scans, when fibrosis is more severe, bronchiectasis tend to follow the convexity of the pleura and to overlap with honeycombing features [21].

Therefore, also in CT scans, traction bronchiectasis observed in IPF subjects is better interpreted as resulting from bronchiolar proliferation rather than from pure mechanical traction of a single airway by scarring tissue. Supporting this point of view is the recent observation by Staats et al. [4] on explanted lungs obtained from patients with IPF. They showed a positive correlation between honeycombing assessed by CT and bronchiolectasis ($p = 0.001$) and respiratory-lined cysts ($p = 0.001$) histologically counted. If we consider traction bronchiectasis as the solely consequence of pure mechanical traction around the airway, this process should result in a relatively stable number of traction "holes" with an enlargement of lumen reaching the periphery, as actually is present only in NSIP. Thus, in IPF, remodeling process appears to be a continuum from traction bronchiectasis to honeycombing and conceptual separation of the two processes may be misleading.

Walsh et Al. [19] reinforced this concept recently. The authors retrospectively reviewed radiological features of 162 biopsy proven cases of UIP and NSIP, delineating a radiological visual score for each case and correlating these radiological data to the fibroblastic foci profusion score and other morphologic aspects. They concluded that in UIP there was a strong correlation between traction bronchiectasis, honeycomb changes and fibroblastic foci profusion. In conclusion, according to the "alveolar stem cell exhaustion" model explaining at least part of the pathogenic events in IPF [14] we suggest that traction bronchiectasis and honeycombing is a unique and continuous process of bronchiolar dysplastic proliferation and to interpret accordingly the HRCT features.

Conclusions

In agreement to the "alveolar stem cell exhaustion pathogenic model" in IPF, we may begin to consider traction bronchiectasis and honeycombing as a unique and continuous process of bronchiolar proliferation also in HRCT scan.

Abbreviations

UIP: Usual Interstitial Pneumonia; NSIP: non specific interstitial pneumonia; IPF: idiopathic pulmonary fibrosis; HRCT: high resolution computed tomography.

Acknowledgements

We are very grateful to Dr Paola Tantalocco, biomedical engineer and data manager of our Institution for her important contribution to our research activity.

Funding

No funders.

Authors' contributions

SP, ST, CR, ChG, CG, AD, AC, MC, TVC, VP : participated in the design of the study. SP, TVC, VP: participated in its design and coordination and helped to draft the manuscript. All authors read and approved the final manuscript.

Competing interests

The authors declare that they have no competing interests.

Consent for publication

Not applicable.

Author details

[1]Department of Radiology, Azienda USL Romagna, Ospedale GB Morgagni, Via C. Forlanini, Forlì FC 34-47121, Italy. [2]Department of Diseases of the Thorax, Azienda USL Romagna, Ospedale GB Morgagni, Forlì, Italy. [3]Department of Pathology, Azienda USL Romagna, Ospedale GB Morgagni, Forlì, Italy. [4]Department of Radiology, Ospedale Santa Maria, Terni, Italy. [5]Department of Pathology and Diagnostics, University of Verona, Verona, Italy. [6]Department of Laboratory Medicine and Pathology, Mayo Clinic, Scottsdale, AZ, USA. [7]Department of Respiratory Diseases & Allergy, Aarhus University Hospital, Aarhus, Denmark.

References

1. Chilosi M, Poletti V, Murer B, Lestani M, Cancellieri A, Montagna L, Piccoli P, Cangi G, Semenzato G, Doglioni C. Abnormal re-epithelialization and lung remodeling in idiopathic pulmonary fibrosis: the role of deltaN-p63. Lab Invest. 2002;82:1335–45.
2. Katzenstein AL. In: Saunders WB, editor. Katzenstein and Askin's Surgical Pathology of Non-Neoplastic Lung Disease: Volume 13; the Major Problems in Pathology Series. 2006.
3. Seibold MA, Smith RW, Urbanek C, Groshong SD, Cosgrove GP, Brown KK, Schwarz MI, Schwarz DA, Reynolds SD. The idiopathic pulmonary fibrosis honeycomb cyst contains a mucocilary pseudostratified epithelium. PLoS One. 2013;8:1–9.
4. Staats P, Kligerman S, Todd N, Tavora F, Xu L, Burke A. A comparative study of honeycombing on high resolution computed tomography with histologic lung remodeling in explants with usual interstitial pneumonia. Pathol Res Pract. 2015;211:55–61.
5. Ryu JH, Moua T, Daniels CE, Hartman TE, Yi ES, Utz JP, Limper AH. Idiopathic pulmonary fibrosis: evolving concepts. Mayo Clin Proc. 2014;89:1130–42.
6. Chilosi M, Carloni A, Rossi A, Poletti V. Premature lung aging and cellular senescence in the pathogenesis of idiopathic pulmonary fibrosis and COPD/emphysema. Transl Res. 2013;162:156–73.
7. Gransner JM, Rosas IO. Telomeres in lung disease. Transl Res. 2013;162:343–52.
8. Selman M, Pardo A, Kaminski N. Idiopathic pulmonary fibrosis: aberrant recapitulation of developmental programs? Plos Medicine. 2008;5:373–80.
9. Chilosi M, Zamò A, Doglioni C, Reghellin D, Lestani M, Montagna L, Pedron S, Ennas MG, Cancellieri A, Murer B, Poletti V. Migratory marker expression in fibroblast foci of idiopathic pulmonary fibrosis. Respir Res. 2006;7:95.

10. Carloni A, Poletti V, Fermo L, Bellomo N, Chilosi M. Heterogeneous distribution of mechanical stress in human lung: A mathematical approach to evaluate abnormal remodeling in IPF. Journal of Theoretical Biology. 2013:32-336.
11. Leslie KO. Idiopathic pulmonary fibrosis may be a disease of recurrent, tractional injury to the periphery of the aging lung: a unifying hypothesis regarding etiology and pathogenesis. Arch Pathol Lab Med. 2012;136: 591–600.
12. Raghu G, Collard HR, Egan JJ, et al. An official ATS/ERS/JRS/ALAT statement: idiopathic pulmonary fibrosis: evidence-based guidelines for diagnosis and management. Am J Respir Crit Care Med. 2011;183:788–824.
13. Sverzellati N. Highlights of HRCT imaging in IPF. Respir Research. 2013;14:S3.
14. Lynch DA, Godwin JD, Safrin S, Starko KM, Hormel P, Brown KK, et al. High-resolution computed tomography in idiopathic pulmonary fibrosis: diagnosis and prognosis. Am J Respir Crit Care Med. 2005;172:488–93.
15. Ley B, Ryerson CJ, Vittinghoff E, Ryu JH, Tomassetti S, Lee JS, et al. A multidimensional index and staging system for idiopathic pulmonary fibrosis. Ann Intern Med. 2012;156:684–91.
16. Walsh SL, Sverzellati N, Devaraj A, Keir GJ, Wells AU, Hansell DM. Connective tissue disease related fibrotic lung disease: high resolution computed tomographic and pulmonary function indices as prognostic determinants. Thorax. 2014;69: 216-222.
17. King Jr TE, Schwarz MI, Brown K, Tooze JA, Colby TV, Waldron Jr JA, et al. Idiopathic pulmonary fibrosis: relationship between histopathologic features and mortality. Am J Respir Crit Care Med. 2001;164:1025–32.
18. Nicholson AG, Fulford LG, Colby TV, du Bois RM, Hansell DM, Wells AU. The relationship between individual histologic features and disease progression in idiopathic pulmonary fibrosis. Am J Respir Crit Care Med. 2002;166:173–7.
19. Walsh SL, Wells AU, Sverzellati N, Deveraj A, Von der Thusen J, Yousem SA, Colby TV, Nicholson AG, Hansell DM. Relationship between fibroblastic foci profusion and high resolution CT morphology in fibrotic lung disease. Medicine. 2015;13:241–9.
20. Edey A, Devaray AA, Barker RP, Nicholson AG, Wells AU, Hansell DM. Fibrotic idiopathic interstitial pneumonias: HRCT findings that predict mortality. Eur Radiol. 2011;21:1586–93.
21. Watadani T, Sakai F, Johkoh T, Noma S, Akira M, Fujimoto K, Bankier AA, Lee KS, Müller NL, Song JW, Park JS, Lynch DA, Hansell DM, Remy-Jardin M, Franquet T, Sugiyama Y. Interobserver variability in the CT assessment of honeycombing in the lungs. Radiology. 2013;266:936–44.

7

Endobronchial ultrasound in real life: primary diagnosis and mediastinal staging of lung cancer in patients submitted to thoracic surgery

João Pedro Steinhauser Motta[1*], Axel Tobias Kempa[2], Alexandre Pinto Cardoso[1], Marcos Eduardo Paschoal[1], Ronir Raggio Luiz[3], José Roberto Lapa e Silva[1] and Franz Stanzel[4]

Abstract

Background: Since the first articles published for over 10 years ago, endobronchial ultrasound (EBUS) has gained a strong scientific backing and has been incorporated into routine medical practice in pulmonology and thoracic surgery centers. How is EBUS performing outside the scientific environment, as a diagnostic and mediastinal staging tool in a subset of patients that undergo thoracic surgery, is an interesting question.

Methods: This study evaluated consecutive patients who, during the period from January 2010 to August 2012, were submitted to EBUS and later to thoracic surgery. The samples obtained by endobronchial ultrasound-guided transbronchial needle aspiration (EBUS-TBNA) were compared to surgical samples. The primary endpoint was the proportion of patients with a final diagnosis of non-small cell lung cancer (NSCLC) by EBUS-TBNA correctly subtyped. The secondary endpoint was the negative predictive value (NPV) of EBUS-TBNA for mediastinal staging of lung cancer.

Results: Two hundred eighty seven patients were studied. Considering 84 patients with a final diagnosis of NSCLC by EBUS-TBNA, 79 % (CI 95 % 70.1–87.3) were correctly subclassified. The NPV of EBUS-TBNA for mediastinal staging was 89 % (IC 95 % 84.9–92.7). From a total of 21 false negative cases of mediastinal staging, 16 (76 %) did not undergo positron emission tomography-computed tomography (PET-CT) before the EBUS and in 15 (71 %) the affected lymph node chain was not punctured by EBUS-TBNA. Ten (47 %) patients had only lymph node metastases not directly accessible by the EBUS.

Conclusions: Performed in hospital routine and in patients submitted to thoracic surgery, EBUS-TBNA proved to be a good tool for proper pathological diagnosis of lung cancer. The negative predictive value of 89 % for mediastinal staging of lung cancer is comparable to that reported in previous studies, but the relatively high number of 21 false negative cases points to the need for standardization of routine strategies before, during and after EBUS.

Background

Lung cancer is the malignant tumor with the highest mortality rate among men and women worldwide, with more than 1,4 million deaths a year [1]. The emergence of endobronchial ultrasound-guided transbronchial needle aspiration (EBUS-TBNA), a minimally invasive technique able to provide valuable information for a primary tumor diagnosis and mediastinal staging, significantly changed the approach to lung cancer [2, 3]. Since the first articles published for over 10 years ago [4], endobronchial ultrasound (EBUS) has gained strong scientific backing [5–7] and has been incorporated into routine medical practice of pulmonology and thoracic surgery centers. Guidelines of respiratory societies reinforce the importance of ultrasound-guided needle techniques in the primary diagnosis and mediastinal staging of lung cancer

* Correspondence: joaosteinhauser@gmail.com
[1]Instituto de Doenças do Torax, Universidade Federal do Rio de Janeiro, Rua Professor Rodolpho Paulo Rocco, 255, 1 andar, sala 01D 58/60, Rio de Janeiro, RJ 21941-913, Brazil
Full list of author information is available at the end of the article

[8–11]. The success of the technique and the spread of its use around the world make it important to revaluate its performance in “real life”, outside the scientific environment, especially in patients undergoing thoracic surgery, in which the sharpest staging tools are required.

The aim of our study is to determine EBUS performance in patients undergoing thoracic surgery in hospital routine. Using surgical pathology as the gold standard, we calculated the proportion of patients with a final diagnosis of non-small cell lung cancer (NSCLC) by EBUS-TBNA correctly subtyped and the performance of EBUS-TBNA for the mediastinal staging of lung cancer.

Methods

Study design

The present work is a single-center, retrospective, observational study. All patients who underwent EBUS and thoracic surgery during the period from January 2010 to August 2012 were selected.

Procedures

The examinations and surgeries took place in the Lungenklinik Hemer, a traditional center for respiratory diseases in Germany. EBUS procedures were performed on hospitalized patients, under general anesthesia. The examination could be accompanied by the presence of a pathologist in the procedure room for rapid on-site evaluation (ROSE) or not. EBUS-TBNA samples were collected using a 22-gauge needle. At least 2 aspirates were obtained from each target lesion. When a pathologist was present, 2 pairs of smears were prepared for ROSE and cytologic examinations. The resulting material (tissue cores, shreds of tissue, cellular components, fluids) was processed using a cell-block technique. If there was no pathologist in the room, all the samples were processed as cell-blocks. Indications for a surgical exploration or resection due to suspicion or confirmation of lung cancer were discussed and had to be approved by a local interdisciplinary clinical session with the mandatory participation of pulmonologists, oncologists, chest surgeons, radiologists and radiotherapists. EBUS-TBNA and surgical samples were analyzed by two different pathology services.

Data collection

Data collection and statistical analysis were conducted at the Federal University of Rio de Janeiro, Brazil. Through the computer program Teamviewer ® (TeamViewer GmbH, Germany) the authors had remote access to a database provided by the Lungenklinik Hemer to access patient data from local electronic medical records.

Inclusion criteria

Patients who underwent EBUS for any indication in the Lungenklinik Hemer from January 2010 to August 2012 and were subsequently subjected to surgical procedures.

Exclusion criteria

Patients with no lymph node sampling by EBUS-TBNA during an EBUS procedure or patients who did not have histopathologic sampling of mediastinal lymph nodes during surgery.

Study population

Patients were identified in the electronic system of the Lungenklinik Hemer by crossing the specific code representing the EBUS with codes representing thoracic surgical procedures such as thoracotomy, thoracoscopy or mediastinoscopy. Patients whose electronic records showed both codes in the same hospital stay were selected. Four hundred thirty-nine patients underwent both an EBUS and thoracic surgery between January 2010 and August 2012 in the Lungenklinik Hemer. One hundred fifty-two cases were excluded for not having mediastinal lymph node sampling from both EBUS and surgery. The remaining 287 patients were studied (Fig. 1).

Endpoints

The primary endpoint was the proportion of patients with a final diagnosis of NSCLC by EBUS-TBNA correctly subtyped as compared to the surgical samples. The secondary endpoint was the negative predictive value (NPV) of EBUS-TBNA for mediastinal staging of lung cancer, according to the 7th edition of the lung cancer staging system of the American Joint Committee on Cancer [12].

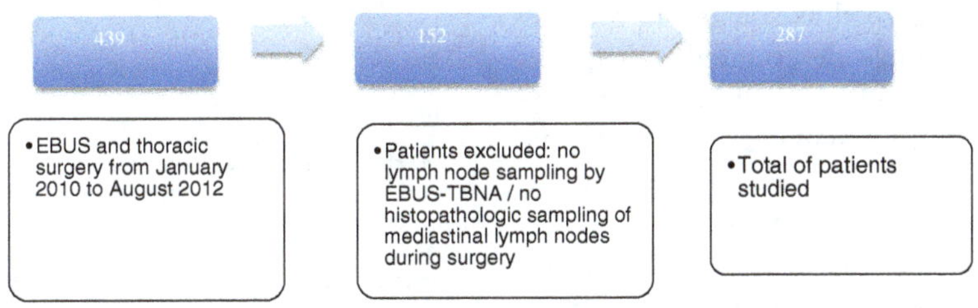

Fig. 1 Flow chart showing selection, exclusion and total of patients studied. EBUS: endobronchial ultrasound. EBUS-TBNA: endobronchial ultrasound-guided transbronchial needle aspiration

Statistical analysis

Patient demographics and disease characteristics were summarized using descriptive statistics. For the primary endpoint, the final result of the pathology after surgical resection was used as the gold standard for comparison to EBUS-TBNA samples. This result takes into account the tumor samples present in the lung parenchyma and/or mediastinum. There was no pairing of samples per lymph node site. For the secondary endpoint, the EBUS-TBNA samples were compared only to mediastinal surgical samples (obtained by mediastinoscopy and/or surgical mediastinal lymphadenectomy). The proportion of NSCLC correctly subclassified, the NPV for mediastinal staging and their 95 % confidence intervals (CI) were calculated using standard definitions. All statistical analyses were performed using SPSS® (IBM SPSS Statistics Version 20, United States of America).

Results

The demographic data, tumor characteristics and details of the procedures performed are summarized in Table 1. The samples obtained by EBUS-TBNA showed no pathological findings in 188 patients (65.5 %) (representative lymph node samples without disease). NSCLC was detected in 84 patients (29.2 %), other malignant diseases in 8 (2.7 %) and benign pathological findings in 7 (2 %) patients (Table 2). Considering the 188 patients without pathological findings in samples of EBUS-TBNA, 156 had a final diagnosis of NSCLC after surgery. Of these, the final surgical mediastinal staging was N0 in 104 patients, N1 in 39 patients and N2 in 13 patients (Fig. 2). In 99 patients it was possible to compare the pathological findings of the EBUS-TBNA samples with the surgical findings. Taking into account NSCLC subtyping analysis, EBUS-TBNA was correct in 67 cases and incorrect or incomplete in 17 cases (Fig. 3). Four patients were diagnosed as NSCLC not otherwise specified (NSCLC-NOS) by EBUS and were determined to be squamous cell carcinoma (3 patients) or adenocarcinoma (1 patient) after the surgical resection; 1 was classified as pulmonary adenocarcinoma and determined to be adenosquamous carcinoma from the surgical sample; 7 were diagnosed as squamous cell carcinoma or adenocarcinoma and the surgical pathology showed large cell carcinoma; 2 cases were subtyped as squamous cell carcinoma and the surgical sample determined a diagnosis of adenocarcinoma; 1 case of adenocarcinoma by EBUS-TBNA was determined to be squamous cell carcinoma by the surgical sample; 1 case classified as adenocarcinoma by EBUS-TBNA and was determined as sarcomatous carcinoma by the surgical sample; and 1 single case of false malignancy of adenocarcinoma with the EBUS-TBNA samples, and surgical resection confirmed a diagnosis of hamartoma. Considering this subclassification,

Table 1 Patient demographics, disease and procedure characteristics

Patients, N	287
Age, mean	64,7
Male gender, N (%)	204 (71.1)
Smoking History, N (%)	126 (43.9)[a]
COPD, N (%)	81 (28.2)
Cardiovascular Disease, N (%)	148 (51.6)
Cancer History, N (%)	42 (14.6)[b]
Lung Cancer History, N (%)	11 (3.8)
Instersticial Lung Disease, N (%)	4 (1.4)
Tumor Location, N, (%)	
Right Superior Lobe	86 (30)
Left Superior Lobe	76 (26.5)
Right Inferior Lobe	47 (16.4)
Left Inferior Lobe	38 (13.2)
Middle Lobe	11 (3.8)
Lymph Node	9 (3.1)
Right Central	10 (3.5)
Left Central	3 (1)
Trachea	2 (0.7)
Bilateral	5 (1.7)
Total Lymph Nodes punctured, N (mean)	849 (2.95)
Number of Lymph Nodes punctured per EBUS, N (%)	
1	30 (10.5)
2	56 (19.5)
3	115 (40.1)
4	70 (24.4)
5	14 (4.9)
6	2 (0.7)
EBUS with ROSE, N (%)	130 (45.3)
Additional Biopsy, N (%)	
Not performed or not diagnostic	153 (53.3)
Endobronchial Biopsie	56 (19.5)
Transbronchial Biopsie	78 (27.2)
Major Surgical Procedure, N (%)	
Right Superior Lobectomy	71 (24.7)
Left Superior Lobectomy	51 (17.8)
Right Inferior Lobectomy	23 (8.0)
Left Inferior Lobectomy	23 (8.0)
Bilobectomy	12 (4.2)
Right Pneumectomy	27 (9.4)
Left Pneumectomy	22 (7.7)
Segmentectomy or wedge resection	48 (16.7)
Mediastinoscopy	4 (1.4)
NSCLC after surgical exploration, N (%)	238 (82.9 %)
Final Tumor Staging, N[c]	242
IA, N (%)	29 (12.0)
IB, N (%)	39 (16.1)
IIA, N (%)	46 (19.0)
IIB, N (%)	43 (17.8)
IIIA, N (%)	66 (27.3)
IIIB, N (%)	12 (5.0)
IV, N (%)	7 (2.9)

COPD chronic obstructive pulmonary disease, *Cardiovascular Disease* coronary arterial disease, arterial hypertension, ischemic or hemorrhagic brain disease, peripheral vascular disease, atrial fibrillation, aortic aneurysm, *EBUS* endobronchial ultrasound, *ROSE* rapid on-set evaluation, *NSCLC* non-small cell lung cancer

[a]smoking history could be assessed only when evidenced in the hospital discharge letter

[b]history of any cancer other than lung cancer

[c]considering 238 patients with NSCLC and 4 patients with Carcinoid Tumor

Table 2 EBUS-TBNA pathological findings

Absence of pathological findings, N (%)[a]	188 (65.5)
Squamous Cell Carcinoma, N (%)	40 (13.9)
Adenocarcinoma, N (%)	38 (13.2)
Large Cell carcinoma, N (%)	1 (0.3)
Adenosquamous Carcinoma, N (%)	1 (0.3)
NSCLC-NOS, N (%)	4 (1.3)
Clear Cell Carcinoma, N (%)	1 (0.3)
Undifferentiated Carcinoma, N (%)	2 (0.7)
Neuroendocrine Tumor, N (%)	1 (0.3)
Thymoma, N (%)	1 (0.3)
Lymphoproliferative Process, N (%)	2 (0.7)
Sarcomatous Process, N (%)	1 (0.3)
Anthracosis and Silica, N (%)	1 (0.3)
Granulomatous Process, N (%)	4 (1.4)
Inflammatory Process, N (%)	2 (0.7)
Total, N (%)	287 (100 %)

NSCLC-NOS non-small cell lung cancer not otherwise specified
[a]representative lymph node samples without disease

the proportion of patients with a final diagnosis of NSCLC by EBUS-TBNA in whom NSCLC subtyping was correct was 79 % (IC 95 % 70.1-87.3).

The EBUS-TBNA performance for the mediastinal staging of lung cancer was calculated by taking into account all 238 patients with NSCLC who had mediastinal lymph node sampling by both EBUS and surgery (Table 3). EBUS staging was correct in 213 cases and incorrect in 25. There were 180 true negative, 33 true positive, 21 false negative and 4 false positive findings. Those findings allowed us to calculate the NPV of 89 % (CI 95 % 84.5-93), the positive predictive value (PPV) of 89 % (72.5–95.7) the sensibility of 61 % (CI 95 % 47.8-72.9) and the specificity of 97 % (CI 95 % 94.5-99.1). From the 21 false negative cases, 16 (76 %)

Table 3 Mediastinal Lymph Node Staging: EBUS-TBNA X Surgery

EBUS-TBNA N stage	Final N stage	Number of cases
Correctly staged		
0 or 1	0 or 1	180
2	2	32
3	3	1
Incorrectly staged		
0 or 1	2	20
2	0 or 1	4
2	3	1

EBUS-TBNA: endobronchial ultrasound-guided transbronchial needle aspiration
Total of patientes with NSCLC: 238
True positive: 33 / True negative: 180 / False positive: 4 / False negative: 21
Sensibility: 61% (CI 95% 47.8-72.9) / Specificity 97% (CI 95% 94.5-99.1) /
Positive predictive value 89% (CI 95% 75.2-95.7) / Negative predictive value: 89 (CI 95% 84.5-93)

did not undergo positron emission tomography-computed tomography (PET-CT) or it was performed after the EBUS. In 15 (71 %) patients the affected lymph node chain was not punctured by EBUS-TBNA. Ten (47 %) patients had only lymph node metastases not directly accessible by the EBUS (lymph node chains 5,6,8 and 9). In 11 (52 %) patients the tumor was located in the left superior lobe. The more often affected lymph node chain was station 5, with 7 false negative cases.

Considering the 4 false positive cases, 2 were surgically classified as N1 and 2 were classified as N0 (all confirmed surgically as NSCLC). In just one of the cases there was a disagreement of the pathological findings of EBUS-TBNA and surgery (EBUS-TBNA suggested adenocarcinoma and surgery confirmed large cell carcinoma). All the 4 cases were submitted to surgical lobectomy and lymph node dissection.

Twenty patients had a mediastinoscopy after the EBUS (4 as the main surgical procedure and 16 as part of the mediastinal staging before surgery). There were 15 true negative, 1 true positive, 4 false negative and no false positive findings comparing mediastinoscopy to final surgical mediastinal staging. Mediastinoscopy did not contribute to a better mediastinal staging than the EBUS in any of the patients. All the 15 true negative cases were also negative by the EBUS. The true positive case was also positive by the EBUS, and one of the 4 false negative mediastinoscopies cases was positive by the EBUS.

Discussion

Our study evaluated the EBUS-TBNA performance in a key subset of patients with lung cancer: those undergoing thoracic surgery. Despite not representing the majority of patients diagnosed with lung cancer, this is the subgroup in which we need to have the sharpest diagnostic and staging tools to ensure an accurate referral to surgery and expectation of cure. To our knowledge, this is the work with the highest number of patients submitted to surgery who had their EBUS-TBNA results directly compared with the surgical sampling. The use of EBUS was evaluated in a hospital routine, without adherence to study protocols influencing the exam.

The primary endpoint of the study was the proportion of patients with a final diagnosis of NSCLC by EBUS-TBNA correctly subtyped. Our results show that NSCLC was correctly subclassified in 79 % of cases. One of the limitations of existing evidence on EBUS diagnostic performance is that many studies included results of the index test and clinical follow-up in a reference standard test and did not account for the surgical sample being the only possible gold standard. This may have overestimated the result of some studies [13]. Esterbrook et al. showed that EBUS-TBNA samples when made into cell-blocks and subjected to a panel of immunohistochemical

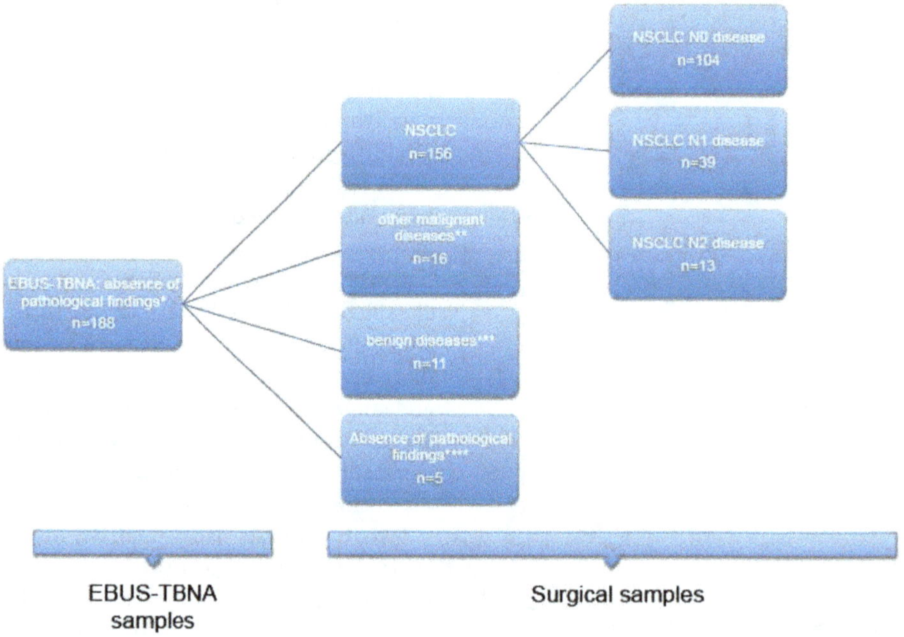

Fig. 2 Flow chart showing the 188 cases with samples without pathological findings by EBUS-TBNA and the final pathological results after surgery. * EBUS-TBNA representative samples without pathological findings. ** surgical samples with malign pathological findings others than NSCLC. *** surgical samples with benign pathological findings. **** surgical samples without pathological findings

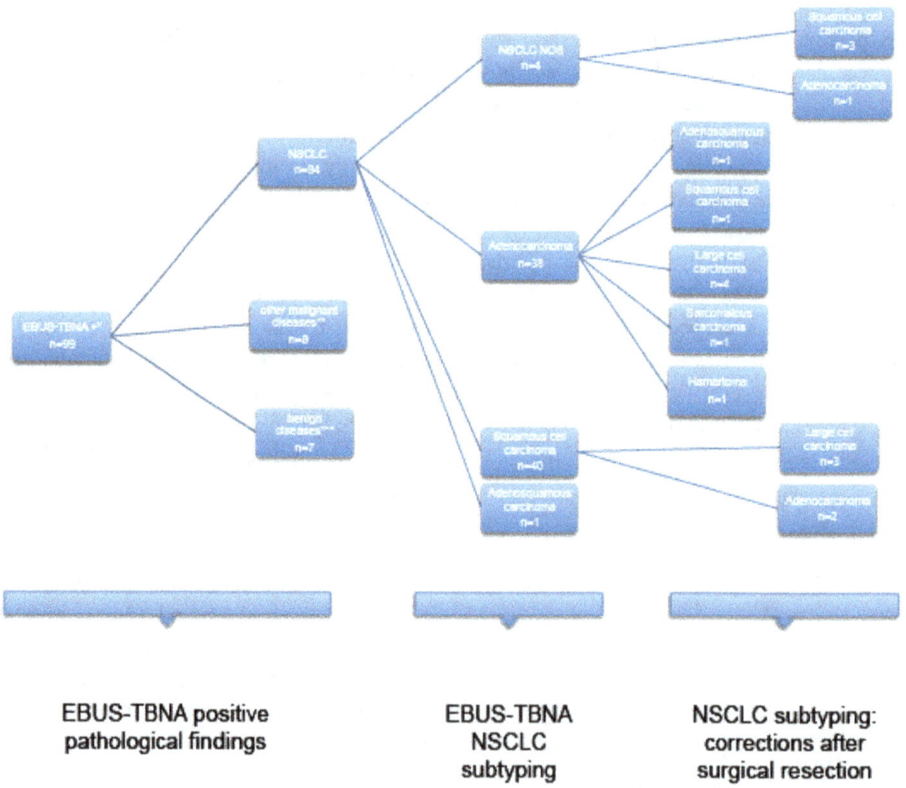

Fig. 3 Flow chart showing pathological findings of the EBUS-TBNA samples; NSCLC subtyping by EBUS-TBNA and corrections after surgical resection. EBUS-TBNA: endobronchial ultrasound-guided transbronchial needle aspiration. NSCLC: non-small cell lung cancer. NSCLC NOS: non-small cell lung cancer not otherwise specified. * EBUS-TBNA samples with positive pathological findings. ** EBUS-TBNA samples with malign pathological findings others than NSCLC. ***EBUS-TBNA samples with benign pathological findings

stains returned adequate tissue for NSCLC subtyping in 79 %, with a NSCLC-NOS reate of 21 % [14]. In a large, multicenter study, Navani et al. demonstrated that samples from EBUS-TBNA provide sufficient information for subtyping NSCLC in 77 % of the cases [15].

We chose the NPV of EBUS-TBNA for the mediastinal staging of lung cancer as the secondary endpoint of our study because we consider it to be the most clinically relevant measure in the subset of patients who undergo thoracic surgery. From a total of 238 patients with NSCLC surgically evaluated, 53 had mediastinal metastatic involvement ipsilateral to the target tumor lesion (N2 disease) and 2 had contralateral mediastinal involvement (N3 disease), representing a prevalence of mediastinal nodal involvement of 23 %. The results of our study showed an NPV of 89 %. Probably some of the most important publications of EBUS and mediastinal lymph node staging in patients with potentially resectable NSCLC are the ASTER trial [16], published in 2010, and the work of Yasufuku et al. [17], published in 2011. The ASTER trial found an NPV for endosonography staging alone without additional surgical staging of 85 % (prevalence of N2/N3 54 %). Yasufuku showed an NPV of 91 % for EBUS-TBNA (prevalence of N2/N3 disease 35 %).

The sensitivity of 61 % in our work was lower than expected and previously reported. This fact is due to the relatively high number of 21 false negative cases. In reviewing such cases we realize that 16 (76 %) did not undergo PET-CT or it was performed after EBUS and in 15 (71 %) the affected lymph node chain was not punctured by EBUS-TBNA. In the ASTER trial [16] all patients underwent PET-CT before EBUS. In the discussion of the Lung-BOOST trial [18], the authors suggest that a PET-CT may not be needed before EBUS-TBNA. In that trial EBUS-TBNA was performed using a systematic aspiration of all visible lymph node stations. Unfortunately, in our study, we are unable to determine if most of the procedures adopted a systematic or selective approach.

In 11 (52 %) patients from the false negative cases, the tumor was located in the left superior lobe and 10 (47 %) had only lymph node metastases not directly accessible by EBUS (lymph node stations 5, 6, 8 and 9). Endoscopic ultrasound (EUS), using the same scope as EBUS, was done in only 6 of our 287 cases. None of the false negative cases underwent also EUS in the same procedure as EBUS. The current consensus is that for a more complete needle-guided ultrasound evaluation of the mediastinum we should associate EBUS and EUS whenever necessary [19, 20]. Perhaps with the more frequent use of EUS in routine practice, some false negative results could have been avoided. However, even though recently showed to be feasible and safe [21], it would still be difficult to access the lymph nodes in chains 5 (the most often affected) and 6. This points to the need for more cautious strategies in patients susceptible to metastases in these chains, such as patients with tumors in the left superior lobe.

The 4 false positive cases represent patients with NSCLC. Unfortunately we do not have follow-up data, so is difficult to affirm that these are really false positive cases or maybe incorrectly surgically staged patients

The small number of 20 mediastinoscopies already reflects the lower use of this technique in our hospital routine. All mediastinoscopies were performed after EBUS to clarify questionable situations before the final surgical decision. Mediastinoscopy did not contribute to better mediastinal staging than EBUS-TBNA in any of those patients. These findings do not reflect the results of the ASTER trial [16] or corroborate the current recommendations of the main guidelines of American and European respiratory societies.

Limitations

Some limitations apply to this study. First, it is a single-center study. We recognize that our results cannot be easily generalized. EBUS was performed in hospitalized patients under general anesthesia. Although this is a standard practice in our service, many procedures, probably the majority, performed in other bronchoscopy services around the world are performed in conscious or moderate sedation. Even tough the World Association for Bronchology and Interventional Pneumology (WABIP) guidelines [22] state that there is not enough evidence to recommend for or against any type of anesthesia, ideally, we should also have data in patients undergoing the procedure under conscious or moderate sedation. Second; two distinct pathology services have analyzed the samples obtained by EBUS-TBNA and surgery, which may have prevented results of one of the tests influencing the analysis of the other test. But it is difficult to clarify if the differences in pathological classification are due to the quality of the samples or a distinct interpretation by the pathologists. Third, at least 2 aspirates were routinely obtained from each target lesion per EBUS. Lee and colleagues [23] showed that, in the absence of ROSE, at least 3 aspirates should be obtained from each target lesion in order to provide optimal results from the test. Unfortunately we are not able to identify the number of aspirates that were used in each examination.

Conclusions

In hospital routine and in the subgroup of patients eligible for surgical resection EBUS-TBNA has been proven to be a good tool for the primary diagnosis of lung cancer. The negative predictive value of 89 % for mediastinal staging of lung cancer is comparable to that reported in previous studies, but the relatively high number of false negative cases points to the need for standardization of routine strategies before, during and after EBUS.

Abbreviations

CI, confidence interval; EBUS, endobronchial ultrasound; EBUS-TBNA, endobronchial ultrasound-guided transbronchial needle aspiration; EUS, endoscopic ultrasound; GIST, gastrointestinal stromal tumor; NPV, negative predictive value; NSCLC, non-small cell lung cancer; NSCLC-NOS, non-small cell lung cancer not otherwise specified; PET-CT, positron emission tomography-computed tomography; PPV, positive predictive value; ROSE, rapid on-site evaluation; WABIP, World Association for Bronchology and Interventional Pneumology

Acknowledgements

We thank all the team of the Lungenklinik Hemer by generous support for the implementation of this study.

Funding

This study was partly funded by a grant (23038.003721/2013-72) from the Coordination for the Improvement of Higher Education Personnel / CAPES, Ministry of Education, Brazil.

Author's contributions

JPSM conceived the study, prepared the first draft of the paper and coordinated the communication between the Lungenklinik Hemer in Germany and the Federal University of Rio de Janeiro in Brazil. FS and AK were responsible for the bronchoscopies in the Lungenklinik Hemer. FS made the supervision of the study in Germany. AK was responsible for the acquisition and organization of the clinical data and eletronical reports. JRLS was responsible for the study design, interpretation of the results and coordination in Brazil. RR made the statistical analysis. MEP contributed to the writing of the introduction and literature revision. APC wrote part of the discussion and conclusion of the study. All authors read and approved the final manuscript.

Competing interests

The authors declare that they have no competing interests.

Consent for publication

Not applicable.

Author details

[1]Instituto de Doenças do Torax, Universidade Federal do Rio de Janeiro, Rua Professor Rodolpho Paulo Rocco, 255, 1 andar, sala 01D 58/60, Rio de Janeiro, RJ 21941-913, Brazil. [2]Klinikum-Stuttgart, Kriegbergstrasse 60, 70174 Stuttgart, Germany. [3]Instituto de Estudos em Saúde Coletiva, Universidade Federal do Rio de Janeiro, Avenida HorácioMacedo, Iha do Fundão - Cidade Universitária, 21941-598 Rio de Janeiro, RJ, Brazil. [4]Lungenklinik Hemer, Theo-Funccius-Straße 1, 58675 Hemer, NW, Germany.

References

1. Jemal A, Bray F, Center MM, et al. Global cancer statistics. CA Cancer J Clin. 2011;61:69–90.
2. Gompelmann D, Herth FJF. Role of endobronchial and endoscopic ultrasound in pulmonary medicine. Respiration. 2014;87:3–8.
3. Kinsey CM, Douglas A. Endobronchial ultrasound-guided transbronchial needle aspiration for non-small cell lung cancer staging. Am J Respir Crit Care Med. 2014;189(6):640–9.
4. Krasnik M, Vilmann P, Larsen SS, et al. Preliminary experience with a new method of endoscopic transbronchial real time ultrassound guided biopsy for the diagnosis of mediastinal and hilar lesions. Thorax. 2003;58(12):183–18.
5. Gu P, Zhuo Y, Jiang LY, et al. Endobronchial ultrasound-guided transbronchial needle aspiration for staging of lung cancer: a systematic review and meta-analysis. Eur J Cancer. 2009;45:1389–96.
6. Adams K, Shah PL, Edmonds L, et al. Test performance of endobronchial ultrasound and transbronchial needle aspiration biopsy for mediastinal staging in patients with lung cancer: systematic review and meta-analysis. Thorax. 2009;64:757–62.
7. Varela-Lema L, Fernandez-Villar A, Ruano-Ravina A, et al. Effectiveness and safety of endobronchial ultrasound-transbronchial needle aspiration: a systematic review. Eur Respir J. 2009;33:1156–64.
8. Rivera MP, Mehta AC, Wahidi MM. Establishing the diagnosis of lung cancer. Chest. 2013;143(5):142–65.
9. Silvestri GA, Gonzales AV, Jantz MA, et al. Methods for staging non-small cell lung cancer. Chest. 2013;143(5):211–50.
10. De Leyn P, Dooms C, Kuzdzal J, et al. Revised ESTS guidelines for preoperative mediastinal lymph node staging for non-small cell lung cancer. Eur J Cardiothorac Surg. 2014;45:787–98.
11. NICE. Lung Cancer Guidelines 2011. https://www.nice.org.uk/guidance/cg121.
12. American Joint Committee on Cancer. Lung Cancer Staging. 7th edition: https://cancerstaging.org/references-tools/quickreferences/Documents/Lung%20Cancer%20Staging%20Poster%20Updated.pdf.
13. Chandra S, Nehra M, Agarwal D, et al. Diagnostic accuracy of endobronchial ultrasound-guided transbronchial needle biopsy in mediastinal lymphadenopathy: a systematic review and meta-analysis. Respir Care. 2012; 57(3):384–91.
14. Esterbrook G, Anathhanam S, Plant PK. Adequacyof endobronchial ultrasound transbronchial needle aspiration samples in the subtyping of non-small cell lung cancer. Lung Cancer. 2013;80:30–4.
15. Navani N, Brown J, Nankivell M, et al. Suitability of endobronchial ultrasound-guided transbronchial needle aspiration specimens for subtyping and genotyping of non-small cell lung cancer. Am J Respir Crit Care Med. 2012;185(12):1316–22.
16. Annema JT, Meerbeeck JP, Rintoul R, et al. Mediastinoscopy vs Endosonography for mediastinal nodal staging of lung cancer. A Randomized trial. JAMA. 2010;304(20):2245–52.
17. Yasufuku K, Pierre A, Darling G, et al. A prospective controlled trial of endobronchial ultrasound-guided transbronchial needle aspiration compared with mediastinoscopy for mediastinal lymph node staging of lung cancer. J Thorac Cardiovasc Surg. 2011;142:1393–400.
18. Navani N, Nankivell M, Lawrence DR, et al. Lung cancer diagnosis and staging with ultrasound-guided transbronchial needle aspiration compared with conventional approaches: an open label, pragmatic, randomized controlled trial. Lancet Respir Med. 2015;3(4):282–9.
19. Annema JT, Rabe KF. Endosonography for lung cancer staging: one scope fits all? Chest. 2010;138:765–7.
20. Hwangbo B, Lee GK, Lee HS. Transbronchial and transesophageal fine needle aspiration using an ultrasound bronchoscope in mediastinal staging of potentially operable lung cancer. Chest. 2010;138(4):795–802.
21. Folch E, Santacruz JF, Fernandez-Bussy S, et al. The feasibility of EBUS-guided TBNA through the pulmonary artery in highly selected patients. J Bronchology Interv Pulmonol. 2016;23(1):7–13.
22. Heijden E, Casal RF, Trisolini R, et al. Guideline for the acquisition and preparation of conventional and endobronchial ultrasound-guided transbronchial needle aspiration specimens for the diagnosis and molecular testing of patients with known or suspected lung cancer. Respiration. 2014;88:500–17.
23. Lee HS, Lee GK, Kim HS, et al. Real time endobronchial ultrasoun-guided transbronchial needle aspiration in mediastinal staging of non-small cell lung cancer: how many aspirations per target lymph node station? Chest. 2008;134:368–74.

8

Re-biopsy by endobronchial ultrasound procedures for mutation analysis of non-small cell lung cancer after EGFR tyrosine kinase inhibitor treatment

Takehiro Izumo*, Yuji Matsumoto, Christine Chavez and Takaaki Tsuchida

Abstract

Background: Re-biopsy for resistant non-small cell lung cancer (NSCLC) after treatment with epidermal growth factor receptor-tyrosine kinase inhibitors (EGFR-TKIs) is important for selection of better therapy, but there have been no reports about the utility of endobronchial ultrasound (EBUS)-guided procedures for such purpose. The aim of this study was to evaluate the utility of EBUS-guided re-biopsy for resistant NSCLC after treatment with EGFR-TKIs.

Methods: From January 2013 to December 2015, 53 consecutive patients who underwent EBUS-guided re-biopsy for mutation analysis of NSCLC after EGFR-TKI treatment were assessed.

Results: Nine patients underwent EBUS-guided transbronchial needle aspiration (EBUS-TBNA) and 44 patients underwent EBUS with a guide sheath (EBUS-GS) transbronchial biopsy. The technical success rates were 100 %. As for mutation analysis, all 9 specimens (100 %) from EBUS-TBNA and 33 specimens (75.0 %) from EBUS-GS were adequate for gene profiling. The remaining 11 specimens from EBUS-GS procedures were inadequate for mutation analysis owing to the absence of tumor component in the sample ($n = 6$) or insufficient specimen ($n = 5$). There were no related severe complications.

Conclusions: Re-biopsy by both EBUS-TBNA and EBUS-GS were useful and safe sampling procedures for mutation analysis of EGFR-TKI resistant NSCLC.

Keywords: EGFR-TKI, EBUS-TBNA, EBUS-GS, T790M, Lung cancer, Re-biopsy

Background

Epidermal growth factor receptor tyrosine kinase inhibitors (EGFR-TKIs) have been demonstrated to be effective in treating non-small cell lung cancer (NSCLC) patients with EGFR mutations [1–3]. EGFR-TKIs offer both good clinical response and survival benefit in NSCLC patients who have EGFR mutation [4]. However, a majority of the responders eventually develop acquired resistance to EGFR-TKIs [5].

Until now, several studies have uncovered several mechanisms of acquired resistance, such as secondary EGFR mutations (T790M mutation), mesenchymal-to-epithelial transition factor receptor (MET) amplification, and human epidermal growth factor receptor 2 (HER2) gene amplification [6]. Among these, a secondary missense T790M mutation was observed in nearly half of all cases that were resistant to EGFR-TKIs [7].

In November 2015, a third generation EGFR-TKI (Osimertinib; Astra Zeneca, London) has been approved by the US Food and Drug Administration (FDA) to treat patients with a type of advanced NSCLC that has a specific EGFR mutation, called T790M, and which has become worse after treatment with other EGFR-TKIs. Osimertinib has shown clinical effectiveness and tolerability in NSCLC patients with T790M mutation of EGFR [8].

* Correspondence: drtake1118@gmail.com
Department of Endoscopy, Respiratory Endoscopy Division, National Cancer Center Hospital, 5-1-1, Tsukiji Chou-ku, Tokyo 104-0045, Japan

Examining T790M is very important in treatment selection. Because EGFR-TKI treatment is indicated for advanced and unresectable NSCLC, examination for T790M mutation is usually performed on small biopsy specimens.

So far, most reports on re-biopsy procedures after EGFR-TKI resistance have been on computed tomography-guided transthoracic needle biopsy (CTNB), which is also the common first method of choice for the initial diagnosis of lung cancer [9]. However, complications, such as pneumothorax and bleeding, after CTNB have been reported [9].

Another biopsy approach is by bronchoscopy, but its use has been limited by a lower diagnostic accuracy compared with CTNB. Recently, endobronchial ultrasound (EBUS) guidance during bronchoscopy procedures, such as EBUS guided-transbronchial needle aspiration (EBUS-TBNA) and EBUS with a guide sheath (EBUS-GS) transbronchial biopsy, have been introduced and improved the diagnostic accuracy of bronchoscopy [10, 11]. However, there have been no reports about the utility of EBUS procedures for re-biopsy.

In this study, we evaluated the efficacy and safety of EBUS procedures for re-biopsy and mutation analysis of EGFR-TKI resistant NSCLC.

Methods

Subjects

This study was approved by the National Cancer Center Institutional Review Board. Written informed consent for the procedure was obtained from all patients. Consecutive patients who underwent re-biopsy by EBUS procedures for mutation analysis of NSCLC after EGFR-TKI treatment at the hospital between January 2013 and December 2015 were enrolled. There were 2907 patients in whom EBUS-guided bronchoscopy procedures were performed during the study period. Among these, 89 patients were for re-biopsy purposes. Among these re-biopsy patients, we selected NSCLC patients who were treated with at least one EGFR-TKI regimen. Disease progression during chemotherapy, based on the RECIST ver1.1 definition, was a criterion for inclusion; 36 patients were ineligible because of the absence of prior EGFR-TKI treatment.

Methods and equipment

All bronchoscopies were performed via the oral route under local anesthesia with mild sedation by intravenous administration of midazolam.

EBUS-GS was performed for patients with peripheral pulmonary lesions (PPLs) without mediastinal and hilar lymphadenopathy; a GS kit (K-201 or K-203; Olympus Ltd, Tokyo, Japan) and a radial EBUS (R-EBUS) probe (UM-S20-20R or UM-S20-17S; Olympus Ltd, Tokyo, Japan) were used. The bronchial route was planned by reviewing the chest CT images before EBUS-GS. Virtual bronchoscopic navigation/simulation systems (Ziostation2, Ziosoft Ltd, Tokyo, Japan; LungPoint, Bronchus Ltd, Mountain View, CA, USA; or Bf-Navi, Olympus Ltd, Tokyo, Japan) were used to detect the bronchial route to the target PPLs. A PPL was defined as an abnormal growth surrounded by normal lung parenchyma and was bronchoscopically invisible. Upon reaching the target bronchus, the GS together with the R-EBUS probe was inserted through the working channel of the bronchovideoscope and was advanced towards the PPL under fluoroscopic guidance (VersiFlex VISTAVR; Hitachi Ltd, Tokyo, Japan). Ultrasound scanning was performed while manipulating the R-EBUS probe until the lesion was localized by the corresponding EBUS image. After confirming the location of the PPLs, the R-EBUS probe was removed while keeping the GS in place for the usual transbronchial sampling using forceps, brush, and/or transbronchial needle aspiration under fluoroscopic guidance. Lesion location was assigned based on a study of Baaklini et al. [12], but with some modifications. With the area around the hilum on CT as reference, lesions in the inner and middle third ellipses were designated as central parenchymal location, whereas lesions in the outer third ellipse were designated as peripheral parenchymal location. The bronchus sign on CT was defined as the presence of a bronchus leading directly to a PPL [13].

EBUS-TBNA was performed for patients who had mediastinal and hilar lymphadenopathy. EBUS–TBNA was performed using either one of the following 22G needles: Vizishot (NA-201SX-4022; Olympus Ltd, Tokyo, Japan) or SonoTip EBUS Pro with stainless steel (GUS-45-18-022; Medi-Globe Ltd, Germany). The convex probe EBUS (CP-EBUS; BF-UC260FW, Olympus Ltd, Tokyo, Japan) was inserted through the oral route in the same way as during usual bronchoscopy. The ultrasound images were generated using a dedicated ultrasound processor (EU-ME1 or EU-ME2; Olympus Ltd, Tokyo, Japan). When the target lesions were visualized by CP-EBUS, the TBNA needle was inserted through the working channel of the bronchoscope and was advanced to penetrate the tracheobronchial wall into the target lesion under real-time EBUS guidance. Aspiration was done by moving the needle back and forth inside the target lesion for 20–30 times, under negative pressure. After sampling, suction was released before retracting the needle from the scope.

Pathologic evaluation and mutation analysis

Cytology and histology specimens were sent for pathologic examination. Positive diagnostic criteria suitable for molecular analysis were defined by the presence of malignant cells based on histologic features or based on class IV/V on cytology examination by Papanicolaou stain. Overall detection rate was based on a positive diagnosis by histology and/or cytology.

EGFR mutation analyses of the genomic DNA extracted from tumor samples were performed using the Scorpion ARMS method.

Statistical analysis

Descriptive statistics were presented as frequency, percentage, and median (range). Univariate analyses were performed using Fisher's exact test. Multivariate analysis using logistic regression was performed to determine the factors associated with the yield. Variables selected via univariate analyses (P value <0.10) were evaluated using multivariate logistic regression analysis. A two-tailed P value <0.05 was considered to indicate statistical significance. Correlation of study variables were performed with EZR (Saitama Medical Center, Jichi Medical University; www.jichi.ac.jp/saitama-sct/SaitamaHP.files/statmed.html), a graphical user interface for R (version 2.13.0, The R Project for Statistical Computing; http://www.r-project.org) and a modified version of R commander (version 1.8-4).

Results

After exclusion, a total of 53 patients were included in this study population. In the 53 patients, the original diagnoses were established by CTNB in 2 cases; by EBUS-TBNA in 5 cases; by EBUS-GS in 39 cases; and by surgical biopsy in 7 cases. There were no cases with positive T790M mutation upon initial diagnosis.

For re-biopsy, EBUS–TBNA was performed in 9 patients, whereas EBUS-GS was performed in 44 patients. The technical success rates of the re-biopsy procedures were 100 %. All 9 specimens (100 %) from EBUS-TBNA and 33 specimens (75.0 %) from EBUS-GS were adequate for gene profiling and mutation analysis. The remaining 11 specimens from EBUS-GS procedures were inadequate for mutation analysis owing to the absence of tumor component in the sample ($n = 6$) or insufficient specimen ($n = 5$).

The baseline characteristics of the study population are summarized in Table 1. Initially, EGFR mutation was detected in 53 cases (exon 19 deletion in 30, L858R point mutation in 22, and L861Q point mutation in 1). Among 42 patients that had adequate samples for gene profiling testing for EGFR mutation, 22 (52.4 %) had EGFR mutation and T790M-resistant mutation (Table 2). One initial EGFR-mutated tissue revealed SCLC transformation.

The adequacy of the re-biopsy specimens for mutation analysis is described in Table 3. The overall detection rate of re-biopsy for malignant cells was 79.2 % (42 of 53); 77.4 % (41 of 53) by cytology and 77.4 % (41 of 53) by histologic examination. The detection rate of re-biopsy by EBUS-TBNA for malignant cells was 100 % (9 of 9), 100 % (9 of 9) by cytology and 88.9 % (8 of 9) by histologic examination. In contrary, the detection rate of re-biopsy by EBUS-GS for malignant cells was 75.0 % (33 of 44);

Table 1 Patient demographics and clinical information ($N = 53$)

Characteristics	
Age (years)	65 (35–85)
Gender	
Male	19 (35.9)
Female	34 (64.1)
ECOG PS	
0	23 (43.4)
1	27 (50.9)
2	2 (3.8)
3	1 (1.9)
4	0 (0)
Histologic diagnosis	
Adenocarcinoma	52 (98.1)
Adenosquamous cell carcinoma	1 (1.9)
Initial EGFR mutation profile	
Del19	30 (56.6)
L858R	22 (41.5)
L816Q	1 (1.9)
EGFR-TKI treatment before re-biopsy	
Gefitinib	29 (54.8)
Erlotinib	7 (13.2)
Afatinib	0 (0)
Gefitinib + Erlotinib	12 (22.6)
Gefitinib + Afatinib	1 (1.9)
Gefitinib + Erlotinib + Afatinib	4 (7.5)

Data are presented as median (range) or number (%)
ECOG PS Eastern Cooperative Group performance status, *EGFR* epidermal growth factor receptor, *EGFR-TKI* EGFR-tyrosine kinase inhibitor

Table 2 Biological profiles of cases that underwent re-biopsy by EBUS procedures ($N = 53$)

Initial EGFR mutation profile		EGFR mutation profile on re-biopsy	
Del19	30	Del19 alone	8
		Del19 + T790M	16
		Re-biopsy failure	6
L858R	22	L858R alone	11
		L858R + T790M	6
		Re-biopsy failure	5
L816Q	1	L816Q alone	1

Data are presented as number
EBUS endobronchial ultrasound, *EGFR* epidermal growth factor receptor

Table 3 Adequacy of re-biopsy samples for molecular analysis ($N = 53$)

		Detection rate of re-biopsy for malignant cells		
		Cytology	Histology	Overall
ALL	53	41 (77.4)	41 (77.4)	42 (79.2)
EBUS-TBNA	9	9 (100)	8 (88.9)	9 (100)
EBUS-GS	44	32 (72.7)	33 (75.0)	33 (75.0)

Data are presented as number (%)
EBUS-TBNA endobronchial ultrasound-guided transbronchial needle aspiration, *EBUS-GS* endobronchial ultrasound with a guide sheath

72.7 % (32 of 44) by cytology and 75.0 % (33 of 44) by histologic examination (Table 3).

The factors affecting re-biopsy by EBUS-GS are shown in Table 4. In the multivariate analysis, central parenchymal location and EBUS probe within were the significant predictors of a successful EBUS-GS re-biopsy.

There were no severe complications after both EBUS-TBNA and EBUS-GS re-biopsy procedures.

Discussion

Currently, the significance of re-biopsy for mutation analysis of NSCLC has been increasing because of a wider range of therapeutic options. The standard cytotoxic chemotherapy for NSCLC patients has limited therapeutic response [14]. Moreover, after treatment with EGFR-TKIs, kinase inhibition frequently leads to the appearance of drug-resistant mutations within the target kinase itself [15, 16]. Recently, a third generation EGFR-TKI (Osimertinib) has been approved by the US FDA to treat patients with a type of advanced NSCLC that has a specific EGFR mutation, called T790M, and which has become worse after treatment with other EGFR-TKIs. Moreover, Osimertinib has shown clinical effectiveness and tolerability in NSCLC patients with T790M mutation of EGFR [8], underscoring the importance of checking for new mutations after EGFR-TKI therapy in advanced NSCLC patients. There have been several reports about the utility of re-biopsy by CTNB for such purpose.

To our best knowledge, this study was the first to demonstrate the utility of bronchoscopic procedures, especially with EBUS guidance, for mutation analysis of NSCLC after EGFR-TKI therapy. EBUS is a very important procedure to determine and collect samples from target sites in the mediastinal, hilar, and peripheral locations under real-time ultrasound [17, 18]. Adequate sampling of histologic specimens is necessary for the development of new treatment options for cancer, especially chemotherapy and gene-targeted therapy; therefore, further improvements of the histologic sampling yield is essential [19, 20].

EBUS-TBNA is an established minimally invasive procedure for proper staging and diagnosis of lung cancer [10, 21]. In this study, EBUS-TBNA was performed successfully and was able to obtain adequate samples in all cases. EBUS-TBNA is useful not only for proper staging and diagnosis of lung cancer, but also to obtain samples for mutation analysis of NSCLC after EGFR-TKI, as demonstrated in this study. Furthermore, EBUS-TBNA was a safe re-biopsy procedure and had no associated severe complications.

In this study, EBUS-GS was able to obtain samples for mutation analysis of NSCLC after EGFR-TKI. However, when compared with EBUS-TBNA, the detection rate

Table 4 Factors affecting the yield of re-biopsy by EBUS-GS ($N = 44$)

	Success ($n = 33$)	Failure ($n = 11$)	Univariate	Multivariate	
			p value	p value	Odds ratio
Age (years)			0.722	–	–
≤70	23 (52.3)	7 (15.9)			
>70	10 (22.7)	4 (9.1)			
Gender			0.282	–	–
Male	13 (29.5)	2 (4.5)			
Female	20 (45.5)	9 (20.5)			
ECOG PS			1.0	–	–
0/1	31 (70.5)	10 (22.7)			
2/3/4	2 (4.5)	1 (2.3)			
Size (mm)			0.139	–	–
≤30	7 (15.9)	5 (11.4)			
>30	26 (59.1)	6 (13.6)			
Location			0.043	0.034	15.7
Central parenchymal	32 (72.7)	8 (18.2)			
Peripheral parenchymal	1 (2.3)	3 (6.8)			
Bronchus sign			0.027	0.239	–
Positive	31 (70.5)	7 (15.9)			
Negative	2 (4.5)	4 (9.1)			
Biopsied pulmonary lesion			0.154	–	–
Primary malignant	30 (68.2)	8 (18.2)			
Metastatic	3 (6.8)	3 (6.8)			
Chest radiograph			0.090	0.080	–
Visible	31 (70.5)	8 (18.2)			
Invisible	2 (4.5)	3 (6.8)			
EBUS			0.016	0.012	10.0
Within	30 (68.2)	6 (13.6)			
Adjacent to/invisible	3 (6.8)	5 (11.4)			

Data are presented as number (%)
EBUS-GS endobronchial ultrasound with a guide sheath, *ECOG PS* Eastern Cooperative Group performance status, *EBUS* Endobronchial ultrasound

for malignancy was only 75 %. The yield of EBUS-GS for primary diagnosis of PPLs has been reported to be about 70–80 % [22], which is similar to the yield for re-biopsy for mutation analysis in this study. The factors that influence the diagnostic yield of EBUS-GS for PPLs have been reported to be the location of the PPL (central parenchymal or peripheral parenchymal), detected EBUS images (within or adjacent to/invisible), and the presence of a bronchus sign. Although central parenchymal location and detection of EBUS image within were significant factors that predicted a successful yield, the number of peripheral parenchymal cases in this study was small. Further study is needed to confirm the usefulness of EBUS-GS according to the location of the lesion. Although there is need for further technical improvement, EBUS-GS was useful to get samples for mutation analysis of NSCLC after EGFR TKI treatment. In addition, EBUS-GS had no severe complications.

CTNB is another diagnostic procedure for PPLs, with a relatively high rate of both diagnostic accuracy and complications, such as pneumothorax. On the contrary, EBUS-GS was a safe method [23]. However, it is important to note that although EBUS-GS might be considered one of the sampling procedures to safely obtain tissues from PPLs for mutation analysis of NSCLC after EGFR-TKI treatment, the detection rate for malignant cells was significantly lower for peripherally located lesions, as shown in this study. In this regard, EBUS-GS should be performed to get samples for mutation analysis of lesions that are in a central parenchymal location.

Another alternative approach, specifically liquid biopsy, now present as a crucial point in the field [24]. Liquid biopsy has grown in importance because the genetic profile of tumors can affect how well they respond to a certain treatment. A recent paper showed that the concordance between re-biopsy and liquid biopsy, including plasma DNA and circulating tumor cell, was 57–60 % [25]. The usefulness of monitoring T790M status in liquid biopsy was already reported [26]. Although liquid biopsy has the potential to detect new mutations after chemotherapy, several reports have demonstrated some difficulties in detecting tumor-derived mutations in plasma [27]. Therefore, liquid biopsy and re-biopsy may be considered to be complementary methods of mutation analysis.

The limitations of this study were its retrospective and single-institution design. Prospective, multi-center trials are ideal and recommended in the future.

Conclusions

EBUS procedures for re-biopsy were useful sampling methods for mutation analysis of NSCLC after EGFR-TKI treatment. This could play an important role in the choice of better targeted therapy and for the development of a novel treatment for advanced lung cancer patients.

Abbreviations

CP-EBUS, convex probe endobronchial ultrasound; CTNB, computed tomography-guided transthoracic needle biopsy; EBUS, endobronchial ultrasound; EBUS-GS, endobronchial ultrasound with a guide sheath; EBUS-TBNA, endobronchial ultrasound guided-transbronchial needle aspiration; EGFR-TKIs, epidermal growth factor receptor-tyrosine kinase inhibitors; NSCLC, non-small cell lung cancer; FDA, Food and Drug Administration; HER2, human epidermal growth factor receptor 2; MET, mesenchymal-to-epithelial transition factor receptor; PPLs, peripheral pulmonary lesions; R-EBUS, radial endobronchial ultrasound

Funding

This work was supported in part by The National Cancer Center Research and Development Fund (28-K-1).

Authors' contributions

TI designed the overall study and performed the statistical analysis. All authors substantially contributed to the acquisition, interpretation, and consolidation of data. All authors wrote the manuscript and approved the final version.

Competing interests

The authors declare that they have no competing interests.

References

1. Watanabe M, Kawaguchi T, Isa S, Ando M, Tamiya A, Kubo A, Saka H, Takeo S, Adachi H, Tagawa T, et al. Ultra-Sensitive Detection of the Pretreatment EGFR T790M Mutation in Non-Small Cell Lung Cancer Patients with an EGFR-Activating Mutation Using Droplet Digital PCR. Clin Cancer Res. 2015;21(15):3552–60.
2. Paez JG, Janne PA, Lee JC, Tracy S, Greulich H, Gabriel S, Herman P, Kaye FJ, Lindeman N, Boggon TJ, et al. EGFR mutations in lung cancer: correlation with clinical response to gefitinib therapy. Science. 2004;304(5676):1497–500.
3. Lynch TJ, Bell DW, Sordella R, Gurubhagavatula S, Okimoto RA, Brannigan BW, Harris PL, Haserlat SM, Supko JG, Haluska FG, et al. Activating mutations in the epidermal growth factor receptor underlying responsiveness of non-small-cell lung cancer to gefitinib. N Engl J Med. 2004;350(21):2129–39.
4. Mitsudomi T, Morita S, Yatabe Y, Negoro S, Okamoto I, Tsurutani J, Seto T, Satouchi M, Tada H, Hirashima T, et al. Gefitinib versus cisplatin plus docetaxel in patients with non-small-cell lung cancer harbouring mutations of the epidermal growth factor receptor (WJTOG3405): an open label, randomised phase 3 trial. Lancet Oncol. 2010;11(2):121–8.
5. Kobayashi S, Boggon TJ, Dayaram T, Janne PA, Kocher O, Meyerson M, Johnson BE, Eck MJ, Tenen DG, Halmos B. EGFR mutation and resistance of non-small-cell lung cancer to gefitinib. N Engl J Med. 2005;352(8):786–92.
6. Yu HA, Arcila ME, Rekhtman N, Sima CS, Zakowski MF, Pao W, Kris MG, Miller VA, Ladanyi M, Riely GJ. Analysis of tumor specimens at the time of acquired resistance to EGFR-TKI therapy in 155 patients with EGFR-mutant lung cancers. Clin Cancer Res. 2013;19(8):2240–7.
7. Ohashi K, Maruvka YE, Michor F, Pao W. Epidermal growth factor receptor tyrosine kinase inhibitor-resistant disease. J Clin Oncol. 2013;31(8):1070–80.
8. Janne PA, Yang JC, Kim DW, Planchard D, Ohe Y, Ramalingam SS, Ahn MJ, Kim SW, Su WC, Horn L, et al. AZD9291 in EGFR inhibitor-resistant non-small-cell lung cancer. N Engl J Med. 2015;372(18):1689–99.

9. Yoon HJ, Lee HY, Lee KS, Choi YL, Ahn MJ, Park K, Ahn JS, Sun JM, Kim J, Kim TS, et al. Repeat biopsy for mutational analysis of non-small cell lung cancers resistant to previous chemotherapy: adequacy and complications. Radiology. 2012;265(3):939–48.
10. Yasufuku K, Chiyo M, Sekine Y, Chhajed PN, Shibuya K, Iizasa T, Fujisawa T. Real-time endobronchial ultrasound-guided transbronchial needle aspiration of mediastinal and hilar lymph nodes. Chest. 2004;126(1):122–8.
11. Kikuchi E, Yamazaki K, Sukoh N, Kikuchi J, Asahina H, Imura M, Onodera Y, Kurimoto N, Kinoshita I, Nishimura M. Endobronchial ultrasonography with guide-sheath for peripheral pulmonary lesions. Eur Respir J. 2004;24(4):533–7.
12. Baaklini WA, Reinoso MA, Gorin AB, Sharafkaneh A, Manian P. Diagnostic yield of fiberoptic bronchoscopy in evaluating solitary pulmonary nodules. Chest. 2000;117(4):1049–54.
13. Gaeta M, Pandolfo I, Volta S, Russi EG, Bartiromo G, Girone G, La Spada F, Barone M, Casablanca G, Minutoli A. Bronchus sign on CT in peripheral carcinoma of the lung: value in predicting results of transbronchial biopsy. AJR Am J Roentgenol. 1991;157(6):1181–5.
14. Schiller JH, Harrington D, Belani CP, Langer C, Sandler A, Krook J, Zhu J, Johnson DH, Eastern Cooperative Oncology G. Comparison of four chemotherapy regimens for advanced non-small-cell lung cancer. N Engl J Med. 2002;346(2):92–8.
15. Uramoto H, Sugio K, Oyama T, Sugaya M, Hanagiri T, Yasumoto K. Resistance to gefitinib. Int J Clin Oncol. 2006;11(6):487–91.
16. Uramoto H, Mitsudomi T. Which biomarker predicts benefit from EGFR-TKI treatment for patients with lung cancer? Br J Cancer. 2007;96(6):857–63.
17. Garcia-Olive I, Monso E, Andreo F, Sanz-Santos J, Taron M, Molina-Vila MA, Llatjos M, Castella E, Moran T, Bertran-Alamillo J, et al. Endobronchial ultrasound-guided transbronchial needle aspiration for identifying EGFR mutations. Eur Respir J. 2010;35(2):391–5.
18. Ishida T, Asano F, Yamazaki K, Shinagawa N, Oizumi S, Moriya H, Munakata M, Nishimura M, Virtual Navigation in Japan Trial G. Virtual bronchoscopic navigation combined with endobronchial ultrasound to diagnose small peripheral pulmonary lesions: a randomised trial. Thorax. 2011;66(12):1072–7.
19. Ikeda N, Nagase S, Ohira T. Individualized adjuvant chemotherapy for surgically resected lung cancer and the roles of biomarkers. Ann Thorac Cardiovasc Surg. 2009;15(3):144–9.
20. Izumo T, Sasada S, Chavez C, Matsumoto Y, Hayama M, Tsuchida T. The diagnostic value of histology and cytology samples during endobronchial ultrasound with a guide sheath. Jpn J Clin Oncol. 2015;45(4):362–6.
21. Izumo T, Sasada S, Chavez C, Matsumoto Y, Tsuchida T. Endobronchial ultrasound elastography in the diagnosis of mediastinal and hilar lymph nodes. Jpn J Clin Oncol. 2014;44(10):956–62.
22. Tamiya M, Okamoto N, Sasada S, Shiroyama T, Morishita N, Suzuki H, Yoshida E, Hirashima T, Kawahara K, Kawase I. Diagnostic yield of combined bronchoscopy and endobronchial ultrasonography, under LungPoint guidance for small peripheral pulmonary lesions. Respirology. 2013;18(5):834–9.
23. Hayama M, Izumo T, Matsumoto Y, Chavez C, Tsuchida T, Sasada S. Complications with Endobronchial Ultrasound with a Guide Sheath for the Diagnosis of Peripheral Pulmonary Lesions. Respiration. 2015;90(2):129–35.
24. Tissot C, Toffart AC, Villar S, Souquet PJ, Merle P, Moro-Sibilot D, Perol M, Zavadil J, Brambilla C, Olivier M, et al. Circulating free DNA concentration is an independent prognostic biomarker in lung cancer. Eur Respir J. 2015;46(6):1773–80.
25. Sundaresan TK, Sequist LV, Heymach JV, Riely GJ, Janne PA, Koch WH, Sullivan JP, Fox DB, Maher R, Muzikansky A, et al. Detection of T790M, the Acquired Resistance EGFR Mutation, by Tumor Biopsy versus Noninvasive Blood-Based Analyses. Clin Cancer Res. 2016;22(5):1103–10.
26. Sueoka-Aragane N, Katakami N, Satouchi M, Yokota S, Aoe K, Iwanaga K, Otsuka K, Morita S, Kimura S, Negoro S, et al. Monitoring EGFR T790M with plasma DNA from lung cancer patients in a prospective observational study. Cancer Sci. 2016;107(2):162–7.
27. Mazurek AM, Fiszer-Kierzkowska A, Rutkowski T, Skladowski K, Pierzyna M, Scieglinska D, Wozniak G, Glowacki G, Kawczynski R, Malusecka E. Optimization of circulating cell-free DNA recovery for KRAS mutation and HPV detection in plasma. Cancer Biomark. 2013;13(5):385–94.

9

Small lung lesions invisible under fluoroscopy are located accurately by three-dimensional localization technique on chest wall surface and performed bronchoscopy procedures to increase diagnostic yields

Chaosheng Deng[1*], Xiaoming Cao[2], Dawen Wu[1], Haibo Ding[1], Ruixiong You[3], Qunlin Chen[3], Linying Chen[4], Xin Zhang[1], Qiaoxian Zhang[1] and Yongquan Wu[2]

Abstract

Background: Nowadays, small peripheral pulmonary lesions (PPLs) are frequently detected and the prognosis of lung cancer depends on the early diagnosis. Because of the high fee and requiring specialized training, many advanced techniques are not available in many developing countries and rural districts.

Methods: Three sets of opaque soft copper wires visible under the fluoroscopy (Flu) in the Flu-flexible bronchoscopy (FB) group ($n = 24$), which determined the three planes of the lesion, were respectively placed firmly on the surface of the chest wall with adhesive tape on the chest wall. The FB tip was advanced into the bronchus toward the crosspoint of the three perpendicular planes under Flu with careful rotation of a C-arm unit. Then the specimen were harvested focusing around the crosspoint for pathologic diagnosis. The rapid on-site evaluation (ROSE) procedure was also performed. The average Flu time during FB procedures were recorded and diagnostic accuracy rates in the Flu-FB group were compared with the other group guided by radial endobronchial ultrasound (R-EBUS) ($n = 23$).

Results: The location of the core point of the lesion, whether it was visible or not under the fluoroscopy could be recognized by three-dimensional localization technique. The accuracy rates of diagnostic yields were 62.5% in the Flu-FB group, and was similar as 65.2% in the R-EBUS group ($P > 0.05$). However, in the Flu-FB group, there was a decreasing tendency on accurate diagnosis rates of lower lobe (LL) lesions when comparing with non-LL lesions (3/8 = 37.5% vs 12/16 = 75%, $P = 0.091$) while in the R-EBUS group it was similar (9/12 = 75% vs 6/11 = 54.6%, $P = 0.278$). In the Flu-FB group, fluoroscopy time was negatively correlated with the lesion length ($r = -0.613$, $P = 0.001$), however, there was no significant difference between the lesions invisible or not (5.83 ± 1.45 min vs 7.67 ± 2.02 min, $P = 0.116$) under the fluoroscopy, as well as no significant difference among SPN, mGGO and GGO (6.12 ± 2.05 min, 7.25 ± 1.33 min and 7.80 ± 2.02 min, $P > 0.05$).

(Continued on next page)

* Correspondence: jasonsci7333@163.com
[1]Division of Respiratory and Critical Care Medicine, First Affiliated Hospital of Fujian Medical University, Fuzhou 350005, Fujian, China
Full list of author information is available at the end of the article

(Continued from previous page)

Conclusions: Small PPL whether it is visible or not under fluoroscopy can be located accurately by our three-dimensional localization technique on chest wall surface and performed bronchoscopy procedures to increase diagnostic yields. It is more convenient, economical and reliable with the similar diagnostic yields than R-EBUS guided method.

Keywords: Small peripheral pulmonary lesions (PPLs), Invisible under fluoroscopy, Three-dimensional localization technique, Opaque soft copper wires, Bronchoscopy, Diagnostic yields, Radial endobronchial ultrasound (R-EBUS), Rapid on-site evaluation (ROSE)

Introduction

Nowadays, with the application of high-resolution computed tomography (CT) imaging techniques to lung cancer screening, small solitary pulmonary nodule (SPN) or ground-glass opacity (GGO) lesions in the lung are frequently detected [1, 2]. For this article, the small peripheral pulmonary lesions (PPLs) are defined as lesions less than 3 cm in length, including the SPN, GGO or mixed GGO (mGGO) and being surrounded by the lung parenchyma without evidence of endobronchial abnormalities. The differential diagnosis of PPN is broad, ranging from benign tumors, edema, infectious lesions to lung cancer and other malignant conditions [3]. Lung cancer is the most common cause of cancer death for both men and women with a 5-year global survival rate in patients in the early stages of the disease of 38–67% and in later stages of 1–8% [4]. Thus, the prognosis of lung cancer depends on the early diagnosis of these lesions. When biopsy is recommended, CT-guided transthoracic fine-needle aspiration (TTNA) or biopsy is currently preferred because it has a diagnostic yield of 90%, although perhaps less with smaller lesions [5]. However, TTNA has limitations such as without bronchoalveolar lavage fluid (BALF), brushing, and with respect to the puncture site, seeding along the needle biopsy tract with malignant cells which are potentially serious, with a risk from 0.06 to 1%, as well as a high risk of complications such as a pneumothorax median 25% (range 4–60%), among which 4% (range 0.2–8%) for pneumothorax requiring chest tube and the median risk of hemorrhage is 12% (range 2–66%), and may be higher in the diffuse lung disease patients with bulla under pleura and those with smaller nodules or nodules deep in the lung parenchyma [6, 7]. Another more complex process video-assisted thoracoscopic surgery (VATS), even CT assisted VATS [8] is also an alternative method to obtain the tissue samples especially for some small PPNs. However, sometimes the techniques need an additional tool such as O-arm CT or some preoperative marking procedures to identify the location of the small lesions [9, 10]. For example, VATS involves hook-wire technique, endoscopic ultrasonography, barium marking through bronchoscopy, and percutaneous injections of dyes, colored collagen, lipiodol, agar, and barium, et al. [7]. These methods may also result in some complications mentioned above, which led to its prohibition in Japan [11]. The diagnostic yields of another diagnostic method, flexible bronchoscopy, for PPLs <2 cm in the published reports have varied from 5 to 28% [12]. Therefore, several guided-bronchoscopy technologies have been developed to improve the yields of transbronchial biopsy for PPLs diagnosis, such as real-time MSCT fluoroscopic guidance with higher radiation doses to the patient and operators [13], ultrathin bronchoscope, electromagnetic navigation bronchoscopy (ENB), virtual bronchoscopy (VB), R-EBUS with guide sheath (GS), and lung point [5, 14]. All these methods have improved the diagnostic yields, for example, the overall diagnostic yield of EBUS-GS-guided transbronchial biopsy (TBB) may be 65.0% when the location of the lesion can be confirmed by EBUS [9].

However, in many patients, the location of target lesion is invisible under the x-ray fluoroscopy and yet can not always be identified so precisely by these guided-bronchoscopy technologies and consequentially affect the diagnostic yields. On the other hand, because of the high fee of guided-bronchoscopy equipments and requiring specialized training doctors, the advanced techniques mentioned above are not always available for the hospitals in many developing countries and rural districts.

Therefore, we are studying for a more convenient, economical and reliable method for accurately locating the small PPLs, then perform the bronchoscopy procedures to improve the diagnostic yields. And we also perform R-EBUS with GS for comparison.

Materials and methods

About the protocol

The protocol was approved by the University Ethics Committee and the Institutional Review Board of the First Affiliated Hospital of Fujian Medical University and the First Hospital of Longyan City in Fujian Province. Written informed consents prior to performing the procedure were obtained from all the enrolled patients with the indications as follows: PPNs less than 30 mm in diameter size. The patients with the contraindications for the flexible bronchoscopy were excluded. All patients were followed-up until achievements of definitive diagnosis.

Groups

Patients from the two hospitals from June 2012 to December 2015 were divided into 3 groups. All patients underwent chest CT scanning using a multidetector CT scanner (Aquilion; Toshiba; Tokyo, Japan) prior to bronchoscopy, in order to locate the lung lesions at full inspiration. Images were reconstructed from helical CT data by one radiologist and transferred to a work site. Our new technique was performed on 24 lesions in 24 patients, we also named as fluoroscopy group, who were classified into 2 groups: group1 ($n = 12$) and group2 ($n = 12$) according to the lesion visible or not under fluoroscopy. The lesion visible or not was confirmed by two radiologists. Visible lesion means the lesion can be recognized under fluoroscopy by the both radiologists and invisible lesion means the lesion can not be recognized under fluoroscopy by the both radiologists. However, if the lesion can not be recognized by one, then should be confirmed invisible by the third radiologist. The group 3 was performed EBUS-GS, namely Radial EBUS-GS group.

Characteristics of patients

Among group 1 and 2, each lung lobe (including left lingular) had lesion for confirming to locate accurately the small PPNs. There were 12 patients with lesion visible under fluoroscopy in the group 1 and also 12 patients with lesion invisible under fluoroscopy in the group 2. There were 23 patients in the group 3. The characteristics of three groups were shown at Table 1.

Table 1 Characteristics of three groups

Characteristics	Group 1 ($n = 12$)	Group 2 ($n = 12$)	Group 3 ($n = 23$)
Age (years)	61 ± 18	58 ± 16	60 ± 15
Sex (cases)			
Female	7	6	9
Male	5	6	14
Lesion size (mm)			
Length	25.25 ± 3.05	13.00 ± 6.00	20.50 ± 5.00
Width	14.42 ± 4.81	9.42 ± 3.61	15.00 ± 4.30
Height	16.42 ± 2.31	7.33 ± 2.78	13.00 ± 6.50
Location and cases of each lobe			
Right (left) upper lobe	2	2	6
Right middle (left lingular) lobe	2	2	5
Right (left) lower lobe	2	2	12
CT findings (Types and Cases)			
GGO	0	5	5
mGGO	4	2	6
SPNs	8	5	12

Group 1: Patients with lung lesion visible under fluoroscopy; Group 2: Patients with lung lesion invisible under fluoroscopy; Group 3: Patients performed EBUS-GS

Bronchoscopy procedures

Bronchoscope was advanced to segment where the lesion located

Local anesthesia of the upper respiratory tract was achieved using 2% lidocaine. Continuous pulse oximetry was performed during FB, and blood pressure was measured every 5 min. Oxygen was administered by a nasal cannula, and the flow was adjusted upward from 2 L/min to maintain the pulse oximetric saturation above 90%. After the FB (BF-1T260, Olympus, Tokyo, Japan) was advanced beyond the vocal cords through the nasal route, all segments of the bronchial tree were visualized. Then the FB was advanced to the lesion segment according to the CT scans. FB procedures were performed by well-trained bronchoscopists who had more than 10 years of experience. The average number of FB procedures performed per year by the bronchoscopist was 200 or greater.

Visible lesion under fluoroscopy

For the patients with PPN visible under fluoroscopy, fluoroscopy-guided bronchoscopy was performed.

Lesions were located accurately by our techniques and performed bronchoscopy procedures

Determing core point L of lesion according to crosspoint of three dimensions of lesion All chest CT scans of the enrolled patients were reviewed to detect the longest diameter of three dimensions: length, width and height of the lesion and the characteristics of the all lesions were carefully analyzed. The CT scans mainly aiming at the lesion were reconstructed again with slices of 1 mm under a deep inspiratory breathhold. The bronchi leading to the lesion were also recorded. A core point of the lesion which we named as point L could be determined according to the crosspoint of the longest diameter of three dimensions, that is length, width and height of the lesion, on CT scans (Fig. 1a and b). Especially, if the branches of bronchi leading into the lesion could be recognized, the end point of the bronchi inside the lesion was determined as point L and also was recorded.

Point L could be reflected by crosspoint determined by three planes lines on surface of chest wall According to the mathematical principle: Three Perpendicular Planes Intersect at ONE Point, this Point can be

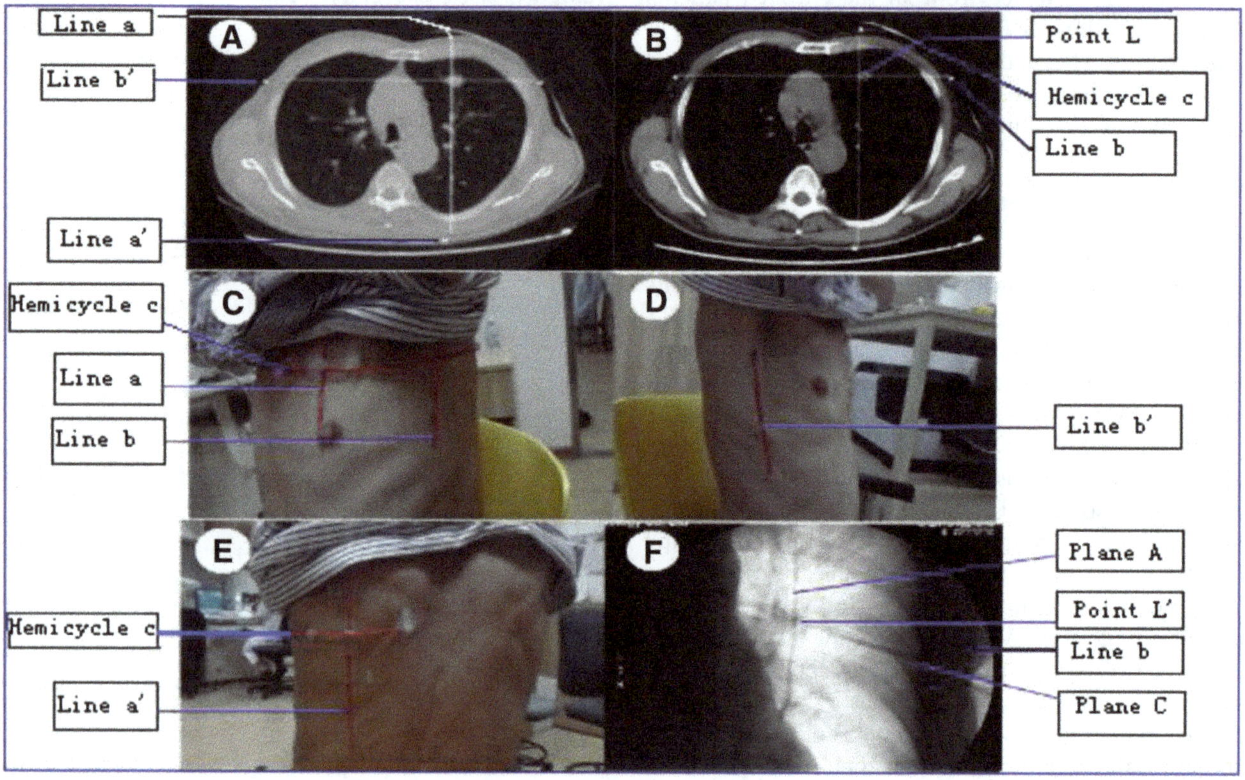

Fig. 1 A core point of the lesion which we named as *point L* could be determined according to the crosspoint of the longest diameter of three dimensions, that is length, width and height of the lesion, on CT scans (shown by **a** and **b**). Opaque soft copper wires were respectively placed firmly on the surface of the chest wall with adhesive tape (shown by **c**, **d** and **e**). Under the fluoroscopy, with the careful rotation of the C-arm machine, the crosspoint *L'* of the three perpendicular planes determined by the three sets copper wires *aa'*, *bb'* and hemicycle *line c* (shown by **a** and **b** with *bright pots* and *lines*, and by **f** with *dark lines*) on the surface of chest wall could reflect and fit accurately with the *Point L* of the lung lesion (shown by **f**)

reflected onto the surface of the chest wall by the three perpendicular planes lines, that is Sagittal Plane A determined by Line a and Line a', Coronal Plane B determined by Line b and Line b' and Horizontal Plane C determined Hemicycle (or Whole Cycle) Line c (Fig. 1a and b). According to the CT parameters scanning the lesion, these three perpendicular planes lines can be marked on the surface of the patients' chest wall (Clearly shown in Model Fig. 2). Opaque soft wires, such as copper wires which were visible under the fluoroscopy, were respectively placed firmly on the surface of the chest wall with adhesive tape according to the marks (Fig. 1c, d, e). Therefore, although the lung lesion can not be recognized under the fluoroscopy, the another crosspoint we named as L' of the three perpendicular planes determined by the three sets of copper wires aa', bb' and hemicycle line c on the surface of chest wall could reflect and fit accurately with the Point L of the lung lesion (Fig. 1f).

Detecting accurately core point L of the lesion under fluoroscopy Fluoroscopic guidance was provided by a multipurpose C-arm type diagnostic unit (Allura Xper FD20; Philipps Company; Amsterdam, the Netherlands). With the careful rotation of a C-arm unit, we can see the wires a and a' overlapped together like one wire named as Line A, and intersected with hemicycle c toward the x-ray anteroposterior direction, which meaned that Plane A intersected with Plane C at Line A. Then, going on rotating the C-arm unit, we can also see the wires b and b' overlapped together like one wire named as Line B, and intersected with hemicycle c toward the x-ray horizontal direction, which meaned that Plane B intersected with Plane C at Line B. As mentioned above, the crosspoint L' was also the crosspoint of Line A and Line B. Therefore, we should advance the bronchoscope tip into the bronchus toward the crosspoint of Line A and Line B, which reflected the core point L of the lesion under the fluoroscopic guidance.

Harvesting specimen focusing around the point L of the lung lesion The brush or forceps exserting from the bronchoscopy reached the crosspoint L' under the fluoroscopy. The specimen were harvested focusing around

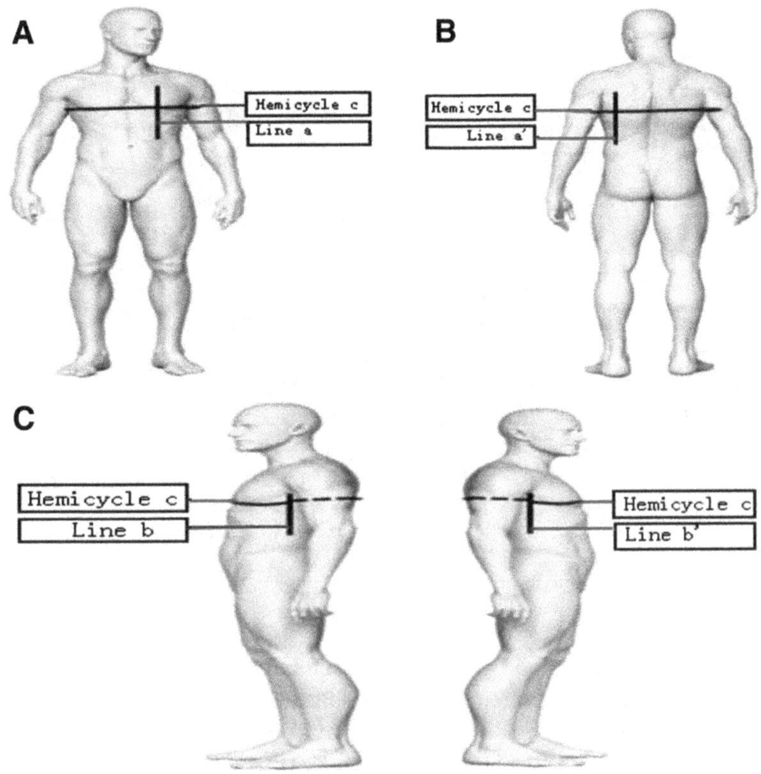

Fig. 2 (model): According to the CT parameters scanning the lesion, the three perpendicular lines: *Line a* and *a'* which determined Sagittal Plane **a**, *Line b* and *b'* which determined Coronal Plane **b**, and Hemicycle *Line c* which determined Horizontal Plane **c** can be marked on the surface of the chest wall

the point L of the lesion through the brushing, forceps biopsy, and BALF.

ROSE

The rapid on-site evaluation (ROSE) procedure was performed by a cytotechnologist after staining the smears from the tissue obtained during the bronchoscopy, enabling immediate cytopathologic evaluation and feedback regarding specimen adequacy and potential diagnosis. At least 2 smears were prepared, one stained immediately with a rapid stain (Diff-Quik, Baxter Diagnostics, Inc) and the other fixed in alcohol for Papanicolaou (PAP) staining later. Cytologic slides were then sent to the pathologist for immediate interpretation of whether the sample was negative (no malignant cells) or positive (definitive cytopathologic evidence of malignancy) [15]. The remaining specimen was placed in 10% formaldehyde for routine histologic examination and diagnosis.

Brief case report involving our techniques

A 75-year-old female with a 5-months' history of recurrent hemoptysis was admitted to the First Affiliated Hospital of Fujian Medical University. The lung CT showed an irregular shape nodule with 2.0 cm*2.0 cm*1.5 cm size in the left posterior basal segment lobe (Fig. 3b, c). As the principles and techniques mentioned above, the core point of the lesion was determined. Then three sets of metal wires were placed on the surface of the patient's chest wall. Although the lesion located behind the heart and was hard to be recognized under the fluoroscopy, the core point of the lesion was detected with the help of our methods of locating lesion (Fig. 3a, d). Subsequently, bronchoscopy procedures under the fluoroscopy were done to harvest the specimen focusing around the core point of the lesion (Fig. 3e, f). The pathology from specimen showed adenocarcinoma in situ with immunohistochemisty: TTF-1, CK7, CK19, Napsina(+); PR, CEA(focal+); Tg, Villion, CR, CK5/6, CDX-2, CA125, ER, GCDFP-15, CK20, CA199(−), KI-67(+, 1%) (Fig. 3g).

EBUS procedures

In the group 3 (patients performed EBUS-GS), equipped with endoscopic ultrasound system (EU-M30S, Olympus, Tokyo, Japan), a 20 MHz radial small-diameter probe (UM-S20–20R Olympus) with guide sheath was inserted through the working channel of the bronchoscope. Once

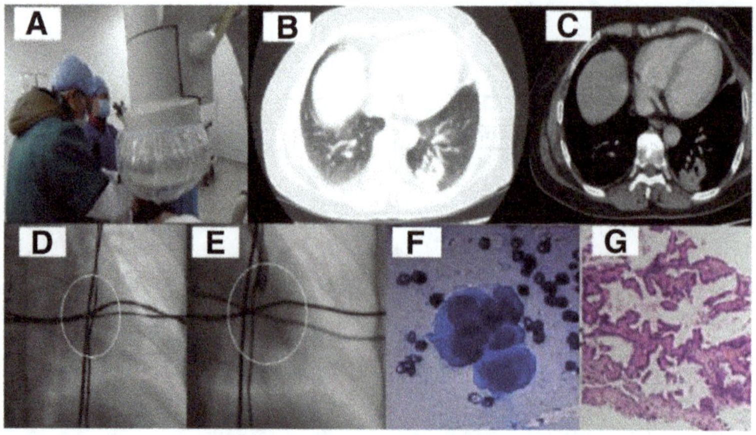

Fig. 3 The lung CT showed an irregular shape nodule with 2.0 cm*2.0 cm*1.5 cm size in the left posterior basal segment lobe (**b**, **c**). Although the lesion located behind the heart and was hard to be recognized under the fluoroscopy, the core point of the lesion was detected with the help of our methods of locating lesion (**a**, **d**, shown within the *white circle*). Bronchoscopy procedures under the fluoroscopy were performed to harvest the specimen focusing around the core point of the lung lesion (**d**, **e**, shown within the *white circle*). The pathology from the specimen showed adenocarcinoma (**f**: ROSE, **g**: Histology)

the precise location of the lesion was identified by EBUS, the probe was withdrawn, leaving the GS in place. Subsequently, the specimen were harvested through the brushing, forceps biopsy, and BALF for ROSE and pathologic diagnosis as other groups.

Statistical analysis

Data were presented as mean ± standard deviation or number (percent) as appropriate. Statistical analysis was performed using $\chi 2$ test or Fisher's exact test and t-test in SPSS statistical software (SPSS version 15; SPSS; Chicago, IL). A two-sided p value of less than 0.05 indicated statistical significance.

Results

Results of patients performed bronchoscopy under fluoroscopy

The location of the core point L of the lesion had been determined in the chest CT scans. The point L whether it was visible or invisible under the fluoroscopy could be recognized by the crosspoint L' of the three perpendicular planes determined by the three sets copper wires aa', bb' and hemicycle line c on the surface of chest wall. The results of the patients performed bronchoscopy under fluoroscopy were showed in Table 2.

Visible lesion under fluoroscopy

Fluoroscopy-guided FB was advanced into the bronchus under fluoroscopic guidance according to the lesion location. The brushing, forceps biopsy and BALF focusing on the lesion were performed in these patients (Fig. 4).

Results of patients performed bronchoscopy with R-EBUS-GS

A total of 23 consecutive patients were included in the study, with 9 female and 14 male. The detail characteristics of this group were shown in group 3 in Table 1. The mean age was 60 ± 15 years (range, 47 to 77 years). The average lesion size in length was 20.50 ± 5.00 mm (range, 10 to 30 mm). Lesion was detected by the R-EBUS-GS through FB according to its location (Fig. 5). The accuracy rates of diagnostic yields were 65.2% (15 in 23 cases).

ROSE results

The cancer cells in the ROSE slides may show as:closter, masslike and overlapped, scattered (Fig. 6). Scattered cancer cells in the slides were prone to be ignored. According to whether the biopsy was successful and adequate diagnostic material was harvested from initial specimens, further specimens collection during bronchoscopy (e.g. brushing, biopsy) will be performed or adjusted the biopsy sites [16].

Accuracy rates of diagnostic cases guided by fluoroscopy guided FB or R-EBUS

The accuracy rates of diagnostic yields were 66.7% in the group 1, 58.3% in the group 2, with average 62.5% in these two groups (both were included in the fluoroscopy group), and was similar as 65.2% in the group 3 (R-EBUS-GS group) ($P > 0.05$). Accurate diagnosis rates were similar among Flu-FB group and EBUS group (15 in 24 patients vs 15 in 23 patients, $P = 0.846$). In the Flu-FB group, there were no significant difference among different CT scan findings ($P = 0.503$) and whether the

Table 2 Results of patients performed bronchoscopy under fluoroscopy were shown

N	Location	CT finding	Size (mm)	Distance to pleura (mm)	Visible or not	Histology results from bronchoscopy	Final diagnosis	Fluoroscopy time (min)
1	RUL	mGGO	30*15*15	15	Visible	Adenocarcinoma	Adenocarcinoma	7.5
2	RLL	SPN	12*10*11	10	Invisible	Negative	Adenocarcinoma	9.0
3	LM(L)L	mGGO	18*15*10	8	Invisible	Inflammation	Inflammation	9.5
4	RLL	SPN	25*15*14	18	Visible	Inflammation?	Adenocarcinoma	7.0
5	RML	GGO	3*4*3	0	Invisible	Negative	Inflammation	10.0
6	LUL	SPN	26*18*16	10	Visible	Caseous necrosis	Caseous necrosis	5.5
7	LUL	SPN	25*11*15	5	Visible	Carcinoma cells	Adenocarcinoma	6.5
8	LLL	SPN	9*8*5	10	Invisible	Negative	AAH	10.0
9	LUL	GGO	4*3*3	15	Invisible	Negative	Inflammation	10.0
10	RML	SPN	25*16*17	22	Visible	Atypical cells	AAH	4.5
11	LULΔ	SPN	10*10*9	15	Invisible	Squamous cell carcinoma	Squamous cell carcinoma	8.0
12	LLL	SPN	20*20*15	0	Visible	Carcinoma cells	Adenocarcinoma	7.5
13	RML	mGGO	22*8*16	10	Visible	Negative	Adenocarcinoma	6.5
14	RUL	SPN	20*8*6	20	Invisible	Squamous cell carcinoma	Squamous cell carcinoma	5.0
15	RUL	mGGO	25*12*16	15	Visible	Negative	Caseous necrosis	5.5
16	RML	GGO	11*13*7	20	Invisible	Carcinomacells	Small cell carcinoma	6.5
17	LM(L)L	mGGO	30*11*20	0	Visible	Poorly differentiated carcinoma	Poorly differentiated carcinoma	7.5
18	RUL	SPN	18*8*10	30	Invisible	Carcinoma cells	Squamous cell carcinoma	4.5
19	RLL	SPN	25*15*22	28	Visible	Small cell carcinoma	Small cell carcinoma	4.0
20	RLL	GGO	19*14*6	30	Invisible	Negative	Squamous cell carcinoma	6.0
21	LLL	SPN	22*10*16	30	Visible	Negative	Inflammation	3.5
22	LM(L)L	SPN	25*12*15	32	Visible	Adenocarcinoma	Adenocarcinoma	4.5
23	LLL*	mGGO	20*10*8	35	Invisible	Carcinoma cells	Adenocarcinoma	7.0
24	LM(L)L	GGO	12*10*10	25	Invisible	Carcinoma cells	Large cell carcinoma	6.5

N Number of cases, Visible:lesion can be recognized under fluoroscopy. Invisible:lesion can not be recognized under fluoroscopy. Visible or not: Visible or not under fluoroscopy. Histology results from bronchoscopy include brushing, BALF and biopsies under fluoroscopy. Final diagnosis: histology pathological diagnosis or diagnosis by following up. *RUL* Right Upper Lobe, *RML* Right Middle Lobe, *RLL* Right Lower Lobe, *LUL* Left Upper Lobe, *LM(L)L* Left Lingular Lobe, *LLL* Left Lower Lobe, *SPN* Solitary Pulmonary Nodules, *(m)GGO* (mix) Ground Glass Opacity, *AAH* Atypical Adenomatous Hyperplasia. *:minor hemorrhage at the biopsy site; Δ:pneumothorax not requiring chest tube

lesion visible or not under the fluoroscopy ($P = 0.50$). However, in the Flu-FB group, there was a decreasing tendency on accurate diagnosis rates of LL lesions when comparing with non-LL lesions (3/8 = 37.5% vs 12/16 = 75%, $P = 0.091$) while in the EBUS group it was similar (9/12 = 75% vs 6/11 = 54.6%, $P = 0.278$). And in the EBUS group, there was a significant difference among different CT scan findings ($P = 0.044$) with SPN vs GGO ($P = 0.028$) and whether the lesion detectable or not by EBUS ($P = 0.008$) (Table 3).

Average fluoroscopy time during bronchoscope procedures

In the fluoroscopy group (Flu-FB group), the average fluoroscopy time was (6.75 ± 1.96) min. There were no significant difference of the fluoroscopy time in lower lobe patients compared with the not lower lobes patients ((6.75 ± 2.24) min vs (6.75 ± 1.88) min, $P > 0.05$). The length of the visible lesion is much larger than the invisible lesion (25.00 ± 2.92 mm vs 13.00 ± 6.00 mm, $F = 8.844$, $P = 0.007$). Fluoroscopy time was negatively correlated with the lesion length ($r = -0.613$, $P = 0.001$). However, about fluoroscopy time, there was no significant difference between visible lesion and the invisible lesion (5.83 ± 1.45 min vs 7.67 ± 2.02 min, $P = 0.116$), as well as no significant difference among SPN, mGGO and GGO (6.12 ± 2.05 min, 7.25 ± 1.33 min and 7.80 ± 2.02 min, $P > 0.05$).

Complications

There was 1 patient with the complication of minor hemorrhage and 1 patient with pheumothorax not requiring chest tube in group 2. No complication was found in other groups.

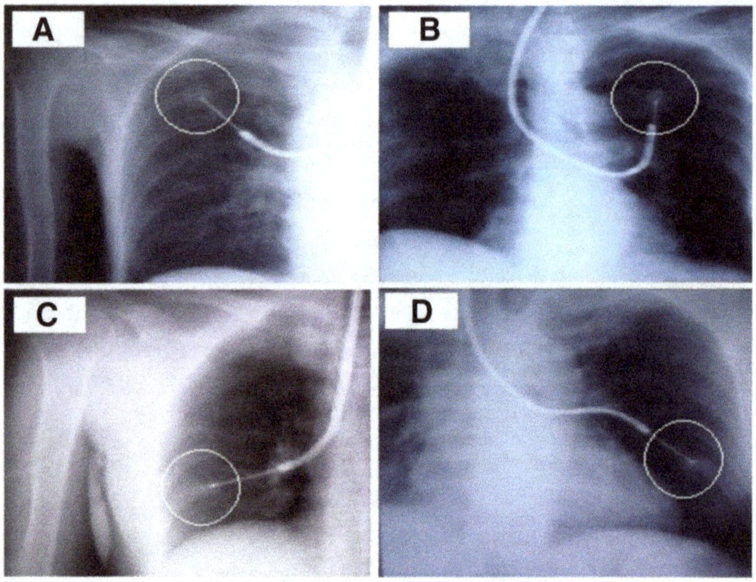

Fig. 4 Bronchoscopy procedures focusing on the visible lesion were performed under fluoroscopic guidance according to the lesion location. **a**, Lesion was showed in Right Upper Lobe within circle. **b**, Lesion was showed in Left Upper Lobe within circle. **c**, Lesion was showed in Right Lower Lobe within circle. **d**, Lesion was showed in Left lower Lobe within circle

Discussion

All of lung lesions shown by chest CT scans can be successfully localized by our techniques

Lung cancer is currently the leading cause of cancer deaths worldwide. The mortality rates have remained high because of the difficulty in detecting early stage of this disease. Fortunately, with the wide application of HRCT, PPLs are frequently detected which made early diagnosis become possible. However, using CT characteristics alone to determine the lesions as benignity, premalignancy or malignancy is often difficult [17]. The tissue samples of the PPNs can be harvested by the FB. The location of the lesion should be determined before harvesting the samples, thus can improve the diagnostic yield. The lung lesion location is estimated by chest radiograph (CXR) or CT of the chest. It is a challenge to determine the location of the small lesion, especially which is invisible under the fluoroscopy.

However, whether the lung lesion is visible or not under the fluoroscopy. The core point of the lesion detected by CT scans can be reflected by the crosspoint of three planes determined by the three sets of opaque soft wires placed

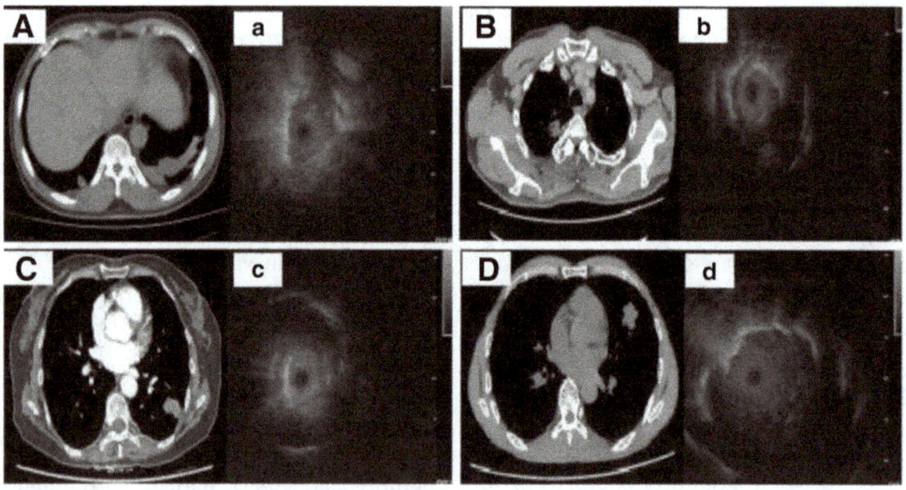

Fig. 5 Lesions were detected by the R-EBUS-GS through bronchoscopy according to their locations in different lobes (Right lower lobe shown in **A** and **a**; Right upper lobe shown in **B** and **b**; Left lower lobe shown in **C** and **c**; Left lingular lobe shown in **D** and **d**)

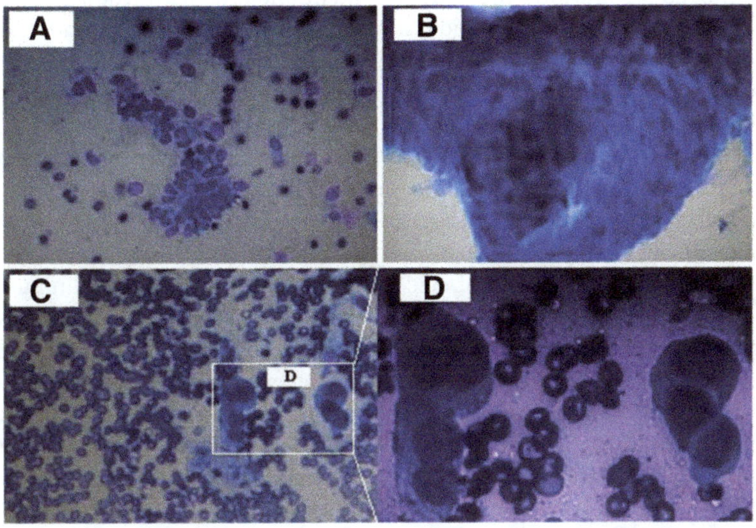

Fig. 6 The cancer cells in the ROSE slides may show as: closter (shown by **a**), masslike and overlapped (shown by **b**), scattered (shown by **c** and **d**)

on the surface of chest wall. According to the mathematical principle: Three Perpendicular Planes Intersect at ONE Point, the lesion can be located accurately by our techniques. Then, under the fluoroscopy, the bronchoscopy procedures can be performed aiming at the crosspoint of the three perpendicular planes and the specimen can be harvested by focusing around the point, which is also the core point of the lung lesion. This technique does not make use of sophisticated equipments, and it is easy to be understood and mastered.

Performing bronchoscopy by our three-dimensional localization technique

Accuracy rates of diagnosis by bronchoscopy whether lesion is visible or not under fluoroscopy are similar

For non-endobronchial peripheral lung lesion, if the lesion is visible under fluoroscopy, the brush and biopsy forceps of the bronchoscopy can be advanced into the bronchus under fluoroscopic guidance according to the lesion location, as been successfully performed in our study. According to Rittirak et al. study, the overall diagnostic yield of Flu-TBLB group may be statistically significantly higher than NFlu-TBLB group (43.8 vs. 32.9%; $P = 0.003$) [18]. However, the diagnostic yields of FB for peripheral pulmonary lesions <2 cm in published reports have varied from 5 to 28%, because some lesions are invisible through conventional flexible bronchoscopy under fluoroscopy [12].

In our study, although lung lesion is invisible under fluoroscopy, we can recognize it by the crosspoint of three perpendicular planes determined by the opaque soft copper wires placed on chest wall surface, therefore, the diagnostic yields have been improved, which is similar as R-EBUS-GS group. And this location method will not be influenced by the different size, whether the lesion visible or not under the fluoroscopy and CT scan characteristics of the lesion, such as SPN, mGGO or GGO.

Accuracy rates of diagnosis by bronchoscopy of non-lower lobe lesion are higher than lower lobe lesion

However, due to the respiratory motion, mainly caused by the diaphragm motion, the lung lesion may be mislocalized [19]. Movement of the lung occurs with respiratory variation during bronchoscopy, and the location of pulmonary nodule during procedures may differ significantly from its location on the initial planning, especially

Table 3 Accuracy rates of diagnostic cases guided by fluoroscopy guided FB or R-EBUS

Methods Cases Items		Lesion location			CT scan findings			Lesion under fluoroscopy or EBUS	
		UL	ML	LL	SPN	mGGO	GGO	Visible	Invisible
Flu-FB	Cases enrolled	8	8	8	13	6	5	12	12
	Accurate diagnosis	6	6	3	9	4	2	8	7
EBUS	Cases enrolled	6	5	12	12	6	5	19	4
	Accurate diagnosis	3	3	9	10	4	1	15	0

UL Upper lobe, *ML* Middle lobe, *LL* Lower lobe. Lesion under fluoroscopy or EBUS

to the lower lobe, which moved significantly more than upper lobe lesion. In the Flu-FB group of our study, a decreasing tendency has been observed on accurate diagnosis rates of LL lesions when comparing with non-LL lesions, while in the EBUS group it was similar. Actually, one of the main challenges for us is hard to find the exact position to perform a biopsy for the lesion located in the lower lobe when respiratory motion. According to the other studies, this movement during bronchoscopy may even significantly affect the diagnostic yield of electromagnetic navigation bronchoscopy procedures [20]. The lesion size and distance from the pleura doesn't significantly impact the movement. Holding a deep breath may manage the respiratory motion problem, but the duration of bronchoscopy procedures which involve BALF, biopsy, brushing et al., may take some longer time. The navigation system with the proposed respiratory motion compensation method and EBUS allow for real time guidance during bronchoscopic interventions, and thus could increase the diagnostic yield [21]. Therefore, combing with other diagnostic techniques may improve diagnostic yields.

Diagnostic yield about R-EBUS

The technique of R-EBUS with a GS has definitely its place in the diagnostic work-up of PPLs, especially for the lesions that can be visualized by EBUS. The diagnostic yield has fluctuated from 53% up to 77% [22], which can be increased by ensuring that TBB is performed at the correct location as identified by the EBUS. Tay et al. performed a retrospective analysis of 196 consecutive patients who underwent investigation with R-EBUS [23]. They found that a definitive diagnosis was established for 109 PPL (56%) using radial EBUS. Visualized lesion by EBUS probe had a higher diagnostic yield (65%) than EBUS-invisible lesions (20%; $P = 0.0001$) and in multivariate analysis, lesion size, malignancy status and distance from hilum to lesion were significant predictors of EBUS visualization yield. In our study, lesions performed R-EBUS were visualized by EBUS probe and there were same diagnostic yields as Tay et al's study. On the other hand, different CT scan findings have been associated with different diagnostic yields bronchoscopy guided by R-EBUS-GS, especially high with SPN lesion and low with GGO lesion. However, the overall diagnostic yields by R-EBUS-GS were similar with that by our three-dimensional localization technique according to our study. What we are concerned about is that the diagnostic yield of EBUS-invisible lesions may be improved according to our three-dimensional localization technique.

CT-guided transthoracic fine-needle aspiration

TTNA or biopsy is widely used currently for its high diagnostic yields [5]. However, TTNA has a limitation mentioned in the introduction part. Tai et al. has evaluated the frequency and severity of pulmonary hemorrhage after transthoracic needle lung biopsy (TTLB) and assess possible factors associated with pulmonary hemorrhage [24]. Tai et al. has found that the pulmonary hemorrhage occurred in 483 of the 1175 TTLBs (41.1%) but rarely requires intervention and higher-grade hemorrhage was more likely to occur with female sex ($P = 0.001$), older age ($P = 0.003$), emphysema ($P = 0.004$), coaxial technique ($P = 0.025$), nonsubpleural location ($P < 0.001$), lesion size of 3 cm or smaller ($P < 0.001$), and subsolid lesions ($P = 0.028$). However, to the lower lobe lesion, because of low accuracy rates of diagnosis by our techniques, we recommend to perform CT-guided TTNA or combine with other motheds to improve the diagnostic yield.

Role of ROSE

As we know, ROSE of tissue obtained by FNA has been first introduced by Washington University investigators in St. Louis, Missouri. Its major advantages have been improvements in health care resource utilization, safety, reduction in the number of sites biopsied, allowing immediate processing and interpretation of the sample in the procedural suite, lowering patient costs, increase of sample adequacy rates and diagnostic yield, decrease x-ray exposure time during radiologically guided interventional procedures and other potential morbidity related to the biopsy procedure [25–28], which has been reported to have 85 to 93% sensitivity and 100% specificity [29]. ROSE can also aim at molecular profiling (optimal lung cancer genotyping) in patients with advanced lung cancer [30]. Therefore, it is recommended to be performed routinely, especially in patients with a suspected diagnosis of lung cancer [31]. In our study, ROSE has been performed in the 3 groups and the cancer cells were found to be mainly distributed as :1) closter, 2) masslike and overlapped, and 3) scattered. Scattered cancer cells in the slides were prone to be ignored. Therefore, the scattered characteristics of cancer cells should be paid much more attention to. However, the main reason for the scarcity of performing ROSE in other practices is oftenly the lack of on-staff cytopathologists [32].

Fluoroscopy time in our study

It takes appropriated procedure time to perform bronchoscope under fluoroscopy. There are a negative correlation between the fluoroscopy time and the lesion length. However, because the lesions can be located accurately by our techniques and performed bronchoscopy procedures, there is no significant difference on fluoroscopy time between visible lesion and the invisible lesion, as well as no significant difference among SPN, mGGO and GGO. Fluoroscopic guidance may be also utilized in many other bronchoscopic procedures, including EBUS for investigation of PPLs. Therefore, x-ray exposure during radiologically guided interventional procedures should be taken into consideration including the medical staffs and patients. The fluoroscopy time in our study was defined as the time from the lesion was nearly reached by the bronchoscope to the biopsy time point. With the help of ROSE in our study, the fluoroscopy time is some shorter, comparing with Fujita Y et al's study [4]. However, Müller et al. reported that the duration of fluoroscopy time correlated with the radiation dose to the hands of the surgeons, and that radiation dose without thyroid protection was 70 times higher than with thyroid protection in a comparison [33]. Therefore, the reduction of fluoroscopy time and proper shielding of radiation doses are recommended.

Adverse effects

It is very convenient for us to use fluoroscopy to check for adverse effects of pneumothorax and hemorrhage, to confirm the position of the brush and forceps with opening or not. Factors that were associated with the increased risk of pneumothorax include patient characteristics (age >60 years; COPD), lesion characteristics (small size, greater distance from pleura), and technical factors (increased number of punctures or aspirates, biopsy performed in supine or lateral rather than prone position). In our study, as one patient with pneumothorax and one patient with minor bleeding, complications do exist [34].

It is recommended to combe with many diagnostic techniques for increasing diagnostic yields

Many advanced bronchoscopy techniques have been studied and performed in the patients with PPL, but as clinicians, we should take these factors into considerations: the choice of optimal investigation, determinants of diagnostic yield for bronchoscopy, complications, and practice pattern variations [34]. As mentioned above, the accuracy of CT-guided lung biopsy is high. However, lesions that are smaller or deeper in the lung result in a higher number of CT scans with increased radiation dose and procedure time, seeding along the needle biopsy tract with malignant cells and the lesions surrounding emphysema, lung bullae or pulmonary vascular, whic are at high risk for pneumothorax or hemorrhage following TTNA. Introducing the biopsy through the bronchus within the target lesion increases the diagnostic yield and also decreases the risk of pneumothorax [35, 36]. When it is more difficult for the biopsy needle to hit the lesion during CT-guided biopsy, it is more likely for specimens to be retrieved and diagnosed from the BALF and brushing guided by the brochoscopy with the help of our three-dimensional localization technique on chest wall surface. On the other hand, measuring and applying the distance between the orifice of bronchus and the lesion could increase the diagnostic yield of EBUS-guided TBBs for PPLs [36]. According to our results, to non-lower lobe PPLs, performing bronchoscopy by our three-dimensional localization technique may be an optional selection, especially its convenient and economical. And to lower lobe, we prefer to perform EBUS-GS procedures.

Limitations of our study

Firstly, the number of the patients is not enough. Secondly, x-ray exposure to the medical staffs and patients during radiologically guided interventional procedures should be taken into much consideration, and the fluoroscopy time may be shorter after our proficiency on performing the related procedures, for example performing the ROSE and manipulating the C-arm unit. Thirdly, there is no data about the combination ulities of diagnostic methods, for example, three-dimensional localization technique plus EUBS or/and CT-guided TTNA or biopsy. Further studies focusing on these limitations are needed.

Conclusions

Small PPNs invisible under fluoroscopy can be located accurately by our three-dimensional localization technique on chest wall surface and performed bronchoscopy procedures to increase diagnostic yields. It is a more convenient, economical and reliable method with the similar diagnostic yields as R-EBUS guided method. This localization technique can also be performed in other organs such as the deep lesion of pancreas etc. The ulities of multiple diagnostic methods are recommended to increase diagnostic yields of PPLs according to the equipments and specialized training available in the hospitals.

Abbreviations

BALF: Bronchoalveolar lavage fluid; CXR: Chest X ray; ENB: Electromagnetic navigation bronchoscopy; FB: Flexible bronchoscopy; Flu: Fluoroscopy; GGO: Ground-glass opacity; GS: Guide sheath; LL: Lower lobe; mGGO: Mixed GGO; PPLs: Small peripheral pulmonary lesions; R-EBUS: Radial endobronchial ultrasound; ROSE: Rapid on-site evaluation; SPN: Small solitary pulmonary nodule; TBB: Transbronchial biopsy; TTLB: Transthoracic needle lung biopsy; TTNA: Transthoracic fine-needle aspiration; VATS: Video-assisted thoracoscopic surgery; VB: Virtual bronchoscopy

Acknowledgements

We are very grateful to Dr. Guiqing Liu from the Hammersmith Hospital, Imperial College Healthcare NHS Trust in London for proofreading and helping revise the manuscript.

Funding

This work was supported by a grant from Key Program of Fujian Provincial Department of Science and Technology (2014Y0020).

Authors' contributions

CSD designed and performed the whole study, discussed and analyzed the findings, and wrote the paper. XMC performed a part of the study, discussed and analyzed a part of the findings, and helped write the paper. DWW, HBD, QXZ and YQW collected data and discussed the findings. XZ helped complete the bronchoscopy procedures. RXY and QLC helped complte the localization of lessions. LYC helped analyze specimens as a pathologist. All authors read and approved the final manuscript.

Competing interests

The authors declare that they have no competing interests.

Consent for publication

All individual materials such private images have been obtained the informed consent before published.

Author details

[1]Division of Respiratory and Critical Care Medicine, First Affiliated Hospital of Fujian Medical University, Fuzhou 350005, Fujian, China. [2]Department of Respiratory Disease, First Hospital of Longyan City, 364000 Fujian, China. [3]Department of Medical Imaging, First Affiliated Hospital of Fujian Medical University, Fuzhou 350005, Fujian, China. [4]Department of Pathology, First Affiliated Hospital, Fujian Medical University, Fuzhou, Fujian Province, China.

References

1. Seo JM, Lee HY, Kim HK, Choi YS, Kim J, Shim YM, et al. Factors determining successful computed tomography-guided localization of lung nodules. J Thorac Cardiovasc Surg. 2012;143(4):809–14.
2. Swensen SJ, Jett JR, Hartman TE, Midthun DE, Mandrekar SJ, Hillman SL, et al. CT screening for lung cancer: five-year prospective experience. Radiology. 2005;235(1):259–65.
3. Murrmann GB, van Vollenhoven FH, Moodley L. Approach to a solid solitary pulmonary nodule in two different settings—common is common, rare is rare. J Thorac Dis. 2014;6(3):237–48.
4. Fujita Y, Seki N, Kurimoto N, Inoue K, Miyazawa T, Abe T, et al. Introduction of Endobronchial Ultrasonography (EBUS) in bronchoscopy clearly reduces fluoroscopy time: comparison of 147 cases in groups before and after EBUS introduction. Jpn J Clin Oncol. 2011;41(10):1177–81.
5. Wang Memoli JS, Nietert PJ, Silvestri GA. Meta-analysis of guided bronchoscopy for the evaluation of the pulmonary nodule. Chest. 2012;142(2):385–93.
6. Wiener RS, Wiener DC, Gould MK. Risks of transthoracic needle biopsy: how high? Clin Pulm Med. 2013;20(1):29–35.
7. Watanabe K, Nomori H, Ohtsuka T, Kaji M, Naruke T, Suemasu K. Usefulness and complications of computed tomography-guided lipiodol marking for fluoroscopy -assisted thoracoscopic resection of small pulmonary nodules: experience with 174 nodules. J Thorac Cardiovasc Surg. 2006;132(2):320–4.
8. Chang SS, Nakano T, Okamoto T. Usefulness of intraoperative computer tomography-assisted thoracoscopic segmentectomy for small-sized lung cancer. Ann Thorac Cardiovasc Surg. 2015;23. [Epub ahead of print] (Article ID: cr. 15–00212)
9. Izumo T, Sasada S, Chavez C, Tsuchida T. The diagnostic utility of endobronchial ultrasonography with a guide sheath and tomosynthesis images for ground glass opacity pulmonary lesions. J Thorac Dis. 2013;5(6):745–50.
10. Ohtaka K, Takahashi Y, Kaga K, Senmaru N, Kotani Y, Matsui Y. Video-assisted thoracoscopic surgery using mobile computed tomography: new method for locating of small lung nodules. J Cardiothorac Surg. 2014;9:110.
11. Sakiyama S, Kondo K, Matsuoka H, Yoshida M, Miyoshi T, Yoshida S, et al. Fatal air embolism during computed tomography-guided pulmonary marking with a hook-type marker. J Thorac Cardiovasc Surg. 2003;126(4): 1207–9.
12. Torrington KG, Kern JD. The utility of fiberoptic bronchoscopy in the evaluation of the solitary pulmonary nodule. Chest. 1993;104:1021–4.
13. Mammarappallil JG, Hiatt KD, Ge Q, Clark HP. Computed tomography Fluoroscopy versus conventional computed tomography guidance for biopsy of intrathoracic lesions: a retrospective review of 1143 consecutive procedures. J Thorac Imaging. 2014;29(6):340–3.
14. Tsushima K, Sone S, Hanaoka T, Takayama F, Honda T, Kubo K. Comparison of bronchoscopic diagnosis for peripheral pulmonary nodule under fluoroscopic guidance with CT guidance. Respir Med. 2006;100(4):737–45.
15. Whitson BA, Groth SS, Odell DD, Briones EP, Maddaus MA, D'Cunha J, et al. True negative predictive value of endobronchial ultrasound in lung cancer: are we being conservative enough? Ann Thorac Surg. 2013;95(5):1689–94.
16. Yarmus L, Van der Kloot T, Lechtzin N, Napier M, Dressel D, Feller-Kopman D. A randomized prospective trial of the utility of rapid on-site evaluation of transbronchial needle aspirate specimens. J Bronchology Interv Pulmonol. 2011;18(2):121–7.
17. Inoue D, Gobara H, Hiraki T, Mimura H, Kato K, Shibamoto K, et al. CT fluoroscopy-guided cutting needle biopsy of focal pure ground-glass opacity lung lesions: diagnostic yield in 83 lesions. Eur J Radiol. 2012;81(2):354–9.
18. Rittirak W, Sompradeekul S. Diagnostic yield of fluoroscopy-guided transbronchial lung biopsy in non-endobronchial lung lesion. J Med Assoc Thai. 2007;90(2):68–73.
19. Liu C, Pierce LA, Alessio AM, Kinahan PE. The impact of respiratory motion on tumor quantification and delineation in static PET/CT imaging. Phys Med Biol. 2009;54(24):7345–62.
20. Chen A, Pastis N, Furukawa B, Silvestri GA. The effect of respiratory motion on pulmonary nodule location during electromagnetic navigation bronchoscopy. Chest. 2015;147(5):1275–81.
21. Gergel I, Hering J, Tetzlaff R, Meinzer HP, Wegner I. An electromagnetic navigation system for transbronchial interventions with a novel approach to respiratory motion compensation. Med Phys. 2011;38(12):6742–53.
22. Durakovic A, Andersen H, Christiansen A, Hammen I. Retrospective analysis of radial EBUS outcome for the diagnosis of peripheral pulmonary lesion: sensitivity and complications. Eur Clin Respir J. 2015;17(2):28947.
23. Tay JH, Irving L, Antippa P, Steinfort DP. Radial probe endobronchial ultrasound: factors influencing visualization yield of peripheral pulmonary lesions. Respirology. 2013;18(1):185–90.
24. Tai R, Dunne RM, Trotman-Dickenson B, Jacobson FL, Madan R, Kumamaru KK, et al. Frequency and severity of pulmonary hemorrhage in patients undergoing percutaneous CT-guided transthoracic lung biopsy: single-institution experience of 1175 Cases. Radiology. 2016;279(1):287–96.
25. Baram D, Garcia RB, Richman PS. Impact of rapid on-site cytologic evaluation during transbronchial needle aspiration. Chest. 2005;128(2):869–75.
26. Diacon AH, Schuurmans MM, Theron J, Louw M, Wright CA, Brundyn K, et al. Utility of rapid on-site evaluation of transbronchial needle aspirates. Respiration. 2005;72(2):182–8.
27. Celik B, Khoor A, Bulut T, Nassar A. Rapid on-site evaluation has high diagnostic yield differentiating adenocarcinoma vs squamous cell carcinoma of non-small cell lung carcinoma, not otherwise specified subgroup. Pathol Oncol Res. 2015;21(1):167–72.
28. Kalluri M, Puttagunta L, Ohinmaa A, Thanh NX, Wong E. Cost analysis of interaprocedural on site evaluation of cytopathology with endobronchial ultrasound. Int J Technol Assess Health Care. 2016;11:1–8.
29. Karnak D, Ciledag A, Ceyhan K, Atasoy C, Akyar S, Kayacan O. Rapid on-site evaluation and low registration error enhance the success of electromagnetic navigation bronchoscopy. Ann Thorac Med. 2013;8(1):28–32.
30. Trisolini R, Cancellieri A, Tinelli C, de Biase D, Valentini I, Casadei G, et al. Randomized trial of endobronchial ultrasound-guided transbronchial needle aspiration with and without rapid on- site evaluation for lung cancer genotyping. Chest. 2015;148(6):1430–7.
31. Walia R, Madan K, Mohan A, Jain D, Hadda V, Khilnani GC, et al. Diagnostic utility of conventional transbronchial needle aspiration without rapid on-site evaluation in patients with lung cancer. Lung India. 2014;31(3):208–11.
32. da Cunha Santos G, Ko HM, Saieg MA, Geddie WR. "The petals and thorns" of ROSE (rapid on-site evaluation). Cancer Cytopathol. 2013;121(1):4–8.

33. Muller LP, Suffner J, Wenda K, Mohr W, Rommens PM. Radiation exposure to the hands and the thyroid of the surgeon during intramedullary nailing. Injury. 1998;29(6):461–8.
34. Ost DE, Ernst A, Lei X, Kovitz KL, Benzaquen S, Diaz-Mendoza J, et al. Diagnostic yield and complications of bronchoscopy for peripheral lung lesions. Results of the AQuIRE registry. Am J Respir Crit Care Med. 2016;193(1):68–77.
35. Huang CT, Ruan SY, Liao WY, Kuo YW, Lin CY, Tsai YJ, et al. Risk factors of pneumothorax after endobronchial ultrasound-guided transbronchial biopsy for peripheral lung lesions. PLoS One. 2012;7(11):e49125.
36. Walsh CJ, Sapkota BH, Kalra MK, Hanumara NC, Liu B, Shepard JA, et al. Smaller and deeper lesions increase the number of acquired scan series incomputed tomography-guided lung biopsy. J Thorac Imaging. 2011;26(3):196–203.

Implementing flexible bronchoscopy in least developed countries according to international guidelines is feasible and sustainable: example from Phnom-Penh, Cambodia

Martin Veaudor[1,2], Sébastien Couraud[1,2,3*], Sophors Chan[4], Chanraksmey Choun[4], Pisethmorokoth Keo[4], Virginie Avrillon[2], Pierre-Jean Souquet[1] and Chanty Ny[4]

Abstract

Background: Flexible bronchoscopy is pivotal for the diagnosis of most respiratory diseases. A flexible bronchoscopy unit (FBU) was created in 2008 in the Preah Kossamak university hospital (Phnom Penh, Cambodia) through a cooperation program between a French and a Cambodian team. In 2009 we conducted an assessment of the compliance of the FBU to international standards and found that most of French and British guidelines were fully applied or adapted to local practice.
The aim of the current work was to assess FBU again 6 years later, in order to determine if compliance to international guidelines was sustainable.

Methods: The 2015 evaluation was conducted identically to 2009. All recommendation items from the French and the British Thoracic Societies guidelines were assessed individually. Each recommendation was assigned a status expressing the level at which it was respected in Cambodia: *applied, adapted, not applied* and *not evaluable*.
An endoscope microbial sampling was performed as recommended by the French Ministry of Health.

Results: Between 2009 and 2015, the pattern of international recommendations in the Cambodian FBU did not change. Notably the rates of *applied* French evaluable recommendations remained stable: respectively 58% vs 57%. Main changes in French guidelines occurred in adapted items that became applied ($n = 5/15$) while 4 previously adapted/applied items became not applied. Furthermore, all microbial analyses showed sterile results.

Conclusions: Our results show that implementation of a high quality FBU in a least-developed country is feasible. In addition, the performance is maintained in the long-term.

Keywords: Bronchoscopy, Cambodia, Guidelines, Least Developed Countries, Pulmonary medicine

* Correspondence: sebastien.couraud@chu-lyon.fr
[1]Service de Pneumologie Aigue Spécialisée et Cancérologie Thoracique, Centre Hospitalier Lyon Sud, Institut de Cancérologie des Hospices Civils de Lyon, 69495 Pierre Bénite, France
[2]Association PRUPET, Centre Hospitalier de Moulin Yzeure, Moulins, France
Full list of author information is available at the end of the article

Background

Cambodia remains one of the poorest countries in the world: in 2014, it ranked 144th (of 188 countries) on the Human Development Index [1]. Lower respiratory tract (LRT) infections are a major public health problem in Cambodia. In 2013, according to the World Health Organization, it had the highest prevalence of documented tuberculosis cases in the world, i.e., 715 cases per 100,000 inhabitants [2]. Furthermore, LRT infections are the second leading cause of premature death in Cambodia [3].

Flexible bronchoscopy (FB) is pivotal for the diagnosis of most respiratory diseases and especially those of infectious or neoplastic origin [4]. However, the deployment and use of FB necessitate advanced equipment and competencies. Through to the mid-2000s, Cambodia had no flexible bronchoscopy unit (FBU) meeting international standards in its public hospitals.

There was however an inter-hospital cooperation program between the Lyon Sud Hospital (Lyon, France) and the Preah Kossamak Hospital (Phnom Penh, Cambodia) [5]. Building upon that ongoing program, a decision was made in 2008 to create a modern FBU in Cambodia.

Toward this goal, two Cambodian physicians had been brought to France for a 2-year training program, and two residents from the Lyon Sud Hospital spent 6 months in Cambodia (between November 2008 and May 2009) to aid the local team with the deployment of the FBU. The materials (endoscope, light source, camera) were provided as a donation by the Lyon University Hospital team. A Cambodian nurse was hired specifically for the FBU and trained during 2 weeks in France then 6 months in Cambodia.

The FBU was designed to conform as much as possible to current international recommendations while nonetheless taking into consideration local sanitary, economic and organizational constraints and conditions. Following upon the launch of the FBU in 2009, we performed and published an evaluation of the unit's first-year conformity to international standards [6]. 54 procedures were performed in 2009. The results of that first study showed that it is possible to deploy a high quality FBU in a least-developed country: we showed that 52% of French recommendations [7] and 46% of British recommendations [8] were strictly applied, whereas respectively only 18 and 23% could not be applied.

Now up and running, the remaining major challenges for the FBU are the appropriation of its daily operation by local teams and the perpetuation of quality standards and optimal use. Considering this, a follow-up study to evaluate the long-term respect of recommendations appeared necessary.

Thus, for the present work, we re-evaluated the FBU to assess its continuing application of international recommendations 6 years after its launch.

Methods

Evaluation protocol

The protocol used for this second evaluation performed in 2015 (2015 evaluation) was the same as that used for the first evaluation in 2009 (2009 evaluation) [6] to enable a comparison of the results of the two evaluations; only the on-site observer (MV) differed. For the present study, like for the first, the on-site observer was a Lyon Sud Hospital resident assigned for 6 months to the Preah Kossamak Hospital in Phnom Penh as part of the cooperation program between the two hospitals. All examinations performed in the FBU between November and December 2015 ($n = 14$) were observed by the resident to assess the application of recommendations. The medical and paramedical teams were not informed of the observation process until after the observation period to avoid bias.

As in the 2009 evaluation, all currently-applicable recommendations were assessed individually. Each recommendation was assigned a status expressing the level at which it was respected:

- *Applied* when the recommendation was entirely respected;
- *Adapted* when the recommendation was not applied as written but as adapted to respond to local conditions or constraints;
- *Not applied* when the recommendation was not respected at all;
- *Not evaluable* when the recommendation could not be evaluated in the setting of FB in Cambodia.

Recommendations used for the assessment

Two sets of recommendations were used as practice standards: those published by the Francophone Endoscopy Group of the Francophone Society of Pulmonology (SPLF) [7] and those published by the *British Thoracic Society (BTS)* [8]. Both documents are similarly structured, with lists of recommendations grouped into a number of specific sections.

The BTS recommendations used in the 2009 evaluation were those first published by the society in 2001 [8]. The BTS updated their recommendations in 2013 [9]. The initial and updated BTS recommendations differ on several points. For the new version, the organization of the existing sections was largely modified, new details were added to some subjects (standards and performances of diagnostic techniques, FB in intensive care units, cleaning and disinfection) and new sections were added (sedation). Some items were reworded or modified. For example, the 2001 version recommended antibiotic prophylaxis in certain conditions (notably for patients with heart valve prosthesis) but the 2013 version does not. Recommendations for cleaning and disinfection also evolved, with the 2013 version insisting on the use of automated endoscope reprocessors (AERs) and disposable materials. For the present 2015 evaluation, we logically chose to use the 2013 version of the BTS recommendations.

The second set of recommendations, those published by the SPLF in 2007 [7], had not been updated as of the launch of the present follow-up study.

To ensure the pertinence and clarity of comparisons with, on one hand, the results from the 2009 evaluation and, on the other, the unchanged French recommendations, we chose to reemploy for the 2015 evaluation the presentation of results used in the 2009 evaluation. Thus, the recommendation items are again grouped in six categories: *patient safety [before/during/after] endoscopy*; *cleaning and disinfection*; *staff safety*; and *standards and performances of diagnostic techniques*. BTS items that were substantially modified between evaluations were marked with an asterisk in the tables of the present study.

Some items present in the recommendations were evaluated neither in the 2009 evaluation nor in the present 2015 evaluation due to economic and organizational conditions that prevent the development and implementation of certain acts. For example, recommendations concerning interstitial pathologies were and remain unevaluable. Also, the 2013 version of the BTS recommendations has a new section on sedation. However, the safety conditions necessary for the intravenous sedation that it proposes are currently not available in Cambodia, and thus this section was not evaluated here. Finally, in 2009, we had deployed a protocol for FB in the intensive care unit. However, that protocol had fallen out of use several years before the 2015 evaluation and thus was not re-evaluated in it.

Microbiological analysis of endoscopes

Endoscope microbial surveillance was performed in accordance with the recommendations of the French Ministry of Health [10]. As specific sampling solutions were not available in Cambodia, we used sterile normal saline (0.9% sodium chloride) as suggested in those recommendations. All three of the endoscopes used at the FBU were controlled as per the global channel evaluation method indicated in the above-mentioned recommendations. A sterile syringe was used to inject the normal saline in all the channels of the endoscope and the resulting flush was passively collected in a unique container. Thereafter, the on-site observer took the samples immediately to the Institut Pasteur in Cambodia for microbiological analyses. Mycobacteria were assessed first by microscopy using Ziehl-Neelsen staining then by culturing both in Löwenstein–Jensen medium and in mycobacteria growth indicator tubes. Cyto-bacteriology was done by cell count (epithelial cells/leukocytes) followed by direct bacteriological and mycological examination and finally bacterial culture on standard media.

Statistical analyses

The number of *applied*, *adapted*, *not applied*, and *not evaluable* items in the French recommendations and in the British recommendations as well as in the 2009 evaluation and in the 2015 evaluation was expressed as a percentage of the total number of recommendations or the number of evaluated recommendations (total - non-evaluable items).

Proportions between the 2009 and 2015 evaluations were compared with the Chi-squared test with n-1° of freedom (n = number in the category) when the expected frequency was greater than five or with a two-tailed Fischer exact test when it was not. Statistical significance was set at $p < 0.05$.

Results

Application of recommendations

Figure 1 provides photos of the FBU at the Preah Kossamak Hospital in 2009 and 2015.

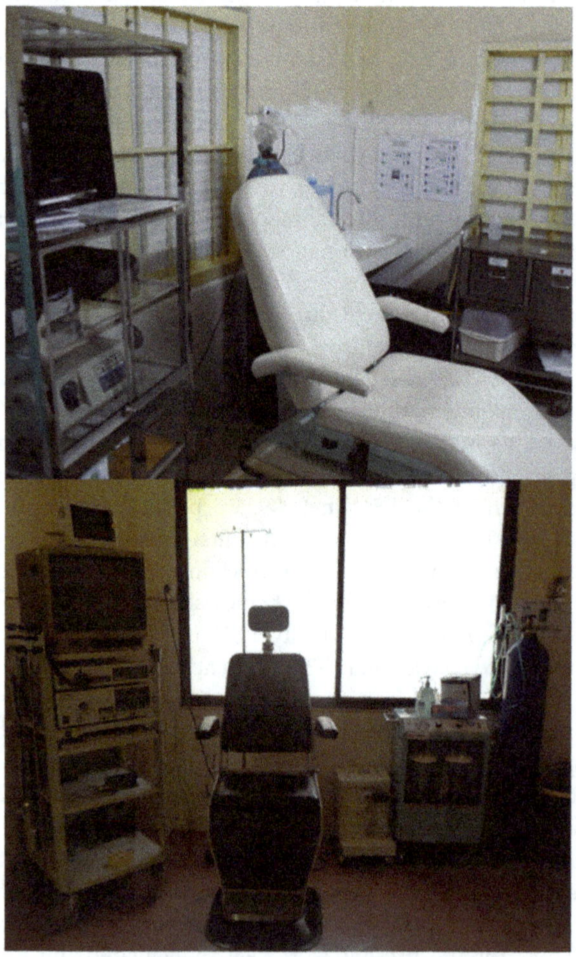

Fig. 1 The bronchoscopy unit at the Preah Kossamak Hospital in Phnom Penh in 2009 (*Up*) and 2015 (*Down*)

Table 1 Results of the 2009 and 2015 evaluations for the then-current French and British recommendations

Recommendations	French guidelines			British guidelines		
Year of evaluation	2009 N (%)	2015 N (%)	*P* value	2009[a] N (%)	2015[b] N (%)	*P* value
Before bronchoscopy						
Applied	11 (69%)	10 (63%)	-	9 (64%)	18 (78%)	-
Adapted	2 (12%)	2 (12%)		1 (7%)	3 (13%)	
Not applied	2 (12%)	1 (6%)		3 (21%)	0 (0%)	
Not evaluable	1 (6%)	3 (19%)		1 (7%)	2 (9%)	
Total	16	16		14	23	
During bronchoscopy						
Applied	8 (89%)	7 (78%)	-	5 (50%)	10 (59%)	-
Adapted	1 (11%)	1 (11%)		2 (20%)	1 (6%)	
Not applied	0	1 (11%)		2 (20%)	4 (23%)	
Not evaluable	0	0 (0%)		1 (10%)	2 (12%)	
Total	9	9		10	17	
After bronchoscopy						
Applied	1 (25%)	1 (25%)	-	1 (20%)	1 (20%)	-
Adapted	1 (25%)	0		2 (40%)	0	
Not applied	0	0		0	1 (20%)	
Not evaluable	2 (50%)	3 (75%)		2 (40%)	3 (60%)	
Total	4	4		5	5	
Cleaning and disinfection						
Applied	4 (33%)	4 (33%)	-	5 (33%)	8 (31%)	-
Adapted	3 (25%)	1 (8%)		4 (27%)	1 (4%)	
Not applied	5 (42%)	7 (58%)		6 (40%)	11 (42%)	
Not evaluable	0	0		0	6 (23%)	
Total	12	12		15	26	
Staff safety						
Applied	3 (30%)	4 (40%)	-	4 (36%)	3 (27%)	-
Adapted	3 (30%)	2 (20%)		3 (27%)	0	
Not applied	4 (40%)	4 (40%)		4 (36%)	5 (45%)	
Not evaluable	0	0		0	3 (27%)	
Total	10	10		11	11	
Standards and performances of diagnostic techniques						
Applied	1 (14%)	2 (28%)	-	0	5 (28%)	-
Adapted	3 (43%)	2 (28%)		2 (50%)	2 (11%)	
Not applied	0	0		0	4 (22%)	
Not evaluable	3 (43%)	3 (43%)		2 (50%)	7 (39%)	
Total	7	7		4	18	
Intensive care unit						
Applied	6 (86%)	0	-	6 (100%)	0	-
Adapted	0	0		0	0	
Not applied	1 (14%)	0		0	0	
Not evaluable	0	7 (100%)		0	17 (100%)	
Total	7	7		6	17	

Table 1 Results of the 2009 and 2015 evaluations for the then-current French and British recommendations *(Continued)*

Sedation						
Not evaluable	-	-	-	-	13 (100%)	-
Total					13	
Total	$n = 65$	$n = 65$	0.64#	$n = 65$	$n = 130$	0.062#
Applied	34 (52%)	28 (43%)		30 (46%)	45 (35%)	
Adapted	13 (20%)	8 (12%)		14 (22%)	7 (5%)	
Not applied	12 (18%)	13 (20%)		15 (23%)	25 (19%)	
Not evaluable	6 (9%)	16 (25%)	0.095$	6 (9%)	53 (41%)	$<10^{-4}$$

% values are calculated within all status (including not-evaluable)
[a]Calculated using 2001 edition of BTS guidelines/[b]Calculated using 2013 edition of BTS guidelines
#*P* value calculated excluding the *not evaluable* status; $*P* value calculated for all statuses (included *not evaluable* status)

Table 1 summarizes the frequencies of recommendation statuses per category and in total for each set of guidelines. Comparing the statuses of the French guidelines between 2009 and 2015, respectively 72% vs 55% were *applied* or *adapted*, 18% vs 20% were *not applied* and 9% vs 25% were *not evaluable*. In 2015, items in the categories *patient safety before* and *patient safety during endoscopy* were *applied* in respectively 63 and 78% of cases. As for the statuses of the British guidelines, 46% of the recommendations were *applied* in 2009 vs 35% in 2015, and 9% were *not evaluable* in 2009 vs 41% in 2015.

Tables S1 through S6 in the Additional file 1 provide the statuses for all the recommendations, grouped within their categories, for both the 2009 and the 2015 evaluations.

Table 2 summarizes the French recommendations for which there was a status change between the 2009 and 2015 evaluations.

Figure 2 summarizes changes in the distribution of the evaluable French recommendations (excluding thus the *not evaluable* status) between the two evaluations: 57% of recommendations were *applied* in 2015 compared to 58% in 2009 ($P = 0.64$).

Microbiological analysis of endoscopes

All three endoscopes passed the microbial surveillance analyses. Particularly, cytology found less than 10 epithelial cells and less than 10 leukocytes per milliliter. The direct bacteriological and mycological examinations were negative as were the ensuing bacterial cultures on standard media. Similarly, mycobacteriological analyses (microscopy and culture) were negative for all samples.

Discussion

Between the 2009 and the 2015 evaluations, the profile for the use of international recommendations in the FBU of the Preah Kossamak Hospital did not significantly change. Notably the rates of *applied* French recommendations remained stable: respectively 52% vs 43%. Furthermore, all microbial surveillance analyses were negative for all of the endoscopes.

To our knowledge, ours study is the first to provide data on recommendation application rates, be it in developing or developed countries. Our work here falls within a dynamic of improvement of care provision quality and aligns with the recommendation for periodic audits of FBUs expressed in the 2013 BTS guidelines.

Several changes in the implementation of recommendations between 2009 and 2015 are to be noted. Considering *patient safety during endoscopy*, the recommendation for having non-invasive ventilation available was *applied* in 2009 but not in 2015. Although the equipment is available, the team lacks training for it and thus it remains unused. Also, certain *cleaning and disinfection* recommendations that had the *adapted* status in 2009 were no longer being implemented in 2015. This was the case for renewed disinfection after prolonged storage of an endoscope, abandoned due to costs and a lack of trained staff. However, this had no apparent impact on endoscope hygiene as illustrated by the good microbial surveillance results. Inversely, the recent acquisition of a new multi-detector CT by the hospital enables pre-bronchoscopy thoracic scans, but the examination is prohibitively expensive (US$100) for many patients. The recommendation concerning CT thus evolved from *not applied* to *adapted*.

The lack of an increase in the rate of *applied* recommendations also appears to point to a lack of spontaneous improvement of practices between 2009 and 2015. We underline however that a status of *adapted* or *not applied* for a given recommendation was usually due to elements independent of the pulmonology service such as the ambient poverty or the organization of the healthcare system. The team itself thus has little leeway to further improve the respect of recommendations.

A major issue in cooperation efforts with least-developed countries is the appropriation of projects by the local teams, a step vital to their durability and effectiveness [11]. In the present work, this appropriation appears to have been attained in 2015: the Cambodian team continued to

Table 2 Focus on changes of statuses of the French recommendations in the 2009 and 2015' evaluations

French recommendations *(some wording summarized for space)*	**2009**	**2015**
Patient safety before bronchoscopy		
Patient is given oral and written information	Applied	Adapted
Fasting time	Adapted	Applied
Patients with suspected COPD must be evaluated and stabilized	Adapted	Applied
Anticoagulant treatments must be stopped or antagonized before performing biopsies	Applied	*Not evaluable*
Premedication may be proposed	Applied	Not applied
Nitrous oxide may be used	Not applied	*Not evaluable*
A chest CT before diagnostic bronchoscopy increases diagnostic yield	Not applied	Adapted
Patient safety during bronchoscopy		
Non-invasive ventilation is useful in hypoxic patients undergoing diagnostic bronchoscopy	Applied	Not applied
Patient safety after bronchoscopy		
Patients who receive sedation must be warned not to drive or make important decisions in the following 24 hours	Adapted	*Not evaluable*
Cleaning and disinfection		
Cleaning and disinfection must be done before and after each endoscopic intervention (British) Disinfection must be renewed when endoscopes are stored for more than 12 hours and less than one week	Adapted	Not applied
Cleaning and disinfection must be done in a dedicated space by trained staff Used materials must be kept separate from cleaned materials	Adapted	Applied
A traceability protocol must be developed so that the bronchoscope and materials used for a given intervention and the decontamination procedures that they underwent can be identified	Adapted	Not applied
Sterile or microfiltered water must be used for final rinsing	Applied	Adapted
Staff safety		
Powder-free latex or non-latex gloves must be worn instead of powdered latex gloves	Adapted	Applied
Standards and performances of diagnostic techniques		
At least 5 biopsies must be taken when endobronchial neoplasia is suspected (4 to 5 for the French recommendations)	Adapted	Applied
Total		
Adapted → Applied	5 (33%)	
Applied → Adapted	2 (13%)	
Not applied → Adapted	1 (7%)	
Adapted → Not applied	2 (13%)	
Applied → Not applied	2 (13%)	
Adapted → Not evaluable	1 (7%)	
Applied → Not evaluable	1 (7%)	
Not applied → Not evaluable	1 (7%)	
Total	15 (100%)	

implement international FB recommendations at a rate comparable to that observed at the launch of the project in 2009, and the number of bronchoscopies per month had increased from 4.5 in 2009 [6] to 7 in November-December 2015. This successful appropriation extends to sanitary issues as well, with the continuing and complete respect of recommendations in the *cleaning and disinfection* category, as illustrated by the good results for microbial surveillance. This latter can be improved by making it systematic and more frequent but cost remains an issue: microbial surveillance analyses are billed at US$50/endoscope whereas the bronchoscopy itself is billed at US$20 (excluding analyses) to the patient. This quality control issue appears essential and will be implemented in the future.

Our study has both strengths and weaknesses. Among the former is the long follow-up for the project. Over

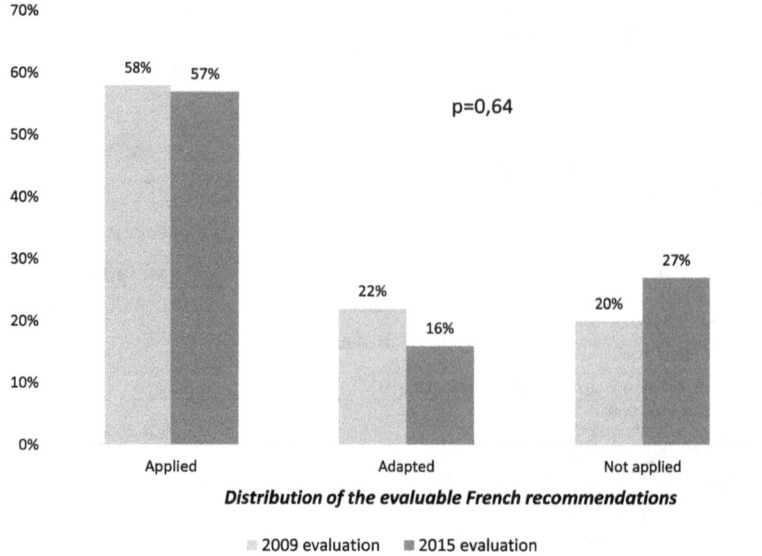

Fig. 2 Changes in the distribution of the evaluable French recommendations between 2009 and 2015

the 6-year period, the Cambodian FBU experienced numerous organizational changes that had the potential to negatively affect the quality of practices: the unit was moved, a new endoscopic nurse was trained and most of the original endoscopists were replaced by new ones. But these events proved to be opportunities. For example, the change of premises enabled improvements to the FBU, with notably the creation of a dedicated decontamination zone immediately next to, but separated from, the examination room. Equally, the peer-to-peer training of the new nurse by the original nurse, who had been trained at the start of the program, was a chance to verify the local team's complete comprehension of FB processes and their ability to transmit that knowledge to new staff. The main weakness of our study resides in the changes made to the BTS guidelines between the 2009 and 2015 evaluations. Consequently, numerous items could not be re-evaluated. Interestingly however, a good proportion of the new items in the 2013 BTS recommendations had already been implemented in the FBU upstream of the 2015 evaluation, illustrating the team's ability to adapt to change. Another weakness is the single-observer nature of the study, which creates a possibility of interpretation and writing biases. And finally, our study is limited by the high number of recommendations that were *not evaluable*. This problem is largely due to the fact that recommendations from developed countries impose increasingly expensive materials (AERs, single-use accessories, etc.) and address indications and techniques that are not currently relevant to Cambodia. For example, such techniques as transbronchial biopsy or fluoroscopy are not yet available in the Preah Kossamak FBU.

Conclusions

Our results show that it is possible not only to create a high quality flexible bronchoscopy unit in a least-developed country, but also, and particularly, to maintain its performance in the long-term. To succeed in this endeavour, international standards and recommendations must often be adapted to local constraints. More than the cost of modern endoscopic equipment, it is the appropriation of techniques and practices by the local teams that is the largest challenge. Over the 6 years between our first and second evaluations, the Preah Kossamak FBU team succeeded in maintaining an optimal level of care, thus ensuring the safety of their bronchoscopy patients. In the future, we intend to develop several more advanced techniques (such as blind transbronchial needle aspiration of carinal nodes) and organize regular microbial surveillance of equipment. Our successful program, built upon the pertinent application and adaptation of international recommendations, constitutes a model for other medical cooperation projects.

Abbreviations

AER: Automated Endoscope Reprocessor; BTS: British Thoracic Society; FB: Flexible bronchoscopy; FBU: Flexible Bronchoscopy Unit; LRT: Lower respiratory tract

Acknowledgments

Authors thank M. Kevin Erwin for expert English rewording.

Funding
Martin Veaudor's training ship in Cambodia was funded by a mobility grant from *Hospices Civils de Lyon*. This work was partially funded by PRUPET NGO. English rewording was supported by a grant from *Bibliothèque Scientifique de l'Association des Internes des Hôpitaux de Lyon*.

Authors' contributions
MV made substantial contributions to conception and design, or acquisition of data, or analysis and interpretation of data; has been involved in drafting the manuscript or revising it critically for important intellectual content; has given final approval of the version to be published; has agreed to be accountable for all aspects of the work in ensuring that questions related to the accuracy or integrity of any part of the work are appropriately investigated and resolved. SéC made substantial contributions to conception and design, or acquisition of data, or analysis and interpretation of data; has been involved in drafting the manuscript or revising it critically for important intellectual content; has given final approval of the version to be published; has agreed to be accountable for all aspects of the work in ensuring that questions related to the accuracy or integrity of any part of the work are appropriately investigated and resolved. SoC has given final approval of the version to be published; has agreed to be accountable for all aspects of the work in ensuring that questions related to the accuracy or integrity of any part of the work are appropriately investigated and resolved. CC has given final approval of the version to be published; has agreed to be accountable for all aspects of the work in ensuring that questions related to the accuracy or integrity of any part of the work are appropriately investigated and resolved. PK has given final approval of the version to be published; has agreed to be accountable for all aspects of the work in ensuring that questions related to the accuracy or integrity of any part of the work are appropriately investigated and resolved. VA has given final approval of the version to be published; has agreed to be accountable for all aspects of the work in ensuring that questions related to the accuracy or integrity of any part of the work are appropriately investigated and resolved. PJS has given final approval of the version to be published; has agreed to be accountable for all aspects of the work in ensuring that questions related to the accuracy or integrity of any part of the work are appropriately investigated and resolved. CN has given final approval of the version to be published; has agreed to be accountable for all aspects of the work in ensuring that questions related to the accuracy or integrity of any part of the work are appropriately investigated and resolved.

Competing interests
The authors declare that they have no competing interests.

Consent for publication
Not applicable.

Author details
[1]Service de Pneumologie Aigue Spécialisée et Cancérologie Thoracique, Centre Hospitalier Lyon Sud, Institut de Cancérologie des Hospices Civils de Lyon, 69495 Pierre Bénite, France. [2]Association PRUPET, Centre Hospitalier de Moulin Yzeure, Moulins, France. [3]EMR 3738 Ciblage thérapeutique en oncologie, Faculté de médecine et de maïeutique Lyon Sud Charles Mérieux, Université Lyon 1, Villeurbanne, France. [4]Service de pneumologie, Hôpital Preah Kossamak, Phnom Penh, Cambodia.

References

1. United Nations, 23 December 2015. United Nations Development Program, Cambodia. http://www.kh.undp.org/content/cambodia/en/home/countryinfo. Accessed 8 Apr 2016.
2. Zumla A, George A, Sharma V, Herbert RHN, Baroness Masham of Ilton, Oxley A, Oliver M. The WHO 2014 global tuberculosis report-further to go. Lancet Glob Health. 2015;3:e10–2.
3. Institute for Health Metrics and Evaluation. Country profiles: Cambodia. http://www.healthdata.org/cambodia. Accessed 28 Dec 2015.
4. Prakash UB, Offord KP, Stubbs SE. Bronchoscopy in North America: the ACCP survey. Chest. 1991;100:1668–75.
5. Couraud S, Chan S, Avrillon V, Souquet P-J, Ny C. Monthly video-assisted web meeting between French and Cambodian team in order to improve management of difficult cases. Rev Pneumol Clin. 2013;69:119–20.
6. Couraud S, Chan S, Avrillon V, Horn K, Try S, Gérinière L, Perrot E, Guichon C, Souquet PJ, Ny C. How practical guidelines can be applied in poor countries? Example of the introduction of a bronchoscopy unit in Cambodia. Rev Pneumol Clin. 2013;69:244–9.
7. Febvre M, Trosini-Desert V, Atassi K, Hermant C, Colchen A, Raspaud C, Vergnon JM, Endoscopy Working Group of the French Society of Pulmonary Medicine. Good practices of diagnostic flexible bronchoscopy. Rev Mal Respir. 2007;24:1363–92.
8. British Thoracic Society Bronchoscopy Guidelines Committee, A subcommittee of the standard of care committee of the British Thoracic Society. British Thoracic Society guidelines on diagnostic flexible bronchoscopy. Thorax. 2001;56:i1–i21.
9. Du Rand IA, Blaikley J, Booton R, Chaudhuri N, Gupta V, Khalid S, Mandal S, Martin J, Mills J, Navani N, Rahman NM, Wrighton JM, Munavvar M, British Thoracic Society Bronchoscopy Guideline Group. British Thoracic Society guideline for diagnostic flexible bronchoscopy in adults: accredited by NICE. Thorax. 2013;68:i1–i44.
10. French Ministry of Health, March 2007. [Elements of quality assurance in hygiene related to the microbiological examination of endoscopes and traceability in endoscopy]. http://social-sante.gouv.fr/IMG/pdf/microbio_endoscopes-2.pdf. Accessed 28 Dec 2015.
11. Food and Agriculture Organization of the United Nations, 1997. [The dynamics of rural societies to participatory rural development projects: Reflections and proposals for action from West Africa experience]. http://www.fao.org/docrep/v9860f/v9860f00.htm. Accessed 14 Jan 2016.

11

End-tidal capnographic monitoring to detect apnea episodes during flexible bronchoscopy under sedation

Tsukasa Ishiwata[1], Kenji Tsushima[1*], Mai Fujie[2], Kenichi Suzuki[1], Kosuke Hirota[1], Mitsuhiro Abe[1], Naoko Kawata[1], Jiro Terada[1] and Koichiro Tatsumi[1]

Abstract

Background: Apnea developing as a result of oversedation is a potential clinical problem in patients undergoing flexible bronchoscopy (FB) under sedation. However, there are no reports of evaluation using a standardized method of the frequency of occurrence of apnea episodes during FB under sedation. The aim of this study was to investigate the frequency of apnea episodes during FB under sedation in the clinical setting by end-tidal capnography.

Methods: This study was a single-institution retrospective review of a prospectively maintained database and medical records, including capnographic data, from April 2015 to March 2016. We enrolled patients who were sedated with midazolam and underwent diagnostic FB under end-tidal capnographic monitoring. Apnea was defined as cessation of airflow for more than 10 s.

Results: Data from a total of 121 eligible patients were analyzed. A total of 131 apnea episodes (median duration 33 s) were recorded in 59 patients (48.8%). Prolonged apnea episodes lasting for more than 30 s occurred in 24 patients (19.8%). Furthermore, 55 apnea episodes (42.0%) were followed by a decline of the SpO_2 by ≥4% from the baseline.

Conclusions: In this study, end-tidal capnography revealed the occurrence of apnea episodes at a high frequency in patients undergoing FB under sedation in the clinical setting.

Background

Sedation is required for relieving the anxiety and calming of patients during a wide variety of medical procedures [1]. However, inadvertent oversedation may sometimes occur, leading to deep sedation and apnea episodes [2]. Bronchoscopic procedures require moderate sedation to alleviate the patient's anxiety and to suppress the cough reflex. However, this is associated with the risk of respiratory depression developing during prolonged procedures, especially diagnostic bronchoscopies, as administration of high doses of sedatives is often necessitated during such procedures. Furthermore, oxygen desaturation is known to occur at a higher frequency during flexible bronchoscopy (FB) than during other endoscopic procedures, e.g., esophagogastroduodenoscopy and colonoscopy, because of the excessive respiratory secretions and endobronchial bleeding encountered during this procedure.

Until date, the frequency of occurrence of apnea episodes during FB under sedation has never been precisely evaluated using a standardized method. Although a previous report referred to the necessity of respiratory monitoring and possible usefulness of end-tidal capnography during FB [3], supportive clinical data have not yet been obtained. The aim of this study was to investigate the actual frequency of occurrence of apnea episodes during FB under sedation by end-tidal capnography.

Methods

This study was a retrospective review of a prospectively maintained database and medical records, including capnographic data, at our institution. This study was conducted at the Chiba University hospital (Chiba, Japan). The study protocol was submitted for Institutional Review Board approval (Chiba #2455). Written informed consent

* Correspondence: tsushimakenji@yahoo.co.jp
[1]Department of Respirology, Graduate School of Medicine, Chiba University, 1-8-1, Inohana, Chuo-ku, Chiba 260-8670, Japan
Full list of author information is available at the end of the article

for the performance of bronchoscopy was obtained from all participants.

Subjects

From April 2015 to March 2016, we enrolled patients who underwent diagnostic FB under midazolam sedation. The performed FB procedures included endobronchial biopsy, bronchial brushing, transbronchial biopsy, transbronchial needle aspiration (including endobronchial ultrasound-guided needle aspiration) and bronchial washing. For each patient, the following medical information was recorded from the medical records: age, gender, body mass index, American Society of Anesthesiologists (ASA) physical status classification [4], frequency of comorbidities, and final diagnosis of the lung disease.

Sedation and patient monitoring

Midazolam was administered by intravenous bolus injection at the starting dose of 1–3 mg, with additional doses of 0.5–1 mg administered as needed for moderate sedation by pulmonologists, not anesthesiologists. Adjustment of the initial and additional doses of midazolam was left to the bronchoscopist's discretion, guided by the criteria for moderate sedation in the ASA clinical practice guidelines [1].

Tracheal intubation was not performed. After spraying 4% lidocaine onto the patient's throat to induce local anesthesia, a FB was inserted through the mouth of the patient lying supine on the bed. An Olympus (Tokyo, Japan) BF-260 videobronchoscope (4.9 mm outer diameter) was used. Additional local anesthesia with 1% lidocaine was used as appropriate. All patients underwent electrocardiographic monitoring and pulse oximetry as standard monitoring procedures. Supplemental oxygen (at a flow rate of 2 L/min through a nasal cannula) was used for each patient, and the oxygen flow rate was increased when the SpO_2 fell below 90%. Decline of the SpO_2 by ≥4% from the baseline was defined as clinically significant.

Capnographic monitoring

For end-tidal capnographic monitoring, we used a device (Smart CapnoLine Guardian, Medtronic, Ireland) consisting of an endoscopic bite block equipped with a cannula designed to sample expired air from both the nostrils and the mouth (Fig. 1a). This was connected to an automated capnographic monitoring device (Capnostream 20P, Medtronic, Ireland) (Fig. 1b) through a sampling tube. This monitoring device can measure the concentrations of carbon dioxide in the expired air continuously. When the capnogram showed a flat line, a clinician made sure that the sample port was not disconnected. The capnographic data and SpO_2 data were routinely collected and recorded in our institutional databank after the procedure. Apnea episodes were defined in this study as cessation of airflow for more than 10 s (Fig. 1c). After identifying both the time of onset and end of the apnea episodes, we calculated the duration of the apnea episodes and the time delay between the onset of an apnea episode and a ≥4% SpO_2 decline from the baseline.

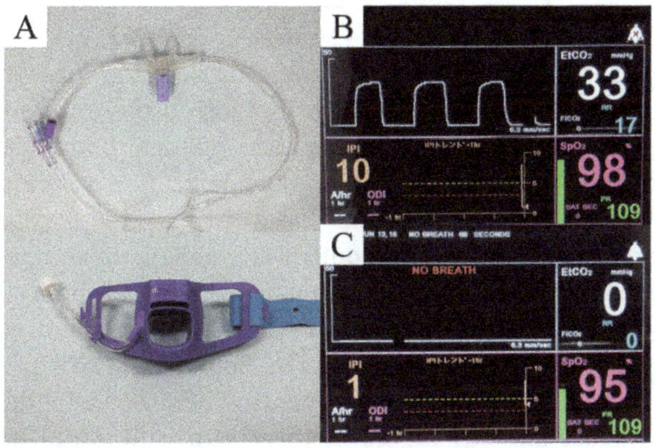

Fig. 1 Devices used in this study for end-tidal capnography. **a** The Smart CapnoLine Guardian™ is an endoscopic bite block equipped with a cannula designed to sample expired air from both the nostril and the mouth for continuous measurement of the carbon dioxide concentration. **b** The automated capnographic monitoring device (Capnostream™ 20P) shows the patient's respiratory airflow as a carbon dioxide concentration curve. **c** Cessation of air flow visualized as a flat line on the capnogram

Data analysis

Descriptive data were expressed as numbers (percentages) and medians (ranges), and continuous data were expressed as means and standard deviations (SD) for normally distributed data, and as medians with interquartile ranges (IQR) for non-normally distributed data. Continuous data were tested for normal distribution using the Kolmogorov–Smirnov test. For statistical comparison, the descriptive data were compared using the chi-square test or Fisher's exact test, and the continuous data were compared using the *t*-test for normally distributed data and the Mann-Whitney test for non-normally distributed data. All *P* values were two sided and the statistical significance level was set at <0.05. Data were entered into an Excel (Microsoft Corp, USA) database. All analysis and interpretations of the data were carried out using SAS, ver. 9.4 (SAS Institute Inc. USA).

Results

Of the 125 eligible patients, four patients were excluded because of missing data. After analysis of the capnographic data from the remaining 121 patients, the patients were divided into a group with apnea episodes (developing at least one apnea episode) and a group without apnea episodes during the FB procedure. There were 59 patients (40 males and 19 females) with a mean age of 71 years (range 23–82) in the group with apnea episodes and 62 patients (42 males and 20 females) with a mean age of 69 years (range 37–81) in the group without apnea episodes. As shown in Table 1, there were no significant differences in the age, gender, body mass index, ASA physical status, frequency of the comorbidities of COPD or interstitial lung disease, and the final diagnosis between the groups with and without apnea episodes. There were no patients with severe obesity or severe obstructive sleep apnea syndrome with abnormality of a neck circumference. The SpO_2 was ≥96% prior to the procedure in all the patients. The mean total dose of midazolam was higher in the group with apnea episodes than in the group without apnea episodes (3.9 mg vs. 2.3 mg, $P < 0.001$). The median minimum SpO_2 during the FB procedure was lower in the group with apnea episodes (89%; IQR 87–93 vs. 96%; IQR 92–97, $P < 0.001$) and the median maximum flow rate of supplemental O_2 required was higher in the group with apnea episodes than in the group without apnea episodes (2 L/min; IQR 2–4 vs. 2 L/min; IQR 2-2, $P < 0.001$).

As shown in Table 2, there were a total of 131 apnea episodes in 59 patients (48.8%). Prolong apnea episodes that lasted for more than 30 s occurred in 24 patients (19.8%). The median duration of the apnea episodes was 33 s (IQR 24–46), and the maximum duration was 97 s. A total of 55 apnea episodes (42.0%) were followed by a decline of the SpO_2 by ≥4% from the baseline. The median time delay between the onset of an apnea episode and decline of the SpO_2 by ≥4% from the baseline was 31 s (IQR 28–42). There were no patients who suffered from massive bleeding or pneumothorax during the FB procedures. None of the patients in this case series required assisted ventilation during/after the FB procedure.

Discussion

Our results revealed that apnea episodes occur at a high frequency during FB under sedation in the clinical setting. In addition, end-tidal capnographic monitoring also allowed earlier detection of the apnea episodes than pulse oximetry.

The present study showed that apnea episodes occurred frequently during FB procedures performed under sedation; apneas occurred in 48.8% of the patients, and especially prolonged apnea episodes, lasting for over 30 s, occurred in 19.8% of the patients. Moreover, as much as 42.0% of the apnea episodes were followed by significant oxygen desaturation. Previous reports may lend support

Table 1 Characteristics of the patient groups with and without apnea episodes ($n = 121$)

Variable	With apnea episodes ($n = 59$)	Without apnea episodes ($n = 62$)	*P* value
Age (years), median (range)	71 (23–82)	69 (37–81)	0.781
Gender (male), *n* (%)	40 (67.8)	42 (67.7)	0.995
BMI (kg/m^2), mean ± SD	22.3 ± 2.8	21.3 ± 2.9	0.061
ASA physical status (I/II/III/IV), *n*	15/36/8/0	25/31/6/0	0.214
Comorbidities and diagnoses, *n* (%)			
COPD	1 (1.7)	4 (6.5)	0.365
ILD	11 (18.6)	8 (12.9)	0.458
Infectious disease	3 (5.1)	3 (4.8)	1.000
Malignancy	41 (69.5)	39 (62.9)	0.565
Others	12 (20.3)	11 (17.7)	0.818
Procedures, (%)			
Endobronchial biopsy	16.9	12.9	0.532
Brushing	42.4	56.5	0.122
TBB	54.2	64.5	0.250
TBNA	25.4	19.4	0.423
Washing	15.3	29.0	0.069
Baseline SpO_2[a] (%), mean ± SD	97.1 ± 1.0	98.0 ± 1.0	0.014
Minimum SpO_2[b] (%), median (IQR)	89 (87–93)	96 (92–97)	<0.001
Maximum O_2 flow (L/min), median (IQR)	2 (2–4)	2 (2-2)	<0.001
Total dose of midazolam (mg), mean ± SD	3.9 ± 1.0	2.3 ± 0.8	<0.001

BMI body mass index, *SD* standard deviation, *ASA* American Society of Anesthesiologists, *COPD* chronic obstructive pulmonary disease, *ILD* interstitial lung disease, *TBB* transbronchial biopsy, *TBNA* transbronchial needle aspiration (including endobronchial ultrasound-guided aspiration), *IQR* interquartile range

[a]Before flexible bronchoscopy in ambient air

[b]During flexible bronchoscopy under supplemental oxygen

Table 2 Apnea profile ($n = 131$)

Apnea episodes per patient, median (range)	2 (1–8)
Duration of the apnea episodes, median (IQR)	33 s (24–46)
Maximum duration time of an apnea episode	97 s
Apnea episodes associated with SpO_2 decline by ≥4%, n (%)	55 (42.0)
Maximum SpO_2 decline	19% in SpO_2
Time delay between the onset of an apnea episode and SpO_2 decline by ≥4%, median (IQR)	31 s (28–42)

IQR interquartile range, *s* seconds

to our results; in the prospective study of 50 patients undergoing colonoscopy under sedation, a total of 29 episodes of anomalous ventilation, including apnea episodes lasting for more than 30 s, were detected in 16 patients by capnographic monitoring [5]. The results of a nationwide survey reported recently from Switzerland showed that apnea episodes requiring bag ventilation occurred at a rate of 0.011% during FB under sedation [6]. However, the results of the end-tidal capnographic monitoring in our present study revealed the occurrence of a number of additional apnea episodes besides those necessitating assisted ventilation. This implies that unintended oversedation occurs in many patients sedated with midazolam in the clinical setting, even though clinicians try to titrate the level of sedation to "moderate" sedation. Moreover, the dose of midazolam used in this study might have been lower than the average dose used at other institutions. A higher number and longer length of apnea episodes can be identified by capnography in patients administered higher doses of midazolam or propofol. Therefore, we suggest that it is necessary to carry out respiratory monitoring during FB under sedation.

This study also showed that end-tidal capnographic monitoring allowed earlier detection of the apnea episodes, not actual measurement values of carbon dioxide, than pulse oximetry. It has been reported that SpO_2 decline to its nadir can be delayed by 45 to 60 s after an apnea episode in patients with obstructive sleep apnea syndrome [7]. Our study showed that the median time delay between the onset of an apnea episode and significant SpO_2 decline was 31 s. This suggests that we can recognize apnea episodes about 30 s earlier by capnographic monitoring than by pulse oximetry alone. This result has a very important implication in relation to the usefulness of capnographic monitoring; end-tidal capnography alerts us of apnea episodes by setting off an alarm and by way of graphics, as shown in Fig. 1c, which allows us to detect apnea episodes early and to promptly implement appropriate corrective measures, such as patient stimulation or oxygen supplementation, before the respiratory depression becomes clinically significant. Furthermore, inappropriate addition of sedatives can also be avoided by early recognition of apnea episodes. Although pulse oximetry is important to evaluate the oxygenation state of a patient and is routinely used for monitoring of respiratory functions during FB [2], it has its limitations. Pulse oximetry can be a delayed indicator of respiratory depression [8]. Especially in sedated patients receiving supplemental oxygen, the decline in the SpO_2 may be delayed even in the presence of severe respiratory insufficiency [9, 10]. Therefore, we need an additional method for the early detection of respiratory depression. End-tidal capnography is a non-invasive method that allows continuous monitoring of ventilation. Although several studies of end-tidal capnographic monitoring during gastrointestinal endoscopy have been conducted, the conclusions remain controversial because of wide differences in the study settings (e.g. in relation to the patients' backgrounds, the type of sedative used, the primary outcome measure, etc.) [11–13]. To investigate the usefulness of end-tidal capnography during FB, prospective comparative trials are warranted in the future.

Various methods for early detection of respiratory depression have been described so far. Monitoring of the chest wall impedance is the most commonly used monitoring method in clinical practice, and recently, the use of acoustic monitoring has also become popular in some countries. However, many factors, including motion artifacts and physiological events unrelated to respiration, such as coughing and swallowing, may generate a high number of false alarms due to inaccurate readings when these two devices are used [14–16]. Moreover, chest wall impedance monitoring may fail to detect apneas secondary to airway obstruction [17]. A previous study demonstrated that transcutaneous capnography is an effective tool for monitoring ventilation during FB [18, 19]. Cutaneous carbon dioxide tension measured with a digital sensor has been reported to show a good correlation with the arterial carbon dioxide concentration. Therefore, currently, end-tidal or transcutaneous capnographic monitoring may be the most reliable for sensitive detection of respiratory depression. However, as there have been no comparative studies to determine the best method for respiratory monitoring, further investigations are awaited.

We need to discuss some limitations of our study here. First, it is possible that flat lines on the capnogram were caused by events other than true apnea episodes. Although we checked for displacement of the sampling tube, we did not record events of continuous suctionings of the airway that may cause a cessation of the waveform on the capnogram. Second, we have to consider multiple causes of SpO_2 decline during FB under sedation. SpO_2 decline can also be caused by conditions such as mucus obstruction of the airways, bronchial bleeding, or pneumothorax. However, there were no cases of massive bleeding or pneumothorax in this case series, and there were no patients who underwent bronchoalveolar lavage. Therefore, most of the SpO_2 declines are presumed to have been associated with apneic episodes in our cases.

Conclusions

End-tidal capnography revealed the occurrence of apnea episodes at a high frequency during FB under sedation. End-tidal capnographic monitoring also allowed earlier detection of the apnea episodes than pulse oximetry. We suggest the possible necessity of respiratory monitoring during FB in the clinical setting.

Abbreviations

ASA: American Society of Anethesiologists; FB: Flexible bronchoscopy; IQR: Interquartile ranges; SD: Standard deviations

Acknowledgements

Not applicable.

Funding

There was no funding of this study.

Authors' contributions

All authors had access to the data. TI and MF participated in the design of the study. TI did performed the statistical analysis and wrote the first draft of the manuscript. KenjiT edited the draft. KenjiT and KoichiroT provided intellectual input. TI, KS, KH, MA, NK and JT performed bronchoscopy and participated in patient care. All authors read and approved the final manuscript.

Competing interests

The authors declare that they have no competing interests.

Consent for publication

Not applicable.

Author details

[1]Department of Respirology, Graduate School of Medicine, Chiba University, 1-8-1, Inohana, Chuo-ku, Chiba 260-8670, Japan. [2]Medical Equipment Control Center, Chiba University Hospital, 1-8-1, Inohana, Chuo-ku, Chiba 260-8670, Japan.

References

1. The American Society of Anesthesiologists Task Force on Sedation and Analgesia by Non-anesthesiologists. Practice guidelines for sedation and analgesia by non-anesthesiologists. Anesthesiology. 2002;96(4):1004–17.
2. Forster A, Gardaz JP, Suter PM, Gemperle M. Respiratory depression by midazolam and diazepam. Anesthesiology. 1980;53(6):494–7.
3. Abdelmalak BB, Wang J, Mehta AC. Capnography monitoring in procedural sedation for bronchoscopy. J Bronchology Interv Pulmonol. 2014;21(4):370–1.
4. The American Society of Anesthesiologists. ASA physical status classification system. 2014. http://www.asahq.org/resources/clinical-information/asa-physical-status-classification-system. Accessed 1 Oct 2016.
5. Cacho G, Perez-Calle JL, Barbado A, Lledo JL, Ojea R, Fernandez-Rodriguez CM. Capnography is superior to pulse oximetry for the detection of respiratory depression during colonoscopy. Rev Esp Enferm Dig. 2010;102(2):86–9.
6. Gaisl T, Bratton DJ, Heuss LT, Kohler M, Schlatzer C, Zalunardo MP, Frey M, Franzen D. Sedation during bronchoscopy: data from a nationwide sedation and monitoring survey. BMC Pulm Med. 2016;16(1):113.
7. Netzer N, Eliasson AH, Netzer C, Kristo DA. Overnight pulse oximetry for sleep-disordered breathing in adults: a review. Chest. 2001;120(2):625–33.
8. Vargo JJ, Zuccaro Jr G, Dumot JA, Conwell DL, Morrow JB, Shay SS. Automated graphic assessment of respiratory activity is superior to pulse oximetry and visual assessment for the detection of early respiratory depression during therapeutic upper endoscopy. Gastrointest Endosc. 2002;55(7):826–31.
9. Fu ES, Downs JB, Schweiger JW, Miguel RV, Smith RA. Supplemental oxygen impairs detection of hypoventilation by pulse oximetry. Chest. 2004;126(5):1552–8.
10. Keidan I, Gravenstein D, Berkenstadt H, Ziv A, Shavit I, Sidi A. Supplemental oxygen compromises the use of pulse oximetry for detection of apnea and hypoventilation during sedation in simulated pediatric patients. Pediatrics. 2008;122(2):293–8.
11. Koniaris LG, Wilson S, Drugas G, Simmons W. Capnographic monitoring of ventilatory status during moderate (conscious) sedation. Surg Endosc. 2003;17(8):1261–5.
12. Beitz A, Riphaus A, Meining A, Kronshage T, Geist C, Wagenpfeil S, Weber A, Jung A, Bajbouj M, Pox C, Schneider G, Schmid RM, Wehrmann T, von Delius S. Capnographic monitoring reduces the incidence of arterial oxygen desaturation and hypoxemia during propofol sedation for colonoscopy: a randomized, controlled study (ColoCap Study). Am J Gastroenterol. 2012;107(8):1205–12.
13. Qadeer MA, Vargo JJ, Dumot JA, Lopez R, Trolli PA, Stevens T, Parsi MA, Sanaka MR, Zuccaro G. Capnographic monitoring of respiratory activity improves safety of sedation for endoscopic cholangiopancreatography and ultrasonography. Gastroenterology. 2009;136(5):1568–76.
14. Gaucher A, Frasca D, Mimoz O, Debaene B. Accuracy of respiratory rate monitoring by capnometry using the Capnomask(R) in extubated patients receiving supplemental oxygen after surgery. Br J Anaesth. 2012;108:316–20.
15. Mimoz O, Benard T, Gaucher A, Frasca D, Debaene B. Accuracy of respiratory rate monitoring using a non-invasive acoustic method after general anaesthesia. Br J Anaesth. 2012;108:872–5.
16. Ramsay MA, Usman M, Lagow E, Mendoza M, Untalan E, De Vol E. The accuracy, precision and reliability of measuring ventilatory rate and detecting ventilatory pause by rainbow acoustic monitoring and capnometry. Anesth Analg. 2013;117:69–75.
17. Wilkinson JN, Thanawala VU. Thoracic impedance monitoring of respiratory rate during sedation–is it safe? Anaesthesia. 2009;64:455–6.
18. Chhajed PN, Rajasekaran R, Kaegi B, Chhajed TP, Pflimlin E, Leuppi J, Tamm M. Measurement of combined oximetry and cutaneous capnography during flexible bronchoscopy. Eur Respir J. 2006;28:386–90.
19. Dreher M, Ekkernkamp E, Storre JH, Kabitz HJ, Windisch W. Sedation during flexible bronchoscopy in patients with pre-existing respiratory failure: Midazolam versus Midazolam plus Alfentanil. Respiration. 2010;79(4):307–14.

12

Airway wall thickness on HRCT scans decreases with age and increases with smoking

Eef D. Telenga[1,2], Matthijs Oudkerk[3], Peter M. A. van Ooijen[3,4], Rozemarijn Vliegenthart[3,4], Nick H. T. ten Hacken[1,2], Dirkje S. Postma[1,2] and Maarten van den Berge[1,2*]

Abstract

Background: To investigate if age, gender and smoking are associated with airway wall thickness (AWT) measured by high resolution computed tomography (HRCT) and if higher AWT is associated with lower levels of pulmonary function in healthy current- and never-smokers with a wide age range.

Methods: HRCT scans were performed in 99 subjects (48 never- and 51 current-smokers, median age 39 years [IQR 22 – 54], 57% males). The AWT at an internal perimeter of 10 mm (AWT Pi10) was calculated as an overall measurement of AWT, based on all measurements throughout the lungs. Extensive pulmonary function testing was performed in all subjects.

Results: Higher age was associated with a lower AWT Pi10 ($b = -0.003$, $p < 0.001$). Current-smokers had a higher AWT Pi10 than never-smokers (mean 0.49 mm versus 0.44 mm, $p = 0.022$). In multivariate analysis, age and current-smoking were independently associated with AWT Pi10 (age $b = -0.002$, $p < 0.001$, current-smoking $b = 0.041$, $p = 0.021$), whereas gender was not ($b = 0.011$, $p = 0.552$). Higher AWT Pi10 was associated with a lower FEV_1, FEV_1/FVC, FEF_{25-75} and higher R5, R20 and X5.

Conclusions: AWT decreases with higher age, possibly reflecting structural changes of the airways. Additionally, current-smokers have a higher AWT, possibly due to remodeling or inflammation. Finally, higher AWT is associated with a lower level of pulmonary function, even in this population of healthy subjects.

Keywords: Airway wall thickness, Computed tomography, Smoking, Age

Background

Chronic inflammatory processes in the airways, like those occurring in asthma and chronic obstructive pulmonary disease (COPD), induce airway remodeling. This is associated with changes in the epithelial layer, reticular basement membrane and smooth muscle, all contributing to thickening of the airway walls [1, 2].

Computed tomography (CT) can be used as a non-invasive tool to assess airway wall thickness (AWT). Using this technique, it has been shown that the airways walls of patients with COPD are significantly thicker than those of healthy non-smoking controls [3]. In addition, it has been shown that higher AWT is associated with more severe airflow obstruction in COPD [3–10]. Although these studies provided important insights, there were also some drawbacks. Most studies performed thus far used transverse CT slices and were therefore only able to measure airways oriented perpendicular to this plane [4–6, 8, 9, 11]. This is an important limitation as it markedly limits the number of airways that can be measured. Further, some studies measured AWT manually [5, 9, 11], which is less accurate than automated measurements and more susceptible to interobserver variation [12]. Advances in multi-detector CT scanners, development

* Correspondence: m.van.den.berge@umcg.nl
[1]Department of Pulmonary Diseases, University of Groningen, University Medical Center Groningen, PO Box 30.001, 9700 RB Groningen, The Netherlands
[2]GRIAC Research Institute, University of Groningen, University Medical Center Groningen, Groningen, The Netherlands
Full list of author information is available at the end of the article

of multiplanar, three-dimensional segmentation of airways and automated measurements of airway walls now make it possible to measure AWT in multiple airways throughout the bronchial tree.

Finally, most previous studies included selective populations of older subjects and often only current- or ex-smokers [13–15]. For this reason, the effects of age and smoking status on AWT are largely unknown. This may be important, since both age and smoking status are likely to affect AWT. Aging has been shown to play a role in remodeling and repair processes in lung parenchyma and similar processes are likely to occur in the airway walls as well [16, 17]. Additionally, smoking is the main risk factor for the development of COPD. It causes airway inflammation and remodeling, both influencing AWT [18–20].

In the present study, we investigated AWT in a group of well characterized healthy subjects. An automated software program was used, measuring a large number of airways perpendicular to the airway direction throughout the lungs. The objectives of this study were to investigate if age, gender and smoking are associated with AWT and whether a higher AWT is associated with lower levels of pulmonary function in healthy current- and never-smokers with a wide age range.

Methods

Study population

In this study, healthy never- and current-smokers were included if they met the following criteria: normal spirometry, no bronchial hyperresponsiveness to methacholine and normal pulmonary health according to the physician. Spirometry was considered to be normal if the forced expiratory volume in 1 s (FEV_1) was ≥80%predicted, the FEV_1/forced vital capacity (FVC) was greater than the lower limit of normal and reversibility to salbutamol was <10% of the predicted value. Never-smokers were defined as subjects who had not smoked during the last year, had never smoked for as long as 1 year, and had not smoked more than 0.5 packyears. The study was approved by the local medical ethics committee (METc 2007/007) and all subjects gave their written informed consent.

High Resolution CT scans and airway measurements

High resolution CT (HRCT) scans were performed using a 64-multidetector CT scanner (Somatom Definition, Siemens, Forchheim, Germany). Scans were performed at full inspiration. Scanning was performed with 20 mAs. The kV setting was determined by weight: 100 kV for subjects <60 kg, 120 kV for subjects ≥60 and <80 kg and 140 kV for subjects >80 kg. Acquired imaging data were reconstructed using a standard soft kernel (B30f), with 1.0 mm slice thickness and 0.7 mm increment. The CT radiation dose was approximately 0.8 mSv (100 kV) to 1.5 mSv (140 kV), the (median CT radiation dose was 0.95 mSv.

Airway measurements were performed with the automated software program MeVis Airway Examiner 1.0 (Fraunhofer Institute for Medical Image Computing MEVIS, Bremen, Germany). The software automatically extracts airway centerlines, re-samples images perpendicular to the airway direction and detects inner and outer airway wall borders in these images (Fig. 1) [21]. The outer wall border is detectable when no adjacent tissue with similar CT density is present. All HRCT scans were visually evaluated for appropriate segmentation and data from lobes that were incorrectly segmented were removed from further analyses. The software calculated AWT, airway wall area percentage (%AWA), i.e. airway wall area/total airway area *100, and the fraction of the airway that was detectable (assessed perimeter fraction, APF) for each location and reported the average AWT and %AWA per lung lobe for airways with predefined external diameters (3.5 mm, 4 mm, 4.5 mm, 5 mm, 6 mm, 8 mm and 10 mm, all ±0.25 mm) from all the separately measured airway locations. The software also reported the cumulative APF per lung lobe for each external diameter measured, i.e. the total number of airway perimeters measured, calculated by adding up the APF of all measured airways with the appropriate external diameter. A higher cumulative APF reflects a higher number of sampling points assessed. The mean AWT and %AWA per lung for each external diameter were calculated as the weighted average of the AWT and %AWA per lobe, with the cumulative APF per lobe as the weighting factor. As an overall measurement of AWT, the AWT at an internal perimeter of 10 mm (AWT Pi10) was estimated based on all measurements at the 7 different diameters, similar to the method of Grydeland et al. [13]. The AWT Pi10 was calculated by plotting the square root of the average area of airway wall per lobe against the internal perimeter of these measurements. The resulting regression line was used to calculate the AWT Pi10. Our method differed slightly from the Grydeland et al. in that they used all measured airways, instead of airways with predefined diameters [13].

Pulmonary function tests

Spirometry was performed before and after 400 µg salbutamol according to current ATS/ERS guidelines [22, 23]. Impulse oscillometry (IOS) was performed to measure resistance at 5 Hz (R5), resistance at 20 Hz (R20), the difference between R5 and R20 (R5-20) and reactance at 5 Hz (X5). Body plethysmography was performed to measure functional residual capacity (FRC), total lung capacity (TLC) and residual volume (RV). The diffusion capacity of the lung for carbon monoxide corrected for hemoglobin level (TLCOc) and TLCOc corrected for the alveolar volume (TLCOc/VA) were measured. Provocation tests

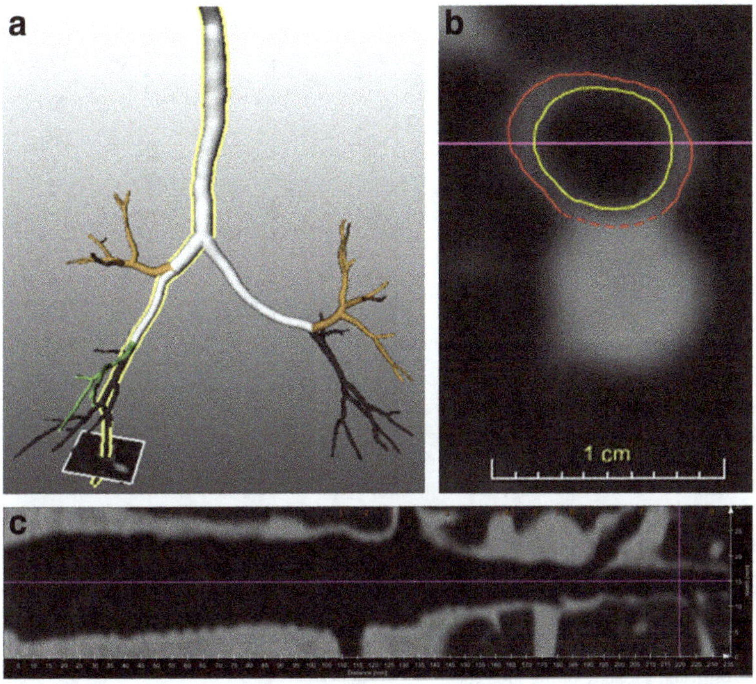

Fig. 1 Airway wall thickness analysis. **a** The airway wall tree as extracted by the software program. The airway highlighted in yellow is stretched to a 2D picture in (**b**). The grey square corresponds to the purple vertical line in (**b**). This is a cross sectional image of the airway oriented perpendicular to the local centerline direction and given in more detail in (**c**). The red line is the outer airway wall perimeter and the yellow line is the inner airway wall perimeter. Airway wall thickness (AWT) and wall area percentage (%AWA) are measured in areas of the continuous red line. Dashed parts of the outer perimeter are interpolated and not used for measurements. The assessed perimeter fraction (APF) is the fraction of the outer perimeter that has a continuous line

were performed with methacholine (0.03 to 16 mg/ml), using a 2-min tidal breathing method, adapted from Cockcroft et al. [24].

Statistical analysis

Differences in AWT Pi10, AWT and %AWA were tested with Student's *t*-test or analysis of variance (ANOVA), with post-hoc Holm's Bonferroni correction for multiple testing. To assess the effect of age on airway wall thickness, linear regressions were performed with either AWT Pi10, AWT or %AWA as the outcome variable and age, gender and smoking status as predictor variables. To assess the effect of airway wall thickness on pulmonary function parameters, multivariate regression analyses with the pulmonary function parameter as outcome variable and AWT Pi10 as predictor variable with adjustment for age, gender and smoking status were performed. If height is part of the formula to calculate the predicted value of a pulmonary function parameter, height was also adjusted for. Similar analyses were performed with the AWT and %AWA transformed to the number of standard deviations (SD) from the mean at the different diameters. All statistical analyses were performed with IBM SPSS version 20 (IBM, Armonk, NY, USA). *P*-values <0.05 were considered statistically significant.

Results

A total of 99 subjects were included. Their baseline characteristics are presented in Table 1. In 25 patients the software was not able to detect the airways correctly in the entire lung and the data from lobes that were incorrectly segmented were removed from further analyses. Data from one lobe was removed from the analysis for 21 patients and data from two lobes was removed in 4 patients. The median cumulative assessed perimeter fractions (APF) per patient and per lung lobe are presented in Additional file 1: Table S1. The median cumulative APF per patient was 146 airways, reflecting that the AWT was measured on a total 146 airway perimeters. The cumulative APF was highest for airways with 5 mm external diameter. At this diameter the software measured a median of 55 airway perimeters. The software was able to measure wall thickness of all subjects between 4.5 and 6 mm. At smaller diameters there were less successful measurements (96 of 99 subjects at 4 mm and 58 of 99 subjects at 3.5 mm). Furthermore the number of airways measured became very limited at 3.5 mm with a cumulative APF of only 0.77 airways. Below 3.5 mm no airways were detected by the software. At higher diameters the APF also decreased to 1.31 airways at 10 mm. The lowest cumulative APF was observed in the right middle lobe, reflecting the smaller size of this lobe.

Table 1 Baseline characteristics of the 99 subjects

Age (years)	39	(22 – 54)
Males (n, %)	56	(57)
Current-smokers (n, %)	51	(52)
Cigarettes/day (n)[a]	15	(3 – 29)
Packyears (n)[a]	15	(10 – 20)
FEV_1 (%predicted)	105	(98 – 113)
FVC (%predicted)	113	(105 – 118)
FEV_1/FVC (%)	79	(76 – 84)
FEF_{25-75} (%predicted)	83	(71 – 99)
RV/TLC (%predicted)	86	(77 – 96)
TLCOc/VA (%predicted)	96	(88 – 104)
R5 (kPa/L/s)	0.30	(0.25 – 0.36)
R20 (kPa/L/s)	0.28	(0.22 – 0.33)
R5-20 (kPa/L/s)	0.02	(0.00 – 0.05)
X5 (kPa/L/s)	−0.07	(−0.10 – −0.06)

Values are presented as medians with interquartile ranges unless stated otherwise
FEV_1 forced expiratory volume in 1 s, *FVC* forced vital capacity, *FEF_{25-75}* forced expiratory flow between 25 and 75% of FVC, *RV/TLC* residual volume/total lung capacity, *TLCOc* diffusion capacity of the lung for carbon monoxide, corrected for hemoglobin level, *VA* alveolar volume, *R5* resistance at 5 Hz, *R20* resistance at 20Hz, *R5-20* difference between R5 and R20, *X5* reactance at 5 Hz, *AX* reactance area
[a]only in current-smokers

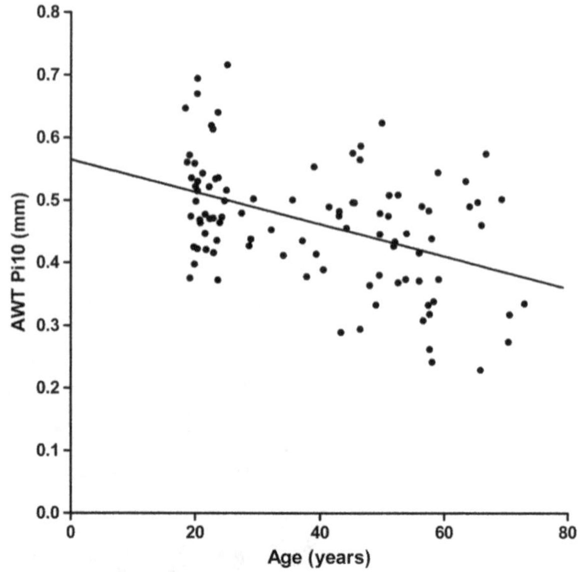

Fig. 2 Association between AWT Pi10 and age. b = −0.003, $p < 0.001$; AWT Pi10 = airway wall thickness at an internal perimeter of 10 mm estimated from all measurements

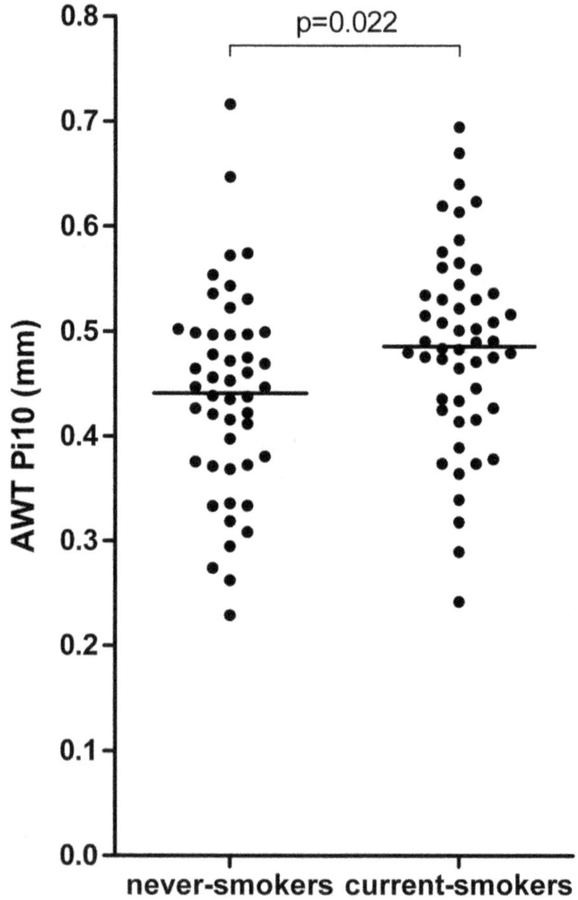

Fig. 3 AWT Pi10 in never- and current-smokers. AWT Pi10 = airway wall thickness at an internal perimeter of 10 mm estimated from all measurements

AWT and %AWA at different diameters and in different lobes

AWT increased linearly with increasing diameter from 0.30 mm to 3.5 mm external diameter to 1.42 mm at 10 mm (Additional file 2: Figure S1a). The %AWA was 29.8% at 3.5 mm external diameter and increased to 45.1% at 6 mm after this the %AWA reached a plateau around 48% (Additional file 2: Figure S1b). The AWT and %AWA were comparable in all lobes for external diameters between 4 and 10 mm (Additional file 2: Figure S1c and d and Additional file 1: Tables S2 and S3). At 3.5 mm the AWT and %AWA were significantly higher in the left lower lobe than in the right upper lobe.

Effect of age, gender and smoking status on AWT Pi10, AWT and %AWA

Higher age was associated with lower AWT, assessed by the overall measure of airway wall thickness, the AWT Pi10 (b = −0.003, $p < 0.001$, Fig. 2). A trend was found towards a lower AWT Pi10 in men compared to women (mean (SD) 0.45 (0.10) mm versus 0.48 (0.09) mm respectively, $p = 0.088$). AWT Pi10 was significantly higher in current- than in never-smokers (mean (SD) 0.49 (0.09) mm and 0.44 (0.10) mm respectively, $p = 0.022$, Fig. 3). AWT and %AWT were also higher in current- than never-smokers at 4 mm, 4.5 mm, 5 mm,

6 mm and 8 mm diameter, but not at 3.5 mm and 10 mm (Additional file 1: Tables S4 and S5). In multivariate linear regression analysis, both age and smoking status were significantly and independently associated with the AWT Pi10. AWT Pi10 was lower at higher age (b = −0.002, $p < 0.001$) and higher in current-smokers (b = 0.041, $p = 0.021$). Gender was not independently associated with AWT Pi10 (b = 0.011, $p = 0.552$). No significant interaction between age and smoking status was found ($p = 0.45$). In similar analyses, age was negatively associated with AWT and %AWA for all predefined diameters, except for 10 mm and current-smoking was associated with a higher AWT and %AWA at 4.5 mm, 5 mm and 6 mm diameter (Additional file 1: Tables S6 and S7).

Association between airway wall thickness and pulmonary function

A higher AWT Pi10 was associated with lower FEV_1, FEF_{25-75}, FVC, FEV_1/FVC and X5 and higher R5 and R20, independently from age, gender, height and smoking status (Table 2). AWT Pi10 was not associated with RV/TLC or R5-20. Additionally, a higher AWT Pi10 was associated with higher TLCOc/VA. Similar associations were seen for AWT and %AWA at the different airway diameters (Additional file 1: Tables S8 and S9). The regression coefficients, representing the change in a pulmonary function test for every standard deviation change in AWT or %AWA, were very similar for the different diameters.

Table 2 Association between AWT Pi10 and pulmonary function parameters

	AWT Pi10	
	b	*p*-value
FEV_1 (L)	−1.697	0.001
FEF_{25-75} (L/s)	−3.215	0.001
FVC (L)	−1.288	0.047
FEV_1/FVC (%)	−13.358	0.018
RV/TLC (%)	3.202	0.468
TLCOc/VA (mmol/min/kPa/L)	0.431	0.029
R5 (kPa/L/s)	0.363	<0.001
R20 (kPa/L/s)	0.288	<0.001
R5-20 (kPa/L/s)	0.075	0.164
X5 (kPa/L/s)	−0.080	0.028

Linear regressions with pulmonary function parameters as outcome and airway wall thickness as predictor variable and age, gender, smoking status and height added as covariates

AWT Pi10 airway wall thickness at an internal perimeter of 10 mm estimated from all measurements, *FEV_1* forced expiratory volume in 1 s, *FVC* forced vital capacity, *FEF_{25-75}* forced expiratory flow between 25 and 75% of FVC, *RV/TLC* residual volume/total lung capacity, *TLCOc* diffusion capacity of the lung for carbon monoxide, corrected for hemoglobin level, *VA* alveolar volume, *R5* resistance at 5 Hz, *R20* resistance at 20Hz, *R5-20* difference between R5 and R20, *X5* reactance at 5 Hz

Discussion

The present study demonstrates that airway wall thickness (AWT) decreases with aging and is higher in current- than never-smokers. In addition, we show that thicker airway walls are associated with lower levels of pulmonary function.

The effect of age on AWT has been previously described by Grydeland et al. in COPD patients and healthy smokers >40 years [13]. In this study, the estimated AWT at an internal perimeter of 10 mm (AWT Pi10) decreased with 0.003 mm per year in the healthy smokers, which is very similar to the results of this study (0.002 mm per year in the multivariate analysis). These findings are partly in agreement with a study by Zach et al. [14]. In this study, age did not contribute to AWT Pi10 in 92 healthy subjects >45 years. However, a higher age was associated with a lower %AWA. We extend the data of Zach et al. by also including younger subjects and never-smokers. This way, we were able to show that airway walls become thinner from early adulthood on throughout life and that this process is independent from smoking. On the other hand, in a study by Matsuoka et al. no differences were found in the ratio of airway wall thickness and the total diameter of the bronchus in healthy subjects aged 21–40, 41–65 and >65 years old [11]. However in this study, only transverse CT slices were used, thereby limiting the number of airways measured. Furthermore, the airways were measured manually, which is less accurate than automated measurements and more susceptible to interobserver variation [12].

Aging has profound influences on the lung. The elastic recoil of the lung decreases significantly with aging, mainly due to alveolar enlargement without alveolar wall destruction, a condition that is also called 'senile lung' [16]. It has been suggested that remodeling of the extracellular matrix (ECM) in the lung parenchyma, with degradation of elastin and collagens, is the main factor in this aging process [16, 17]. However, there is limited knowledge of the effects of aging on changes in the airway walls. Animal studies suggest that aging of Clara cells, the progenitor cells of the airway epithelium, may impair airway regeneration, which could lead to thinning of the airway walls [25]. It is also possible that, similar to the parenchyma, ECM proteins are degraded in the airway walls with aging. ECM proteins also degrade with age in many other structures in the human body, for instance the skin [26]. Interestingly, in the aging skin, an altered function of fibroblasts has been observed, resulting in a decreased production of collagen and increased production of collagen-degrading matrix metalloproteinases. It is tempting to speculate that comparable changes may occur in aging airway fibroblasts. Alternatively, inflammatory cells and other residential cells, like epithelial and smooth muscle cells, may have similar effects.

This study demonstrates that current-smokers have a higher AWT than never-smokers, independently from age. Donohue et al. did not find higher thickness of airway walls in current-smokers than in never- or ex-smokers in a large cohort of ex-, current- and never-smokers [15]. However, they did show that airway walls were thicker with more cigarette exposure, i.e. more packyears smoked and that current-smoking was associated with a narrower airway lumen. In the study by Matsuoka et al. the in the ratio of airway wall thickness and the total diameter of the bronchus was higher in smokers aged >65 than never-smokers aged >65. No differences were seen between smokers and never-smokers <65 years [11]. Thicker airway walls in current-smokers may be due to the effects of continuous smoke exposure on the epithelium, causing the epithelium to produce pro-inflammatory cytokines that induce remodeling [18–20]. In line with this, a study in 25 smokers and 14 non-smokers showed more goblet cell metaplasia, more smooth muscle hypertrophy and more inflammation in the walls of airways in current-smokers [27]. Thus, smoking may affect AWT in several different ways. It is not possible to distinguish between the different causes of airway wall thickening on HRCT scans.

An increase in AWT may be of clinical relevance, since it is associated with lower levels of pulmonary function, independent of age, gender, height and smoking status. Correlations between pulmonary function and wall thickness have previously been demonstrated in studies with COPD patients and older healthy controls [3, 5–9]. In this study, associations between AWT and pulmonary function are demonstrated in a population of subjects who were specifically selected to be asymptomatic and have normal spirometry. Interestingly, AWT was associated not only with large airway parameters like the FEV_1, FVC and FEV_1/FVC, but also with small airway parameters like the FEF_{25-75} and X5. This is remarkable since the small airways have an internal diameter <2 mm and are therefore too small to be measured on HRCT scans at the moment. Additionally, an increase of 1 SD in AWT in airways with smaller diameters (e.g. 4 or 4.5 mm) or larger diameters (e.g. 6 or 8 mm) had similar effects on pulmonary function tests measuring large and small airways (Additional file 1: Tables S8 and S9). These results suggest that thickening of airway walls in current-smokers occurs not only in the airways that were measured, but throughout the lungs. Advances in ultra-high resolution imaging, like cone beam CT imaging, may provide more information about the AWT in the small airways in the future [28, 29]. Unexpectedly, thicker airway walls were associated with a higher TLCOc/VA. As it is unlikely that subjects with thicker airway walls truly have a higher diffusion capacity, we hypothesize that the increased diffusion capacity in subjects with thicker airway walls most likely results from underestimation of the alveolar volume due to ventilation inhomogeneity [30].

There are several strengths to our study. First, we used a software program automatically detecting the bronchial tree and measuring AWT perpendicular to the airway direction. Using this method, we were able to measure a median of 146 airway perimeters (combined from partial airway perimeters) per patient. These measurements were performed at different airway diameters, ranging from 3.5 to 10 mm external diameter, in all lung lobes. Second, all HRCT scans were performed in the same center, using the same acquisition device settings. Finally, all subjects were extensively characterized with pulmonary function tests, smoking and medical history. There are also limitations to this study. As AWT was measured at pre-defined external airway parameters, it is not possible to determine if increases in AWT are due to actual thickening of the wall or due to reduction in the luminal diameter. This is a general problem with measuring AWT. A possible solution could be to assess airways per generation. However, currently, it is still difficult to do this and labeling of airway generation is prone to error.

Conclusions

In conclusion, airway wall thickness measured with HRCT scans is a feasible technique to investigate anatomical changes of the airways. We showed that airway wall thickness decreases with age, possibly reflecting structural changes of the airways during aging. Additionally, current-smokers have thicker airway walls than never-smokers, and this increased airway wall thickness is associated with lower levels of pulmonary function.

Additional files

Additional file 1: Table S1. Cumulative APF at the different airway diameters per lung lobe. **Table S2.** Airway wall thickness per lobe. **Table S3.** Airway wall area per lobe. **Table S4.** Airway wall thickness according to smoking status. **Table S5.** Airway wall area according to smoking status. **Table S6:** Associations between airway wall thickness and age, gender and smoking status. **Table S7.** Associations between airway wall area and age, gender and smoking status. **Table S8.** Association between pulmonary function parameters and airway wall thickness, independent of age, gender, smoking status and height. **Table S9.** Association between pulmonary function parameters and airway wall area, independent of age, gender, smoking status and height. (DOCX 51 kb)

Additional file 2: Figure S1. AWT and %AWA at different external airway diameters. AWT = airway wall thickness; %AWA = airway wall area percentage.

Abbreviations

%AWA: Airway wall area percentage; APF: Assessed perimeter fraction; AWT: Airway wall thickness; AWT: Pi10 airway wall thickness at an internal perimeter of 10 mm; COPD: Chronic obstructive pulmonary disease; CT: Computed tomography; ECM: Extracellular matrix; FEF_{25-75}: Forced expiratory flow between 25 and 75% of FVC; FEV_1: Forced expiratory volume in 1 s; FRC: Functional residual capacity; FVC: Forced vital capacity; HRCT: High resolution computed tomography; IOS: Impulse oscillometry; R20: Resistance at 20 Hz; R5: Resistance at 5 Hz; R5-20: Difference between R5 and R20; RV: Residual volume; TLC: Total lung capacity; TLCOc: Diffusion capacity of the lung for carbon monoxide corrected for hemoglobin level; TLCOc/VA: TLCOc corrected for the alveolar volume; X5: Reactance at 5 Hz

Acknowledgements
Not applicable.

Funding
This study was funded by the Royal Netherlands Academy of Arts and Sciences and the Stichting Astmabestrijding (Dutch Foundation Against Asthma).

Authors' contributions
EDT conceived & designed the study, performed clinical study, analysed results, drafted the manuscript and approved the final version of the manuscript. MO helped design the study, critically revised the manuscript and approved the final version of the manuscript. PMAO helped design the study, critically revised the manuscript and approved the final version of the manuscript. RV helped in acquisition of data, critically revised the manuscript and approved the final version of the manuscript. NHTH conceived the study, critically revised the manuscript and approved the final version of the manuscript. DSP conceived & designed the study, supervised the clinical study, critically revised the manuscript and approved the final version of the manuscript. MvdB conceived & designed the study, supervised the clinical study, helped analyse the data, helped drafting the manuscript and approved the final version of the manuscript.

Competing interests
EDT, MO, PMAO, RV, and NHTtH, have no conflicts of interest to declare. The University of Groningen has received money for Professor Postma regarding an unrestricted educational grant for research from Chiesi. Travel to ERS and/or ATS has been partially funded by Astra Zeneca, Chiesi, GSK, Takeda. Fees for consultancies were given to the University of Groningen by Astra Zeneca, Boehringer Ingelheim, Chiesi, GSK, Takeda and TEVA. Travel and lectures in China paid by Chiesi.
The University of Groningen has received money for Dr. van den Berge regarding research grants from Chiesi, Astra Zeneca and TEVA pharma, outside the submitted work.

Author details
[1]Department of Pulmonary Diseases, University of Groningen, University Medical Center Groningen, PO Box 30.001, 9700 RB Groningen, The Netherlands. [2]GRIAC Research Institute, University of Groningen, University Medical Center Groningen, Groningen, The Netherlands. [3]Center for Medical Imaging North East Netherlands, University of Groningen, University Medical Center Groningen, Groningen, The Netherlands. [4]Department of Radiology, University of Groningen, University Medical Center Groningen, PO Box 30.0019700 RB Groningen, The Netherlands.

References
1. Nagai A, West WW, Thurlbeck WM. The National Institutes of Health Intermittent Positive-Pressure Breathing trial: pathology studies. II. Correlation between morphologic findings, clinical findings, and evidence of expiratory air-flow obstruction. Am Rev Respir Dis. 1985;132(5):946–53.
2. Bosken CH, Wiggs BR, Pare PD, Hogg JC. Small airway dimensions in smokers with obstruction to airflow. Am Rev Respir Dis. 1990;142(3):563–70.
3. Kurashima K, Hoshi T, Takayanagi N, Takaku Y, Kagiyama N, Ohta C, Fujimura M, Sugita Y. Airway dimensions and pulmonary function in chronic obstructive pulmonary disease and bronchial asthma. Respirology. 2012;17(1):79–86.
4. Berger P, Perot V, Desbarats P, Tunon-de-Lara JM, Marthan R, Laurent F. Airway wall thickness in cigarette smokers: quantitative thin-section CT assessment. Radiology. 2005;235(3):1055–64.
5. Arakawa H, Fujimoto K, Fukushima Y, Kaji Y. Thin-section CT imaging that correlates with pulmonary function tests in obstructive airway disease. Eur J Radiol. 2011;80(2):e157–63.
6. Nakano Y, Muro S, Sakai H, Hirai T, Chin K, Tsukino M, Nishimura K, Itoh H, Pare PD, Hogg JC, Mishima M. Computed tomographic measurements of airway dimensions and emphysema in smokers. Correlation with lung function. Am J Respir Crit Care Med. 2000;162(3 Pt 1):1102–8.
7. Hasegawa M, Nasuhara Y, Onodera Y, Makita H, Nagai K, Fuke S, Ito Y, Betsuyaku T, Nishimura M. Airflow limitation and airway dimensions in chronic obstructive pulmonary disease. Am J Respir Crit Care Med. 2006;173(12):1309–15.
8. Patel BD, Coxson HO, Pillai SG, Agusti AG, Calverley PM, Donner CF, Make BJ, Muller NL, Rennard SI, Vestbo J, Wouters EF, Hiorns MP, Nakano Y, Camp PG, Nasute Fauerbach PV, Screaton NJ, Campbell EJ, Anderson WH, Pare PD, Levy RD, Lake SL, Silverman EK, Lomas DA, International COPD Genetics Network. Airway wall thickening and emphysema show independent familial aggregation in chronic obstructive pulmonary disease. Am J Respir Crit Care Med. 2008;178(5):500–5.
9. Orlandi I, Moroni C, Camiciottoli G, Bartolucci M, Pistolesi M, Villari N, Mascalchi M. Chronic obstructive pulmonary disease: thin-section CT measurement of airway wall thickness and lung attenuation. Radiology. 2005;234(2):604–10.
10. Xie X, de Jong PA, Oudkerk M, Wang Y, Ten Hacken NH, Miao J, Zhang G, de Bock GH, Vliegenthart R. Morphological measurements in computed tomography correlate with airflow obstruction in chronic obstructive pulmonary disease: systematic review and meta-analysis. Eur Radiol. 2012;22(10):2085–93.
11. Matsuoka S, Uchiyama K, Shima H, Ueno N, Oish S, Nojiri Y. Bronchoarterial ratio and bronchial wall thickness on high-resolution CT in asymptomatic subjects: correlation with age and smoking. AJR Am J Roentgenol. 2003;180(2):513–8.
12. Reinhardt JM, D'Souza ND, Hoffman EA. Accurate measurement of intrathoracic airways. IEEE Trans Med Imaging. 1997;16(6):820–7.
13. Grydeland TB, Dirksen A, Coxson HO, Pillai SG, Sharma S, Eide GE, Gulsvik A, Bakke PS. Quantitative computed tomography: emphysema and airway wall thickness by sex, age and smoking. Eur Respir J. 2009;34(4):858–65.
14. Zach JA, Newell Jr JD, Schroeder J, Murphy JR, Curran-Everett D, Hoffman EA, Westgate PM, Han MK, Silverman EK, Crapo JD, Lynch DA, on behalf of the COPDGene Investigators. Quantitative Computed Tomography of the Lungs and Airways in Healthy Nonsmoking Adults. Invest Radiol. 2012;47(10):596–602.
15. Donohue KM, Hoffman EA, Baumhauer H, Guo J, Budoff M, Austin JH, Kalhan R, Kawut S, Tracy R, Graham Barr R. Cigarette smoking and airway wall thickness on CT scan in a multi-ethnic cohort: The MESA Lung Study. Respir Med. 2012;106(12):1655–64.
16. Fukuchi Y. The aging lung and chronic obstructive pulmonary disease: similarity and difference. Proc Am Thorac Soc. 2009;6(7):570–2.
17. Knudson RJ, Clark DF, Kennedy TC, Knudson DE. Effect of aging alone on mechanical properties of the normal adult human lung. J Appl Physiol. 1977;43(6):1054–62.
18. Takizawa H, Tanaka M, Takami K, Ohtoshi T, Ito K, Satoh M, Okada Y, Yamasawa F, Nakahara K, Umeda A. Increased expression of transforming growth factor-beta1 in small airway epithelium from tobacco smokers and patients with chronic obstructive pulmonary disease (COPD). Am J Respir Crit Care Med. 2001;163(6):1476–83.
19. Vignola AM, Chanez P, Chiappara G, Merendino A, Pace E, Rizzo A, la Rocca AM, Bellia V, Bonsignore G, Bousquet J. Transforming growth factor-beta expression in mucosal biopsies in asthma and chronic bronchitis. Am J Respir Crit Care Med. 1997;156(2 Pt 1):591–9.
20. Morris DG, Huang X, Kaminski N, Wang Y, Shapiro SD, Dolganov G, Glick A, Sheppard D. Loss of integrin alpha(v)beta6-mediated TGF-beta activation causes Mmp12-dependent emphysema. Nature. 2003;422(6928):169–73.
21. Weinheimer O, Achenbach T, Bletz C, Duber C, Kauczor HU, Heussel CP. About objective 3-d analysis of airway geometry in computerized tomography. IEEE Trans Med Imaging. 2008;27(1):64–74.
22. Miller MR, Hankinson J, Brusasco V, Burgos F, Casaburi R, Coates A, Crapo R, Enright P, van der Grinten CP, Gustafsson P, Jensen R, Johnson DC, MacIntyre N, McKay R, Navajas D, Pedersen OF, Pellegrino R, Viegi G, Wanger J, ATS/ERS Task Force. Standardisation of spirometry. Eur Respir J. 2005;26(2):319–38.

23. Quanjer PH, Tammeling GJ, Cotes JE, Pedersen OF, Peslin R, Yernault JC. Lung volumes and forced ventilatory flows. Work Group on Standardization of Respiratory Function Tests. European Community for Coal and Steel. Official position of the European Respiratory Society. Rev Mal Respir. 1994;11 Suppl 3:5–40.
24. Cockcroft DW, Killian DN, Mellon JJ, Hargreave FE. Bronchial reactivity to inhaled histamine: a method and clinical survey. Clin Allergy. 1977;7(3):235–43.
25. Aoshiba K, Nagai A. Senescence hypothesis for the pathogenetic mechanism of chronic obstructive pulmonary disease. Proc Am Thorac Soc. 2009;6(7):596–601.
26. Naylor EC, Watson RE, Sherratt MJ. Molecular aspects of skin ageing. Maturitas. 2011;69(3):249–56.
27. Cosio MG, Hale KA, Niewoehner DE. Morphologic and morphometric effects of prolonged cigarette smoking on the small airways. Am Rev Respir Dis. 1980;122(2):221–65.
28. King GG. Tomographic imaging of small airways. Respiration. 2012;84(4):265–74.
29. Miracle AC, Mukherji SK. Conebeam CT of the head and neck, part 1: physical principles. Am J Neuroradiol. 2009;30(6):1088–95.
30. Cotton DJ, Mink JT, Graham BL. Nonuniformity of diffusing capacity from small alveolar gas samples is increased in smokers. Can Respir J. 1998;5(2):101–8.

13

Combined cumulative sum (CUSUM) and chronological environmental analysis as a tool to improve the learning environment for linear-probe endobronchial ultrasound-guided transbronchial needle aspiration (EBUS-TBNA) trainees

Yasuhiro Norisue[1*], Yasuharu Tokuda[2], Mayrol Juarez[3], Ryo Uchimido[4], Shigeki Fujitani[5] and David A. Stoeckel[6]

Abstract

Background: Cumulative sum (CUSUM) analysis can be used to continuously monitor the performance of an individual or process and detect deviations from a preset or standard level of achievement. However, no previous study has evaluated the utility of CUSUM analysis in facilitating timely environmental assessment and interventions to improve performance of linear-probe endobronchial ultrasound-guided transbronchial needle aspiration (EBUS-TBNA). The aim of this study was to evaluate the usefulness of combined CUSUM and chronological environmental analysis as a tool to improve the learning environment for EBUS-TBNA trainees.

Methods: This study was an observational chart review. To determine if performance was acceptable, CUSUM analysis was used to track procedural outcomes of trainees in EBUS-TBNA. To investigate chronological changes in the learning environment, multivariate logistic regression analysis was used to compare several indices before and after time points when significant changes occurred in proficiency.

Results: Presence of an additional attending bronchoscopist was inversely associated with nonproficiency (odds ratio, 0.117, 95% confidence interval, 0–0.749; $P = 0.019$). Other factors, including presence of an on-site cytopathologist and dose of sedatives used, were not significantly associated with duration of nonproficiency.

Conclusions: Combined CUSUM and chronological environmental analysis may be useful in hastening interventions that improve performance of EBUS-TBNA.

Keywords: CUSUM analysis, Quality improvement, Endobronchial ultrasound-guided transbronchial needle aspiration, EBUS-TBNA, CUSUM analysis, Quality improvement

* Correspondence: norisue.yasuhiro@gmail.com
[1]Department of Pulmonary and Critical Care Medicine, Tokyo Bay Urayasu-Ichikawa Medical Center, 3-4-32 Toudaijima, Urayasushi, Chiba 279-0001, Japan
Full list of author information is available at the end of the article

Background

Cumulative sum (CUSUM) analysis is a method of monitoring the performance of an individual or process and detect deviations from a preset or standard level of achievement [1, 2]. It has been used in medical disciplines, particularly in monitoring and characterizing trainee learning curves. In theory, CUSUM analysis is an ideal tool to improve the quality of medical procedures, as it can alert observers to performance declines or improvements among workers, thus facilitating timely assessment of the learning environment. However, no previous study has examined the utility of combining CUSUM analysis with assessment of the learning environment for medical procedures.

Linear-probe endobronchial ultrasound-guided transbronchial needle aspiration (EBUS-TBNA) is a bronchoscopic technique that uses ultrasound to visualize and guide sampling of mediastinal and hilar lymph nodes [3, 4]. Kemp et al. used CUSUM analysis to plot learning curves for EBUS-TBNA and found that the curves varied widely among bronchoscopists [5]. Differences in learning speed among bronchoscopists at the same institution are mostly attributable to variation in their individual characteristics. However, if a bronchoscopist has an unexpected important change in proficiency in CUSUM analysis, investigating the learning environment and current performance characteristics of the bronchoscopist could help in implementing appropriate early interventions.

This study investigated whether CUSUM analysis could be used to monitor individual and institutional proficiency in linear EBUS-TBNA and improve the quality of the learning environment for EBUS-TBNA. CUSUM analysis was used to monitor EBUS-TBNA performance of bronchoscopists during training and investigate the relationship between change in performance and changes in the characteristics of the learning environment in the bronchoscopy suite.

Methods

Study design and setting

Linear-probe EBUS-TBNA bronchoscopy has been performed since March 2008 at our institution, the Saint Louis University Hospital. All attending bronchoscopists had more than 5 years of experience in bronchoscopy without EBUS and had received less than 1 week of EBUS-TBNA training before EBUS-TBNA was initiated at our center. We analyzed data from 131 patients evaluated from March 2008 to September 2010 by 3 bronchoscopists (bronchoscopist A: 47 patients with 84 lymph nodes sampled; bronchoscopist B: 50 patients with 89 lymph nodes sample; and bronchoscopist C: 34 patients with 49 lymph nodes sampled). All procedures utilized 22G needles.

Charts and procedure notes were examined to collect information on patient demographics, EBUS-TBNA indications, the procedures (date, operator(s), sampled lymph nodes, complications), final cytology results of transbronchial needle aspiration for each node, pathology results for mediastinoscopy, CT-guided lymph node biopsy, video-assisted thoracic surgery and thoracotomy, findings of subsequent imaging studies, and final clinical diagnosis.

Information on bronchoscopy suite conditions that was available retrospectively included the name of the main attending bronchoscopist (resident and fellow physicians were not included in the analysis), the names of attending bronchoscopists who assisted the main bronchoscopist, the doses of sedatives and opiates used during each procedure, and the presence of cytopathologists for rapid on-site evaluation of specimens. Two bronchoscopy nurses were present for all procedures. This observational chart review was approved by the Institutional Review Board at Saint Louis University.

Kemp et al. defined success on EBUS-TBNA as a true positive or true negative for malignancy, and failure as a false positive or false negative for malignancy. However, a procedure that successfully samples a lymph node but yields a false negative should not be defined as operator failure, as it represents a limitation of the EBUS-TBNA technique itself rather than a lack of operator skill. We believe that procedure failure should instead be defined as absence of lymphocytes, malignant cells, or granuloma in a specimen. In other words, a procedure is successful when the lymph node is adequately visualized and sampled, as determined by the presence of diagnostic cells or lymphocytes in the sample.

Statistical analysis

The primary outcome was sampling failure or success. Each sampled lymph node was used as the unit for determining success or failure. A lymph node sampling was defined as successful if 1 or more cytology slides showed lymphocytes, granulomas, or malignant cells.

CUSUM analysis has been used to continuously monitor procedural outcomes of trainees, to determine if performance is acceptable [2]. In this study, we used the presentation format and parameters for CUSUM scoring used by Kemp et al. [5, 6] Briefly, the CUSUM value was plotted on the y axis against the attempt on the x axis [2, 5, 6]. The CUSUM value is the running sum of a mixture of increments (for each failure) and decrements (for each success). An acceptable success rate is indicated by a declining trend in CUSUM score, whereas a lower-than-expected success rate is indicated by an increasing trend in CUSUM score. For EBUS-TBNA, the designated acceptable failure rate (p0) was 10% and the unacceptable failure rate (p1) was 20%. *s* is the CUSUM score given for each success and is calculated using the equation:

$$P = \ln(p1/p0)\ Q = \ln((1-p0)/(1-p1))\ s = Q/(P+Q)$$

Thus:

$$p0 = 0.1\ p1 = 0.2\ s = 0.14\ 1{-}s = 0.86$$

On CUSUM analysis, a trainee was considered "proficient" when the line on the graph descended and crossed 2 boundary lines on a downward slope. A trainee was considered "nonproficient" if the line ascended and crossed 2 boundary lines on an upward slope, which could prompt an intervention such as retraining of the operator. The assessment was considered "inconclusive" if the line remained between the 2 boundary lines. In such cases, additional attempts are necessary in order to determine competence [6, 7]. H0 denotes the value between each acceptable decision interval, and H1 indicates the value between each unacceptable decision level. To determine H, one needs to set the type 1 error (odds of falsely deeming an operator nonproficient, designated as α below) and type 2 error (odds of falsely deeming an operator proficient, designated as β below). We set both to 0.1 in the present analysis. H0 and H1 were calculated as follows:

$$a = \ln((1-\beta)/\alpha)b = \ln((1-\alpha)/\beta)H0 = b/(P+Q)H1 = a/(P+Q)$$

Thus, in our series:

$$H0 = 2.71\ H1 = 2.71$$

To investigate chronological changes in learning environment, multivariate logistic regression analysis was used to compare each index before and after time points when significant proficiency changes occurred. To evaluate factors associated with a worsening interval, a multivariate-adjusted logistic regression model was constructed by including the presence of additional attending bronchoscopists or on-site cytopathologists, sedative dose (midazolam dose of ≥10 mg vs a lower dose), and opiate dose (fentanyl dose of ≥300 μg vs a lower dose). For measures of association, 95% confidence intervals were computed, and statistical significance was set at a *P* value of <0.05 (2-tailed). STATA 12.0 software was used for all analyses.

Results

Figure 1 shows CUSUM graphs depicting operator learning curves. Failed sampling attempts are indicated by upward deflections in the plot, and successful sampling attempts are indicated by downward deflections. The interval until the line exhibits a stable horizontal or downward direction, without crossing the boundary above it, can be regarded as the time required for an operator to become proficient in EBUS-TBNA. Operator A showed nonproficiency until the 30th sampling attempt, after which he or she exhibited proficiency (Fig. 1). Operator B was proficient from the start of observation until the 36th sampling, after which he or she became nonproficient until the 45th sampling (Fig. 1b). Operator C was proficient throughout the observation period and never crossed the unacceptable boundary (Fig. 1c). Fig. 2 shows the CUSUM learning curve for the institution as a whole. It shows significant chronological changes in proficiency before and after sampling numbers 61, 102, and 142, which correspond to cases 26, 51, and 73, respectively. Institutional proficiency was attained at case 27. However, the success rate started to decline to an unacceptable level after case 51 until proficiency was again attained, starting at case 73.

In the analysis of institutional EBUS-TBNA proficiency, we divided the study period into 4 intervals, namely, the intervals between cases 1 and 26 (learning interval), between cases 27 and 51 (proficiency interval), between cases 52 and 73 (worsening interval), and after case 73 (proficiency interval). To identify factors associated with success rate, we compared indices during the worsening interval (between cases 52 and 73) with those during the other intervals. A multivariate-adjusted logistic regression model was used to analyze the effects of the presence of additional attending bronchoscopists and on-site cytopathologists and higher doses of sedatives (≥10 mg of midazolam) and opiates (≥300 microgram of fentanyl). Comparison of the worsening interval with the other intervals revealed that presence of an additional attending bronchoscopist was inversely associated with nonproficiency (odds ratio [OR], 0.117; 95% confidence interval [CI], 0–0.749; $P = 0.019$). Other factors were not significantly associated with nonproficiency, including presence of on-site cytopathologists (OR, 0.365; 95% CI, 0.0369-1.835; $P = 0.322$), use of a midazolam dose of ≥10 mg (OR, 0.847; 95% CI, 0.167-3.512; $P = 0.999$, $n = 38$), and use of a fentanyl dose of ≥200 μg (OR, 2.786; 95% CI, 0.562-15.471; $P = 0.2588$, $n = 22$). The numbers of procedures performed by operators A and B did not significantly differ in any interval. Operator C performed fewer procedures than the other operators during intervals 1 ($P < 0.016$), 3 (worsening interval) ($P < 0.045$), and 4 ($P < 0.075$).

Discussion

Summary of results

A previous study using CUSUM analysis of the EBUS-TBNA learning curve found that the learning rate varied, even among experienced bronchoscopists [5]. In addition, our data suggest that chronological analysis and comparisons of variables before and after time points when significant proficiency changes occurred could be useful in improving the EBUS-TBNA learning environment.

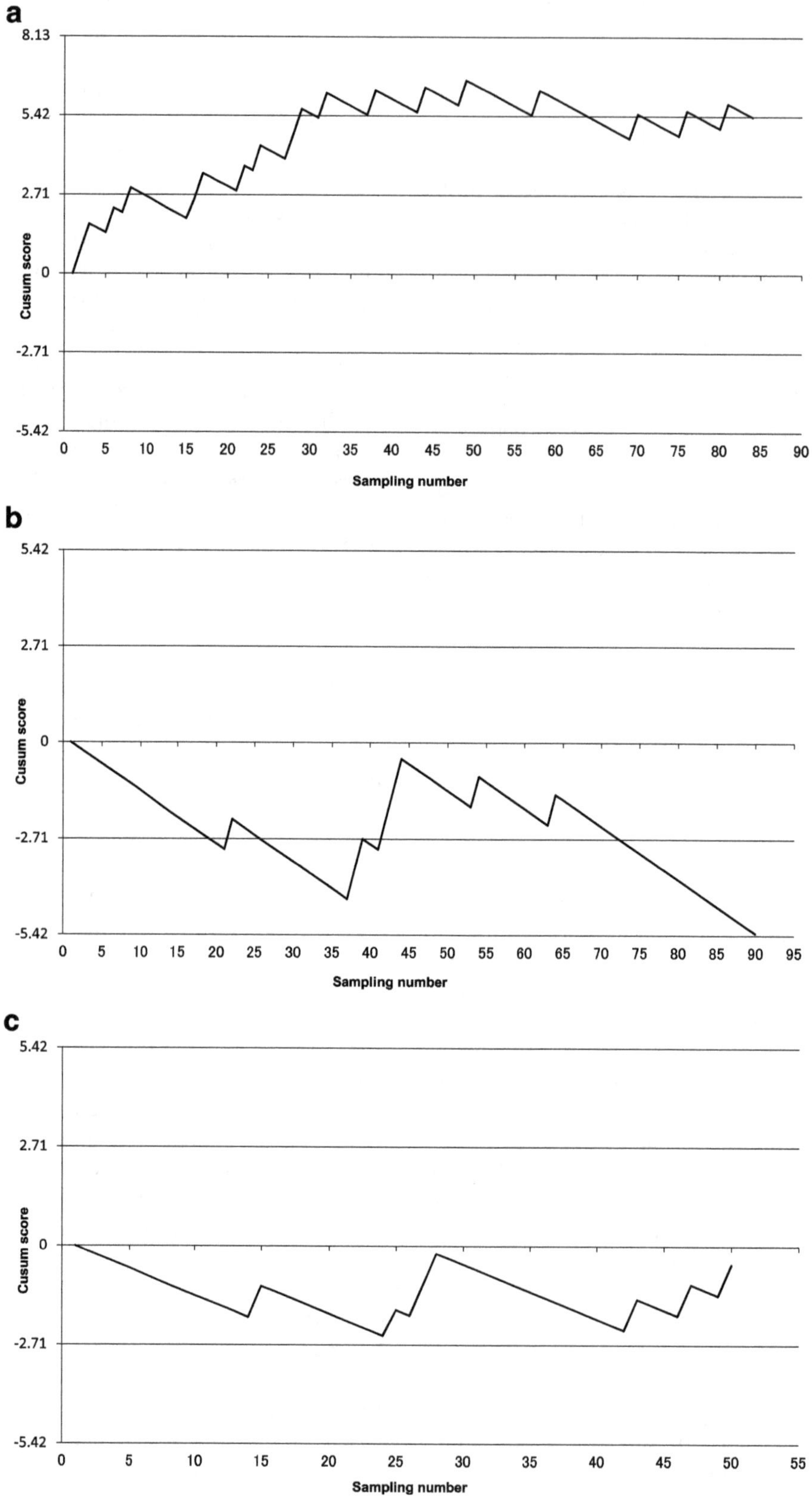

Fig. 1 **a** CUSUM Graphs of learning curves for operator A. **b** CUSUM Graphs of learning curves for operator B. **c** CUSUM Graphs of learning curves for operator C

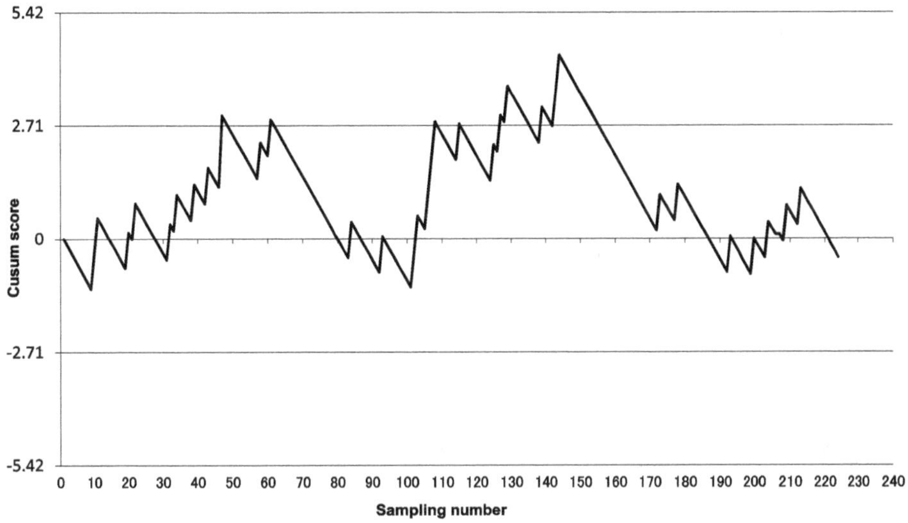

Fig. 2 CUSUM Graph of institutional learning curve

The findings of this pilot study indicate that CUSUM analysis was useful in detecting deviations in bronchoscopist performance and identifying environmental factors associated with such performance. This is the first study to show that CUSUM analysis could be used to investigate the EBUS-TBNA learning environment and identify possible causes for performance declines. We believe that CUSUM analysis can hasten intervention when changes in performance levels are detected.

Both individual and institutional factors affect successful performance of EBUS-TBNA. In this study, we found that presence of additional assisting attending bronchoscopists was associated with successful performance of EBUS-TBNA, which suggests that having an assisting attending bronchoscopist was associated with successful procedures during the institutional learning phase at our center. During the study period, additional attending physicians assisted in identifying target lymph nodes and needle activation. When an assisting attending physician was not present, a respiratory therapist or fellow physician assisted with the procedures. It is possible that the presence of an assisting attending physician resulted in better identification of target lymph nodes, better sampling technique, or both. Operator B exhibited the steepest learning curve, while operator A had the slowest learning curve among the operators. Further quality improvement efforts could attempt to use the present results for detailed investigation and comparison of the learning environments of these 2 operators. For example, operator B might have had greater input from other bronchoscopists. Interestingly, the presence of cytopathologists for rapid on-site evaluation in the bronchoscopy suite did not seem to affect the likelihood of a successful procedure. This finding contradicted our expectations, as we had assumed that the availability of a cytopathologist for rapid on-site evaluation would positively affect performance because lymph node sampling could then be repeated until satisfactory samples were obtained. The change in proficiency during the worsening interval did not appear to coincide with the change in the ratio of procedures performed by the bronchoscopist.

We used new definitions of EBUS-TBNA success and failure. We believe that these definitions are better for determining bronchoscopic proficiency than those used by Kemp et al. [5], as our definitions do not penalize bronchoscopists for the inherent limitations of the FNA procedure.

Study limitations and implications

This study has several limitations, which are mainly the result of its retrospective design. We were able to obtain information on only a limited number of environmental factors in our bronchoscopy suite. In particular, we lacked data on the technique and performance-based factors. We also had no information on changes in bronchoscopist lifestyle that might have affected performance. Additionally, we had no way of determining the "degree of difficulty" for each attempted sample. The presence of subcentimeter lymph nodes in less accessible locations might decrease success rate, even for a moderately proficient bronchoscopist. To address these limitations and increase the feasibility of this method for quality improvement, our next investigation will be a prospective study. The variables assessed will be more comprehensive, including bronchoscopist work hours, sleep hours, technique and performance-based factors, teaching methods, location and size of lymph nodes, and factors involved in specimen processing.

Conclusions

Combined CUSUM and environmental analysis is a promising method for monitoring and improving performance in EBUS-TBNA.

Abbreviations

CUSUM: Cumulative sum; EBUS-TBNA: Endobronchial ultrasound-guided transbronchial needle aspiration

Acknowledgements

The authors wish to thank David Kipler for reviewing the language of the manuscript.

Funding

This study received no external funding.

Authors' contributions

YN and MJ designed the study. DS supervised the project. MJ collected the data. YT, RU and SF analyzed the data. YN, RU and SF wrote the manuscript. All authors read and approved the final manuscript.

Competing interests

The authors declare that they have no competing interests.

Consent for publication

Not applicable.

Author details

[1]Department of Pulmonary and Critical Care Medicine, Tokyo Bay Urayasu-Ichikawa Medical Center, 3-4-32 Toudaijima, Urayasushi, Chiba 279-0001, Japan. [2]Japan Community Healthcare Organization, 3-22-12, Takanawa, Tokyo 108-0074, Japan. [3]Mercy Hospital, 1235 E Cherokee St, Springfield, MO 65804, USA. [4]Beth Israel Deaconess Medical Center, 330 Brookline Ave, Boston, MA 02215, USA. [5]Department of Emergency and Critical Care Medicine, St. Marianna University Hospital, 2-16-1, Miyamae, Kawasaki, Kanagawa, Japan. [6]Division of Pulmonary, Critical Care and Sleep Medicine, Saint Louis University, 1402S. Grand Avenue, Saint Louis, MO 63104-1004, USA.

References

1. Page E. Continuous inspection schemes. Biometrika. 1945;41:100–15.
2. Bolsin S, Colson M. The use of the Cusum technique in the assessment of trainee competence in new procedures. Int J Qual Health Care. 2000;12(5):433–8.
3. Hurter T, Hanrath P. Endobronchial sonography: feasibility and preliminary results. Thorax. 1992;47(7):565–7.
4. Dhooria S, Gupta N, Bal A, Sehgal IS, Aggarwal AN, Sethi S, et al. Role of Xpert MTB/RIF in differentiating tuberculosis from sarcoidosis in patients with mediastinal lymphadenopathy undergoing EBUS-TBNA: a study of 147 patients. Sarcoidosis Vasc Diffuse Lung Dis. 2016;33(3):258–66.
5. Kemp SV, El Batrawy SH, Harrison RN, Skwarski K, Munavvar M, Rosell A, et al. Learning curves for endobronchial ultrasound using cusum analysis. Thorax. 2010;65(6):534–8.
6. Kestin IG. A statistical approach to measuring the competence of anaesthetic trainees at practical procedures. Br J Anaesth. 1995;75(6):805–9.
7. Sivaprakasam J, Purva M. CUSUM analysis to assess competence: what failure rate is acceptable? Clin Teach. 2010;7(4):257–61.

Electromagnetic navigation bronchoscopy to access lung lesions in 1,000 subjects: first results of the prospective, multicenter NAVIGATE study

Sandeep J. Khandhar[1†], Mark R. Bowling[2], Javier Flandes[3], Thomas R. Gildea[4], Kristin L. Hood[5], William S. Krimsky[6], Douglas J. Minnich[7,14], Septimiu D. Murgu[8], Michael Pritchett[9], Eric M. Toloza[10,11], Momen M. Wahidi[12], Jennifer J. Wolvers[5], Erik E. Folch[13*†] and for the NAVIGATE Study Investigators

Abstract

Background: Electromagnetic navigation bronchoscopy (ENB) is an image-guided, minimally invasive approach that uses a flexible catheter to access pulmonary lesions.

Methods: NAVIGATE is a prospective, multicenter study of the superDimension™ navigation system. A prespecified 1-month interim analysis of the first 1,000 primary cohort subjects enrolled at 29 sites in the United States and Europe is described. Enrollment and 24-month follow-up are ongoing.

Results: ENB index procedures were conducted for lung lesion biopsy ($n = 964$), fiducial marker placement ($n = 210$), pleural dye marking ($n = 17$), and/or lymph node biopsy ($n = 334$; primarily endobronchial ultrasound-guided). Lesions were in the peripheral/middle lung thirds in 92.7%, 49.7% were <20 mm, and 48.4% had a bronchus sign. Radial EBUS was used in 54.3% (543/1,000 subjects) and general anesthesia in 79.7% (797/1,000). Among the 964 subjects (1,129 lesions) undergoing lung lesion biopsy, navigation was completed and tissue was obtained in 94.4% (910/964). Based on final pathology results, ENB-aided samples were read as malignant in 417/910 (45.8%) subjects and non-malignant in 372/910 (40.9%) subjects. An additional 121/910 (13.3%) were read as inconclusive. One-month follow-up in this interim analysis is not sufficient to calculate the true negative rate or diagnostic yield. Tissue adequacy for genetic testing was 80.0% (56 of 70 lesions sent for testing). The ENB-related pneumothorax rate was 4.9% (49/1,000) overall and 3.2% (32/1,000) CTCAE Grade ≥2 (primary endpoint). The ENB-related Grade ≥2 bronchopulmonary hemorrhage and Grade ≥4 respiratory failure rates were 1.0 and 0.6%, respectively.

Conclusions: One-month results of the first 1,000 subjects enrolled demonstrate low adverse event rates in a generalizable population across diverse practice settings. Continued enrollment and follow-up are required to calculate the true negative rate and delineate the patient, lesion, and procedural factors contributing to diagnostic yield.

(Continued on next page)

* Correspondence: efolch@mgh.harvard.edu

Prior Presentation: Presented at the IASLC 17th World Conference on Lung Cancer, December 5, 2016: Folch E, Flandes J, Khandhar S. MA05.02 Electromagnetic Navigation Bronchoscopy: A Prospective, Global, Multicenter Analysis of 1000 Subjects with Lung Lesions. Journal of Thoracic Oncology. 2017;12:S365.

†Equal contributors
[13]Division of Pulmonary and Critical Care Medicine, Massachusetts General Hospital, Harvard Medical School, 55 Fruit Street, Bulfinch 148, Boston, MA 02114, USA
Full list of author information is available at the end of the article

(Continued from previous page)

Keywords: Image-Guided Biopsy, Lung Cancer, Lung Neoplasms, Neoplasm Staging, Solitary Pulmonary Nodule

Background

Guidelines for lung nodule evaluation recommend the least invasive approach given each patient's clinical presentation [1]. Utilization of electromagnetic navigation bronchoscopy (ENB) has increased over the past ten years as a minimally invasive approach to complement traditional bronchoscopy, endobronchial ultrasound (EBUS), and image-guided transthoracic biopsy. Selection of the most appropriate diagnostic modality based on patient comorbidities and lesion location is critical to provide the fastest, safest, and most complete diagnosis possible.

Seventeen published studies of ENB use have been summarized in three recent meta-analyses [2–4]. Pneumothorax is the most common complication, occurring in approximately 3% of patients [2], lower than the pooled 20% rate reported for transthoracic needle biopsy [5]. However, published studies have typically been small, single-center, retrospective, and mostly conducted by expert users. The safety, usage profile, and clinical utility of ENB in a large, prospective, multicenter, generalizable population is unknown. The pragmatic design [6] of NAVIGATE maximizes patient eligibility, usual care settings, flexibility of adherence, and a relevant primary outcome for clinical practice. The detailed prospective collection of data also minimizes retrospective bias and allows future multivariate analyses to provide more meaningful information on the variable utilization of this technology into real-world practice and its impact on measurable outcomes, such as diagnostic yield and risk. Furthermore, a heterogeneous dataset will be instructive for the design of potential comparative studies with respect to operator training, subject inclusion criteria, data to be collected, definitions, and expected complication rates.

The primary objectives of this protocol-specified 1,000-subject, 1-month interim analysis of the NAVIGATE study [7] are to present the preliminary safety, clinical usage patterns, and performance of ENB in a large, unrestricted, generalizable population across diverse practice settings. The interim data will provide an early look at typical patient and lesion characteristics and procedural standard-of-care, generating questions for future NAVIGATE analyses and new clinical studies. Enrollment and continued follow-up are ongoing.

Methods

NAVIGATE is a prospective, multicenter, global, single-arm, cohort study in subjects undergoing ENB procedures. Enrollment of up to 1,500 subjects is planned at 37 sites in the United States and Europe. Subjects evaluations occur at baseline (within 30 days of the procedure), on the procedure day, and at 1 month, 12 months, and 24 months post-procedure. This manuscript describes the results of a prespecified 1-month interim analysis of the first 1,000 subjects enrolled at 29 sites in the United States and Europe. Enrollment and 12- and 24-month follow-up are ongoing. Brief methods are included below. A full list of study assessments and definitions is included in Additional files 1 and 2. The study design has been published [7].

Inclusion criteria are intentionally broad to ensure external validity. All consecutive, consented adult patients, who are not pregnant or nursing, and who are candidates for an elective ENB procedure based on physician discretion per recommended guidelines and institutional standard-of-care, are eligible. A maximum of 75 subjects is allowed per site. All investigators must have prior ENB experience. Investigators without extensive experience may enroll a maximum of five "roll-in" cases, which are excluded from this interim analysis. Roll-in cases will be included in the 1-year and 2-year analyses of the full enrollment when a more complete evaluation of the impact of user experience on diagnostic yield and other outcomes can be conducted.

All ENB procedures use the superDimension™ navigation system [8, 9] version 6.0 or higher (Medtronic, Minneapolis, MN) per product instructions and institutional standard practice. All complementary tools and procedures, including choice of catheter and biopsy tools, order of biopsy tool use, and strategy for staging and diagnostic bronchoscopy were performed at clinician discretion and were captured prospectively for data analysis.

The primary endpoint is pneumothorax related to the ENB index procedure rated Grade ≥2 according to the validated Common Terminology Criteria for Adverse Events (CTCAE) scale [7, 10], as adjudicated by an independent medical monitor. Pneumothorax was protocol-specified as the primary endpoint because it is applicable to all ENB procedures, including lung lesion biopsy, lymph node biopsy, fiducial placement, and pleural dye marking. Major secondary endpoints were all ENB-related pneumothorax, bronchopulmonary hemorrhage, and respiratory failure. Other secondary endpoints reported at 1 month were subject self-reported satisfaction with the procedure; adequacy of samples for molecular testing and mutation type; accurate fiducial placement as assessed by follow-up imaging;

and success rate of pleural dye marking demonstrated by surgical resection [7].

Diagnostic yield of the ENB index procedure will be calculated at the 12- and 24-month follow-up as the proportion of subjects with a definitive diagnosis (final pathology of the ENB-aided sample). One-month follow-up in this interim analysis is not sufficient to calculate the true negative rate or diagnostic yield. All lung nodules evaluated during the ENB index procedure will be followed for confirmation. Sensitivity, specificity, negative predictive value, and positive predictive value will be published beginning with the 12-month follow-up.

No sample size calculations were conducted for this single-arm, observational study. Analyses were performed using SAS® Version 9.4 (SAS Inc., Cary, NC). Data are summarized by descriptive statistics, including frequency distributions and cross-tabulations for discrete variables and mean, standard deviation, median, minimum, and maximum values for continuous variables. At least 10% of the data are verified against source files by the sponsor using risk-based monitoring.

Results

Participants

This prespecified interim analysis includes the first 1,000 primary cohort subjects enrolled at 29 clinical sites in the United States (27 sites) and Europe (two sites) from April 16, 2015 to June 27, 2016 (Fig. 1, and Additional file 3). Enrollment ranged from 2 to 75 subjects per site. Site types include academic centers (11 sites), private practice (11 sites), and mixed academic/private practice (seven sites). One-month follow-up was completed in 93.3% of subjects. Chronic obstructive pulmonary disease was present in 44.8%. Approximately one-third of subjects had a history of prior invasive lung procedures (Table 1).

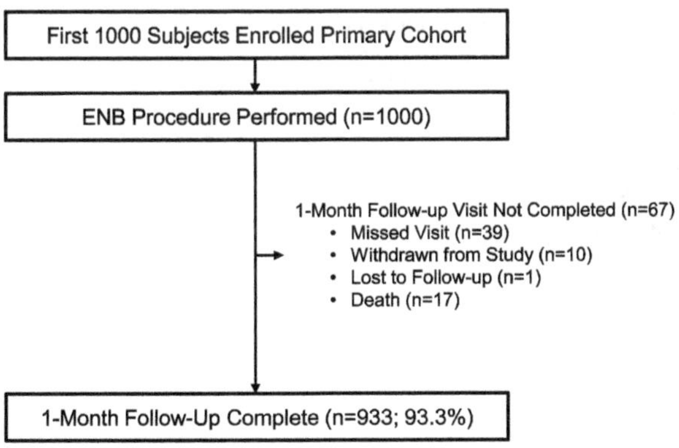

Fig. 1 Flow Diagram. As of June 27, 2016, 1,000 primary cohort subjects had been enrolled into the NAVIGATE study and comprise the first protocol-specified interim analysis of the 1-month results. The primary cohort is defined per protocol as those subjects who undergo an ENB index procedure minus roll-in subjects [7]. One-month follow-up is complete in 933/1,000 subjects (93.3%)

Table 1 Subject demographics (all primary cohort subjects)

	N = 1000 Subjects
Age at consent (years)	67.7 ± 11.3 (1000) [69.0] (21.0–93.0)
Female/Male	49.1%/50.9%
Race	
White	85.5% (855/1000)
Black or African American	12.5% (125/1000)
Asian	0.6% (6/1000)
American Indian or Alaska Native	0.4% (4/1000)
Native Hawaiian or Other Pacific Islander	0.1% (1/1000)
Unknown	0.8% (8/1000)
Unable To Report	0.1% (1/1000)
Hispanic or Latino Ethnicity	4.4% (44/1000)
Tobacco History (Current or Former)	80.8% (807/999)
COPD	44.8% (448/999)
FEV_1 (% of predicted)	74.8 ± 25.6 (332) [75.5] (20.0–140.0)
FEV_1/FVC Ratio	0.9 ± 0.2 (331) [0.9] (0.3–1.9)
DLCO (% of predicted)	66.4 ± 24.9 (225) [66.0] (6.0–141.0)
Asthma	12.6% (126/999)
Prior Invasive Lung Procedures[a]	30.6% (306/1000)
Bronchoscopy	20.4% (204/1000)
Standard Bronchoscopy	12.3% (123/1000)
Image-guided Bronchoscopy[b]	9.7% (97/1000)
Transthoracic Needle Aspiration	5.1% (51/1000)
Surgery	11.1% (111/1000)
Other	3.0% (30/1000)
Personal History of Cancer	45.8% (458/999)
Family History of Cancer	61.3% (612/999)
Subject taking Antithrombotic Medications[c]	45.8% (458/1000)
Anticoagulant	10.2% (102/1000)
Prescription Antiplatelet	6.8% (68/1000)
Aspirin	32.5% (325/1000)
Other	1.4% (14/1000)

Data are presented as n/N (%) or mean ± standard deviation (n) [median] (range)
Acronyms: *COPD* chronic obstructive pulmonary disease, *DLCO* diffusing capacity of the lung for carbon monoxide, *FVC* forced vital capacity, FEV_1 forced expiratory volume in 1 s, *EBUS* endobronchial ultrasound, *ENB* electromagnetic navigation bronchoscopy
[a]Each subject could have multiple prior procedures
[b]Includes 2.3% (23/1000) standard bronchoscopy with EBUS, 2.8% (28/1000) superDimension ENB, 2.6% (26/1000) superDimension ENB with EBUS, 0.8% (8/1000) other navigation bronchoscopy, and 1.8% (18/1000) other navigation bronchoscopy with EBUS
[c]Subjects could have multiple antithrombotic medications. "Other" includes nonsteroidal anti-inflammatory drugs, fish oil, and vitamins

Procedural characteristics

One thousand ENB index procedures were conducted in 1,000 subjects. Procedures were conducted for one or more purposes, including lung lesion biopsy (*n* = 964 subjects), fiducial marker placement ($n = 210$), pleural dye marking ($n = 17$), and/or lymph node biopsy ($n = 334$; primarily guided by linear EBUS), as shown in Fig. 2. General anesthesia was used in 79.7% of subjects. Radial EBUS was used during the ENB index procedure in 54.3% (543/1,000) and fluoroscopy was used in 90.1% (1,017/1,129) of lesions. The median ENB procedure time was 25.0 min (interquartile range 14.0–41.0 min). See Table 2 for other procedural characteristics. Overall, 94.8% (827/872) of subjects reported that their expectations for the procedure we adequately met.

Safety

Pneumothorax CTCAE Grade ≥2 occurred in 32/1,000 subjects (3.2%; Table 3). Any-grade pneumothorax occurred in 49 subjects (4.9%). Bronchopulmonary hemorrhage was 1.0% CTCAE Grade ≥2 (10/1,000) and 2.3% overall (23/1,000). CTCAE Grade ≥4 respiratory failure occurred in 6/1,000 (0.6%). As of the 1-month follow-up (which allowed a visit window up to 37 days post-ENB), 23 subjects had died (six completed the 1-month visit; 17 did not). No deaths were considered related to the ENB device or associated tools by either the clinical investigator or the independent medical monitor. There was one procedure-related death due to Grade 5 hypoxic respiratory failure 9 days after the ENB index procedure, deemed related to complications of general anesthesia, in a patient with multiple comorbidities, including cirrhosis, hepatocellular carcinoma, small cell carcinoma, and ovarian cancer.

Lung lesion biopsies

Among the 964 subjects (1,129 lesions) undergoing lung lesion biopsy, the median lesion size was 20.0 mm (interquartile range: 16.0 mm [Q1: 14.0, Q3: 30.0]), and 49.7% of lesions were <20 mm in diameter (Table 4). Most lesions were in the peripheral (62.6%) or middle (30.1%) lung thirds. An airway to the lesion was visible on pre-procedure CT (bronchus sign) in 48.4%.

ENB was able to navigate successfully to allow a tissue biopsy (according to subjective operator assessment) in 910 subjects (94.4%) and 1,036 lesions (91.8%; Table 5). Rapid on-site evaluation (ROSE) for immediate peri-procedural feedback on pathology specimens was conducted in 66.1% (601/909) of subjects. Among 247 lesions diagnosed with primary lung adenocarcinoma or non-small-cell lung cancer not otherwise specified, molecular genetic testing was attempted in 70/247 (28.3%), with adequate tissue in 56/70 (80.0%; Table 5).

Based on the final pathology results of the ENB index procedure, tissue was interpreted as malignant in 417/910 (45.8%) subjects (Table 6). Primary lung cancer was diagnosed in 40.1% of subjects. Preliminary clinical stage [11] in subjects diagnosed with primary lung cancer was 52.9% Stage I, 10.7% Stage II, 18.9% Stage III, and 17.3% Stage IV (Fig. 3), to be confirmed with follow-up. Lymph node biopsies were attempted during the ENB index procedure (same anesthetic event) in 33.4% of cases (334/1,000). In 322/334 (96.4%) of these cases, mediastinal staging was conducted using linear EBUS. Lymph node biopsy was guided by ENB in 42 cases (alone or in combination with linear EBUS).

Based on site-reported assessments of the ENB-aided final pathology sample, tissue was interpreted as non-malignant in 372/910 (40.9%) subjects (Table 6). An additional 121/910 (13.3%) were interpreted as inconclusive. Longer follow-up is required to confirm true

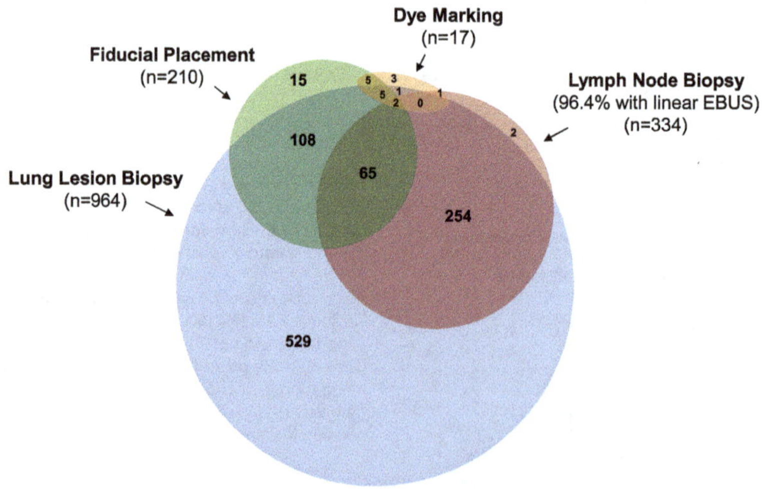

Fig. 2 Reasons for Conducting ENB on a Per Subject Basis. The NAVIGATE ENB index procedure could be conducted for more than one purpose in the same anesthetic event, including lung lesion biopsy, fiducial marker placement, pleural dye marking, or lymph node biopsy. Not drawn to scale. Not shown in graph: ENB-guided fiducial marker placement plus lymph node biopsy ($n = 10$); ENB-guided fiducial marker placement plus lymph node biopsy plus ENB-guided pleural dye marking ($n = 0$)

Table 2 General procedural characteristics (all primary cohort subjects)

	N = 1000 Procedures
General Anesthesia	79.7% (797/1000)
Moderate Sedation	20.3% (203/1000)
ENB Software Version	
Version 6	18.4% (184/1000)
Version 7	81.6% (816/1000)
Radial EBUS used During ENB Procedure[a]	54.3% (543/1000)
Cone Beam CT used	5.4% (54/1000)
Total Procedure Time (Bronchoscope In/Out), min	52.0 (36.0 [35.0–71.0])
ENB Procedure Time (Locatable Guide In/Out), min[b]	25.0 (27.0 [14.0–41.0])

Data are presented as n/N (%) or median (interquartile range [Q1-Q3])
Acronyms: *CT* computed tomography, *EBUS* endobronchial ultrasound, *ENB* electromagnetic navigation bronchoscopy
[a]Other than for lymph node biopsy but including all biopsy, fiducial, and pleural dye marking procedures
[b]Data only available for 499 subjects, because question was added to case report forms after enrollment had begun

versus false negatives and calculate diagnostic yield. At this time, the true prevalence of malignancy in the patient population is unknown.

Fiducial placement and pleural dye marking

A total of 417 fiducial markers were placed in 210 subjects. Subjective operator assessment of accurate fiducial placement was 208/210 (99.0%) and fiducial markers were still present at follow-up imaging in 192/205 (93.7%). In subjects undergoing fiducial marker placement, ENB-related adverse events included eight pneumothoraces CTCAE Grade ≥2 (3.8%), three respiratory failures CTCAE Grade ≥4 (1.4%), and one bronchopulmonary hemorrhage Grade 1. Pleural dye marking was conducted in 17 subjects, of which 15 (88.2%) were considered adequate for surgical resection.

Table 3 Adverse events related to the ENB index procedure or devices (1 Month Follow-up)[a]

	N = 1000 Subjects
Pneumothorax	
CTCAE Grade 2 or Higher	3.2% (32/1000)
All Grades	4.9% (49/1000)
Bronchopulmonary Hemorrhage	
CTCAE Grade 2 and Higher	1.0% (10/1000)
All Grades	2.3% (23/1000)
Respiratory Failure, CTCAE Grade 4 or Higher	0.6% (6/1000)
Death (anesthesia-related respiratory failure 9 days post-ENB)[b]	0.1% (1/1000)

Data are presented as % (n/N subjects)
Acronyms: *CTCAE* Common Terminology Criteria for Adverse Events, *ENB* electromagnetic navigation bronchoscopy
[a]Other than expected observations associated with anesthesia (e.g., common or expected post-procedure pain, transient nausea, transient emesis, post-procedure constipation)
[b]Grade 5 hypoxic respiratory failure 9 days after the ENB index procedure, deemed related to complications of general anesthesia, in a patient with multiple comorbidities, including cirrhosis, hepatocellular carcinoma, small cell carcinoma, and ovarian cancer. As of 1-month follow-up, a total of 23 subjects had died (6 completed 1-month follow-up visit; 17 did not). As of the 1-month follow-up, no other deaths were considered related to the ENB device or associated tools by either the clinical investigator or the independent medical monitor

Table 4 Lung lesion characteristics (subjects undergoing ENB-aided biopsy)

	N = 1129 Lesions in 964 Subjects
Pre-test probability of malignancy (physician estimation)	67.1 ± 26.5 (790) [75.0] (0.0–100.0)
Pre-test probability of malignancy (Swenson's equation)[a]	61.6 ± 29.4 (789) [67.1] (2.9–100.0)
Average Lung Lesion Size, mm	
Mean ± SD (N)	23.6 ± 14.4 (1129)
Median, Range (min-max)	20.0 (3.0–118.0)
Interquartile Range (Q1-Q3)	16.0 (14.0–30.0)
< 20 mm	49.7% (561/1129)
≥ 20 mm	50.3% (568/1129)
Lesion Location	
Right Upper Lobe	31.7% (358/1129)
Right Middle Lobe	8.1% (91/1129)
Right Lower Lobe	19.0% (215/1129)
Left Upper Lobe	25.9% (292/1129)
Left Lower Lobe	15.3% (173/1129)
Lung Zone[b]	
Peripheral third of lung on CT	62.6% (707/1129)
Middle third of lung on CT	30.1% (340/1129)
Proximal third of lung on CT	7.3% (82/1129)
Lesion Visible on Fluoroscopy	60.0% (610/1017)
Ground Glass Lesions (Suzuki Class 1 or 2) [28]	6.3% (71/1123)
Spiculated Lesion Border	60.9% (687/1128)
Bronchus Sign Present on CT	48.4% (546/1129)
Lesion PET Positive (≥2.5 standard uptake value)	80.9% (479/592)

Data are presented as n/N (%) or mean ± standard deviation (n) [median] (range)
Acronyms: *CT* computed tomography, *PET* positron emission tomography, *SD* standard deviation
[a]Pre-test probability of malignancy (calculated): x = −6.8272 + (0.0391 * "age") + (0.7917 * "tobacco history") + (1.3388 * "history of extrathoracic cancer") + (0.1274 * "diameter in mm") + (1.0407 * "spiculation") + (0.7838 * "upper lobe"). Not applicable to patients with a diagnosis of cancer that has been made within the previous 5 years or to patients with previous lung cancer [29]
[b]See Folch et al. 2016 for definitions [7]

Discussion

Lung cancer causes one quarter of all cancer deaths, representing a significant public health problem [12].

Table 5 Procedural characteristics in lung lesion biopsy cases

	N = 1129 Lesions in 964 Subjects
Navigation Success (per lesion)[a]	91.8% (1036/1129)
Navigation Success (per subject)[a]	94.4% (910/964)
Number of Lesions Biopsied (per subject)	1.2 ± 0.5 (964) [1.0] (1.0–5.0)
Biopsy Tools Used During ENB Index Procedure[b]	
Aspiration Needle	52.2% (503/964)
Biopsy Forceps	81.2% (783/964)
Cytology Brush	47.0% (453/964)
Needle-Tipped Cytology Brush	20.2% (195/964)
Triple Needle-Tipped Cytology Brush	23.4% (226/964)
GenCut™ Core Biopsy Tool	18.9% (182/964)
Bronchoalveolar Lavage or Washing	37.8% (364/964)
Rapid on-site evaluation (ROSE) used[c]	66.1% (601/909)
Molecular/genetic testing attempted[d]	28.3% (70/247)
Molecular/genetic testing successful	80.0% (56/70)
Inadequate Sample	20.0% (14/70)
Molecular/genetic testing not attempted[d]	71.7% (177/247)
Not Necessary	49.2% (87/177)
Not Standard Practice	41.2% (73/177)
Other	9.6% (17/177)

Data are presented as n/N (%) or mean ± standard deviation (n) [median] (range)
[a]Able to navigate successfully and allow a tissue biopsy (according to subjective operator assessment)
[b]More than one tool used per procedure
[c]Per subject, among subjects with an ENB-aided tissue sample obtained. Data missing for 1 subject
[d]Per lesion, among 247 lesions with primary adenocarcinoma ($n = 233$) or primary non-small-cell lung cancer not otherwise specified ($n = 14$). More than one reason could be chosen per lesion

Table 6 Pathology result aided by the index ENB procedure[a]

N = 910 subjects with navigation complete and tissue sample obtained	
Malignant	45.8% (417/910)
Lung cancer	40.1% (365/910)
Non-Small Cell Lung Cancer (NSCLC)	36.4% (331/910)
Adenocarcinoma	23.5% (214/910)
Squamous Carcinoma	11.4% (104/910)
Other NSCLC	1.5% (14/910)
Small Cell Carcinoma	2.9% (26/910)
Neuroendocrine Carcinoma	1.1% (10/910)
Metastatic Carcinoma of Extrathoracic Origin	4.4% (40/910)
Lymphoma	0.2% (2/910)
Malignant Cells (unable to characterize)	0.9% (8/910)
Other	0.3% (3/910)
Site-Reported Non-Malignant or Inconclusive Results	
Non-Malignant	40.9% (372/910)
Normal Lung Tissue/Bronchial Epithelium	10.4% (95/910)
Benign Non-Specific	21.9% (199/910)
Benign Inflammation	15.3% (139/910)
Other[b]	6.7% (61/910)
Infection	2.9% (26/910)
Bacterial	1.8% (16/910)
Fungal	0.9% (8/910)
Viral	0.2% (2/910)
Granuloma	1.4% (13/910)
Atypical Cells	1.9% (17/910)
Lymphocytes	1.1% (10/910)
Organizing Pneumonia	0.8% (7/910)
Interstitial Lung Disease	0.4% (4/910)
Other[c]	1.0% (9/910)
Inconclusive	13.3% (121/910)

Data are presented as n/N (%) or mean ± standard deviation (n) (range)
Acronym: *ENB* electromagnetic navigation bronchoscopy
[a]Preliminary 1-month results, to be confirmed by subsequent surgery, biopsy, or radiographic follow-up through 2 years as appropriate per clinician's assessment of the patient's probability of malignancy. One-month follow-up in this interim analysis is not sufficient to calculate the true negative rate or diagnostic yield
[b]Includes reactive bronchial cells and other nonspecific "benign" diagnoses
[c]Reported as 1 case each of: (1) fibroelastic scar, (2) squamous dysplasia, (3) squamous metaplasia, (4) radiotherapy changes, (5) blood clots post-FNA, (6) asbestos fibrosis, (7) benign metastasizing leiomyoma, (8) focally anthracotic alveolated pulmonary parenchyma, and (9) iron pill aspiration

While the incidence has declined in concert with decreased smoking prevalence, survival rates have improved little over the past 50–60 years, largely due to a high proportion of late-stage diagnoses with a 5-year survival rate of only 4% [12]. Earlier-stage diagnoses will lead to more meaningful improvements in survival and will require modalities that allow the accurate sampling of smaller, more peripheral lung lesions. The National Lung Screening Trial [13] and screening coverage in select high-risk patients [14] has been projected to increase low-dose CT utilization by over ten million procedures annually [15]. However, an extremely high percentage (96%) of false positive screening results [13, 16] and the risk of unnecessary procedures requires the judicious use of minimally invasive options and a careful balance of the risk-to-benefit ratio for further diagnosis and management [17].

Several current technologies can provide minimally invasive diagnostic evaluation in appropriately selected patients, although each has limitations. PET-CT is often considered the second-line diagnostic option for nodules detected on CT [18], but is typically not reimbursed for screening and does not provide tissue diagnosis. Conventional bronchoscopy is safe but is limited to proximal lesions and has a high non-diagnostic rate, potentially leading to unnecessary invasive procedures in 20–25% of patients, including the use of thoracoscopy for diagnostic wedge resection [19–21]. Image-guided transthoracic biopsy provides high diagnostic accuracy but at the cost of pneumothorax rates averaging 20% (range 4 to 62%)

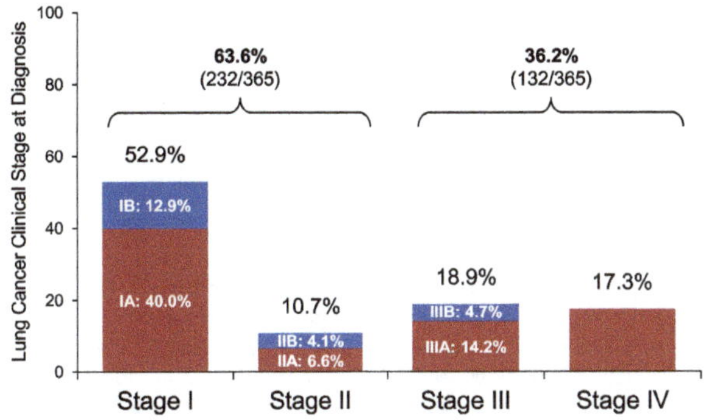

Fig. 3 Lung Cancer Clinical Stage at Diagnosis in Subjects with Primary Lung Cancer (365 subjects with 395 lesions). Not shown in graph: One subject had a diagnosis of Stage 0

[5] and the need for additional procedures to diagnose and stage mediastinal lymph nodes. ENB provides a minimally invasive platform for peripheral lung lesion sampling, concurrent lymph node staging with linear EBUS, preparation for treatment via fiducial placement or localization via pleural dye marking in a single procedure.

The primary objective of this interim NAVIGATE analysis was to evaluate ENB safety. While published pneumothorax rates are low (3.1% [range 0–13%]) [2], most prior studies are single-center with fewer than 100 subjects [4, 7]. The current analysis demonstrates low pneumothorax, bronchopulmonary hemorrhage, and respiratory failure rates in the context of a large, diverse study cohort and a wide range of user experience levels, confirming the safety of advanced bronchoscopy for the access and sampling of all pulmonary nodules. Pneumothorax was also infrequent following fiducial placement (3.8%), in contrast to rates ranging from 22 to 67% following percutaneous fiducial marking [22], Despite the advanced stage of some of the enrolled subjects, there were only 23 deaths within the 1-month follow-up time-frame, further substantiating the safety of the procedure. Only one death was considered related to the ENB index procedure, due to general anesthesia in a patient with multiple comorbidities, and none were related to the ENB device or associated tools. These results suggest a highly favorable risk-to-benefit ratio for the use of ENB to aid in lung lesion biopsies, particularly given the risk profile of the patients included, with approximately 45% COPD incidence and a relatively high rate of Stage III-IV disease.

A second objective of this analysis was to explore the real-world usage patterns and clinical utility of ENB. The interim results elucidate the rates of general anesthesia use (79.7%), ROSE utilization (66.1%), and concurrent fluoroscopic (90.1%) and radial EBUS (54.3%) guidance. Of note, nearly half of ENB index procedures were conducted for multiple purposes, including 33.4% with lymph node staging (primarily EBUS-guided) and 21.0% with fiducial markers placed. Tissue adequacy for molecular genetic testing was also high (80.0%) and similar to prior studies [23]. These results suggest that, in unrestricted practice settings, ENB is used to diagnose peripheral lung nodules and perform concurrent linear EBUS-guided mediastinal lymph node staging in a single anesthetic event, facilitating a multidisciplinary, comprehensive patient care approach.

A third objective of this interim analysis was to provide a preliminary look at ENB performance. From a patient perspective, all important follow-up cadence and treatment decisions are made within the 30-day window after the diagnostic procedure. At the 1-month time-point, ENB provided a preliminary malignant diagnosis in 45.8% of subjects, including 40.1% with lung cancer. The initial 45.8% malignancy rate in NAVIGATE is consistent with other recent ENB publications reporting malignancy rates of 35–60% [24–27], and is expectedly higher than the 3.7% positive malignancy rate seen in the National Lung Screening Trial [13].

One-month follow-up is not sufficient to calculate the true versus false negative rate or diagnostic yield, as the true prevalence of lung cancer in this population is unknown at this time. All non-malignant pathology findings require confirmation with longer-term follow-up or additional diagnostic procedures, depending upon the pretest probability of malignancy and in accordance with society guidelines [1, 18]. All follow-up procedures and final diagnoses will be captured and reported. Early indicators of clinical stage in NAVIGATE subjects diagnosed with lung cancer also suggest a 64% rate of Stage I-II diagnoses, which are more amenable to surgical intervention for curative intent. In this observational study with consecutive enrollment, approximately 36% of NAVIGATE subjects had Stage III-IV lung cancer. Diagnostic testing of late-stage patients in NAVIGATE may reflect not only a lack of standardization for patient selection but also the changing landscape of personalized medicine and treatment options for Stage III-IV disease. Patient selection for ENB, as well as multivariate predictors of safety and effectiveness, will be explored in future NAVIGATE analyses of the full cohort. This will include an analysis of Stage III-IV cases to explore the patient, lesion, and operator/center factors leading to the inclusion of these cases in the study.

The final objective of this preliminary analysis was to generate questions for future NAVIGATE analyses and comparative studies. Unexpected observations included a high percentage of lesions without a CT bronchus sign (52%) and a relatively low proportion of subjects in whom genetic testing was attempted (28%). While current guidelines recommend genetic testing for only late-stage disease, there is extensive variation between institutions. Tissue requirements for comprehensive molecular testing and the practice of personalized medicine will continue to evolve.

Future analyses will describe molecular genetic evaluation in the NAVIGATE cohort in more detail. Other future questions include multivariate predictors of safety and diagnostic yield, factors affecting the need for concurrent radial EBUS or other fluoroscopic guidance, usage patterns of fiducial and pleural dye marking, success rates of various biopsy tools, and cost effectiveness. In this way, NAVIGATE will help to set the benchmark for the ideal ENB patient, and define the procedural techniques contributing to enhanced performance. Whether ENB truly enables a shift to an earlier stage diagnosis, and the impact on long-term patient survival, healthcare utilization, and costs, will also be topics for future NAVIGATE analyses.

Limitations

This is a nonrandomized, single-arm analysis of 1-month interim results. Longer-term follow-up is required to determine the accuracy of ENB-aided diagnoses, and calculate diagnostic yield. Follow-up through 24 months is in progress. This analysis also evaluates only one navigational bronchoscopy system; other systems are currently available for clinical use.

Conclusions

This early look at the NAVIGATE results provides information about usage patterns and utility of ENB in a large, unrestricted, generalizable population across diverse practice settings. In the first 1,000 subjects enrolled, 1-month follow-up demonstrates low adverse event rates among a heterogeneous cohort. Continued enrollment and follow-up will demonstrate the negative predictive value and delineate the patient, lesion, and procedural characteristics contributing to diagnostic yield. This preliminary analysis generates questions to be explored in future controlled clinical studies. Further follow-up will also help define objective endpoints to guide future population-based guidelines for intervention.

Abbreviations

CT: Computed tomography; CTCAE: Common Terminology Criteria for Adverse Events; EBUS: Endobronchial ultrasound; ENB: Electromagnetic navigation bronchoscopy; PET: Positron-emission tomography; TTNA: Transthoracic needle aspiration

Acknowledgements

The study is sponsored and funded by Medtronic (Minneapolis, MN). Medical writing support was provided by Kristin L. Hood PhD, a full-time employee of Medtronic and coauthor on this paper. The authors wish to thank Haiying Lin (Medtronic) for biostatistics support. The authors also wish to thank the investigators and staff of all participating clinical sites (see Additional file 3).

Funding

The study is sponsored and funded by Medtronic (Minneapolis, MN), which contributed to the study design, data collection, and data analysis, and assisted with manuscript writing. The lead authors (EF and SK) had full access to all study data and final responsibility for the decision to submit for publication.

Authors' contributions

All authors made substantial contributions to all aspects of the study conduct and manuscript development beginning with the initial study conception, including study design (SJK, MRB, TRG, KLH, WSK, SDM, MP, EMT, MMW, EEF), data acquisition (MRB, JF, TRG, WSK, DJM, SDM, MP, MMW), data analysis (SJK, KLH, JJW, EEF), data interpretation (SJK, MRB, TRG, SDM, MMW, EEF), manuscript writing (SJK, KLH, EEF), critical revisions (all authors), final approval of the manuscript for submission (all authors); and agreement to be accountable for the accuracy and integrity of the work (all authors).

Competing interests

Financial disclosures related to the submitted work: SJK, MRB, TRG, WSK, SDM, EMT, MMW, and EEF serve on the Clinical Advisory Board for Medtronic and received travel funds and fees for participation; SJK, JF, DJM, SDM, and EEF serve on the NAVIGATE Steering Committee and have received fees for participation; KLH and JJW are full-time employees and stockholders of Medtronic, MMW received consulting fees from Medtronic. Financial disclosures outside the submitted work: MRB and MP received consulting fees from Medtronic; KLH is a stockholder of Boston Scientific; WSK is a part-time employee of Medtronic (employment began after study enrollment was complete) and has received consulting fees from Medtronic with intellectual property rights; SDM received consulting fees from Boston Scientific, Olympus, Concordia, and Auris Robotics; EMT received travel funds and honoraria from Medtronic as a member of their Speakers' Bureau; EEF is on the Scientific Advisory board for Boston Scientific and the Education Advisory Board for Olympus.

Consent for publication

Not applicable. This paper presents aggregate data.

Author details

[1]Inova Health System, Fairfax Hospital, Falls Church, VA, USA. [2]East Carolina University, Greenville, NC, USA. [3]Pulmonary Department, IIS-Fundacion Jimenez Diaz University Hospital, CIBERES, Madrid, Spain. [4]Department of Pulmonary, Allergy, and Critical Care Medicine and Transplant Center, Cleveland Clinic, Cleveland, OH, USA. [5]Medtronic, Minneapolis, MN, USA. [6]Pulmonary and Critical Care Associates of Baltimore, Baltimore, MD, USA. [7]Division of Cardiothoracic Surgery, University of Alabama at Birmingham, Birmingham, AL, USA. [8]Interventional Pulmonology Fellowship Program, The University of Chicago Medicine, Chicago, IL, USA. [9]Pulmonary Department, Pinehurst Medical Clinic and FirstHealth Moore Regional Hospital, Pinehurst, NC, USA. [10]Department of Thoracic Oncology, Moffitt Cancer Center, Tampa, FL, USA. [11]Department of Surgery and Department of Oncologic Sciences, University of South Florida Morsani College of Medicine, Tampa, FL, USA. [12]Department of Medicine, Duke University Medical Center, Durham, NC, USA. [13]Division of Pulmonary and Critical Care Medicine, Massachusetts General Hospital, Harvard Medical School, 55 Fruit Street, Bulfinch 148, Boston, MA 02114, USA. [14]Present Address: Princeton Baptist Medical Center, Birmingham, AL, USA.

References

1. Rivera MP, Mehta AC, Wahidi MM. Establishing the diagnosis of lung cancer: Diagnosis and management of lung cancer, 3rd ed: American College of Chest Physicians evidence-based clinical practice guidelines. Chest. 2013; 143:e142S–65.
2. Gex G, Pralong JA, Combescure C, Seijo L, Rochat T, Soccal PM. Diagnostic yield and safety of electromagnetic navigation bronchoscopy for lung nodules: a systematic review and meta-analysis. Respiration. 2014;87:165–76.
3. Wang Memoli JS, Nietert PJ, Silvestri GA. Meta-analysis of guided bronchoscopy for the evaluation of the pulmonary nodule. Chest. 2012;142:385–93.
4. Zhang W, Chen S, Dong X, Lei P. Meta-analysis of the diagnostic yield and safety of electromagnetic navigation bronchoscopy for lung nodules. J Thorac Dis. 2015;7:799–809.
5. DiBardino DM, Yarmus LB, Semaan RW. Transthoracic needle biopsy of the lung. J Thorac Dis. 2015;7:S304–16.
6. Ford I, Norrie J. Pragmatic Trials. N Engl J Med. 2016;375:454–63.
7. Folch EE, Bowling MR, Gildea TR, Hood KL, Murgu SD, Toloza EM, et al. Design of a prospective, multicenter, global, cohort study of electromagnetic navigation bronchoscopy. BMC Pulm Med. 2016;16:60.
8. Reynisson PJ, Leira HO, Hernes TN, Hofstad EF, Scali M, Sorger H, et al. Navigated bronchoscopy: a technical review. J Bronchology Interv Pulmonol. 2014;21:242–64.
9. Seijo L. Electromagnetic navigation bronchoscopy: clinical utility in the diagnosis of lung cancer. Lung Cancer. 2016;7:111–8.
10. National Cancer Institute, Cancer Therapy Evaluation Program, United States Department of Health and Human Services, National Institutes of Health. Common Terminology Criteria for Adverse Events (CTCAE) Version 4.0. http://ctep.cancer.gov/protocolDevelopment/electronic_applications/ctc.htm#ctc_40. Accessed 16 Dec 2016.
11. Hari DM, Leung AM, Lee JH, Sim MS, Vuong B, Chiu CG, et al. AJCC Cancer Staging Manual 7th edition criteria for colon cancer: do the complex modifications improve prognostic assessment? J Am Coll Surg. 2013;217:181–90.
12. Siegel RL, Miller KD, Jemal A. Cancer statistics, 2016. CA Cancer J Clin. 2016; 66:7–30.
13. Aberle DR, Adams AM, Berg CD, Black WC, Clapp JD, Fagerstrom RM, et al. Reduced lung-cancer mortality with low-dose computed tomographic screening. N Engl J Med. 2011;365:395–409.
14. Centers for Medicare & Medicaid Services, United States Department of Health and Human Services. Decision Memo for Screening for Lung Cancer with Low Dose Computed Tomography (LDCT) (CAG-00439 N, 5 Feb 2015). https://www.cms.gov/medicare-coverage-database/details/nca-decision-memo.aspx?NCAId=274. Accessed 16 Dec 2016.
15. Roth JA, Sullivan SD, Goulart BH, Ravelo A, Sanderson JC, Ramsey SD. Projected Clinical, Resource Use, and Fiscal Impacts of Implementing Low-Dose Computed Tomography Lung Cancer Screening in Medicare. J Oncol Pract. 2015;11:267–72.
16. McWilliams A, Tammemagi MC, Mayo JR, Roberts H, Liu G, Soghrati K, et al. Probability of cancer in pulmonary nodules detected on first screening CT. N Engl J Med. 2013;369:910–9.
17. Tanoue LT, Tanner NT, Gould MK, Silvestri GA. Lung cancer screening. Am J Respir Crit Care Med. 2015;191:19–33.
18. Gould MK, Donington J, Lynch WR, Mazzone PJ, Midthun DE, Naidich DP, et al. Evaluation of individuals with pulmonary nodules: when is it lung cancer? Diagnosis and management of lung cancer, 3rd ed: American College of Chest Physicians evidence-based clinical practice guidelines. Chest. 2013;143:e93S–120.
19. Silvestri GA, Vachani A, Whitney D, Elashoff M, Porta Smith K, Ferguson JS, et al. A Bronchial Genomic Classifier for the Diagnostic Evaluation of Lung Cancer. N Engl J Med. 2015;373:243–51.
20. Detterbeck FC, Mazzone PJ, Naidich DP, Bach PB. Screening for lung cancer: Diagnosis and management of lung cancer, 3rd ed: American College of Chest Physicians evidence-based clinical practice guidelines. Chest. 2013; 143:e78S–92.
21. Grogan EL, Weinstein JJ, Deppen SA, Putnam Jr JB, Nesbitt JC, Lambright ES, et al. Thoracic operations for pulmonary nodules are frequently not futile in patients with benign disease. J Thorac Oncol. 2011;6:1720–5.
22. Hagmeyer L, Priegnitz C, Kocher M, Schilcher B, Budach W, Treml M, et al. Fiducial marker placement via conventional or electromagnetic navigation bronchoscopy (ENB): an interdisciplinary approach to the curative management of lung cancer. Clin Respir J. 2016;10:291–7.
23. Vanderlaan PA, Yamaguchi N, Folch E, Boucher DH, Kent MS, Gangadharan SP, et al. Success and failure rates of tumor genotyping techniques in routine pathological samples with non-small-cell lung cancer. Lung Cancer. 2014;84:39–44.
24. Loo FL, Halligan AM, Port JL, Hoda RS. The emerging technique of electromagnetic navigation bronchoscopy-guided fine-needle aspiration of peripheral lung lesions: promising results in 50 lesions. Cancer Cytopathol. 2014;122:191–9.
25. Odronic SI, Gildea TR, Chute DJ. Electromagnetic navigation bronchoscopy-guided fine needle aspiration for the diagnosis of lung lesions. Diagn Cytopathol. 2014;42:1045–50.
26. Garwood SK, ClenDening P, Hevelone ND, Hood KL, Pidgeon S, Wudel LJ. Navigational bronchoscopy at a community hospital: clinical and economic outcomes. Lung Cancer Manag. 2016;5:131–40.
27. Bowling MR, Kohan MW, Walker P, Efird J, Ben OS. The effect of general anesthesia versus intravenous sedation on diagnostic yield and success in electromagnetic navigation bronchoscopy. J Bronchology Interv Pulmonol. 2015;22:5–13.
28. Suzuki K, Kusumoto M, Watanabe S, Tsuchiya R, Asamura H. Radiologic classification of small adenocarcinoma of the lung: radiologic-pathologic correlation and its prognostic impact. Ann Thorac Surg. 2006;81:413–9.
29. Swensen SJ, Silverstein MD, Ilstrup DM, Schleck CD, Edell ES. The probability of malignancy in solitary pulmonary nodules. Application to small radiologically indeterminate nodules. Arch Intern Med. 1997;157:849–55.

Chronic hypersensitivity pneumonitis: identification of key prognostic determinants using automated CT analysis

Joseph Jacob[1*], Brian J. Bartholmai[2], Ryoko Egashira[3], Anne Laure Brun[1], Srinivasan Rajagopalan[4], Ronald Karwoski[4], Maria Kokosi[5], David M. Hansell[1] and Athol U. Wells[5]

Abstract

Background: Chronic hypersensitivity pneumonitis (CHP) has a variable disease course. Computer analysis of CT features was used to identify a subset of CHP patients with an outcome similar to patients with idiopathic pulmonary fibrosis (IPF).

Methods: Consecutive patients with a multi-disciplinary team diagnosis of CHP ($n = 116$) had pulmonary function tests (FEV1, FVC, DLco, Kco, and a composite physiologic index [CPI]) and CT variables predictive of mortality evaluated by analysing visual and computer-based (CALIPER) parenchymal features: total interstitial lung disease (ILD) extent, honeycombing, reticular pattern, ground glass opacities, pulmonary vessel volume (PVV), emphysema, and traction bronchiectasis. Mean survival was compared between both CHP and IPF patients ($n = 185$).

Results: In CHP, visual/CALIPER measures of reticular pattern, honeycombing, visual traction bronchiectasis, and CALIPER ILD extent were predictive of mortality ($p < 0 \cdot 05$) on univariate analysis. PVV was strongly predictive of mortality on univariate ($p < 0 \cdot 0001$) and multivariate analysis independent of age, gender and disease severity (represented by the CPI [$p < 0 \cdot 01$]). CHP patients with a PVV threshold >6 · 5% of the lung had a mean survival (35 · 3 ± 6 · 1 months; $n = 20/116$ [17%]) and rate of disease progression that closely matched IPF patients (38 · 4 ± 2 · 2 months; $n = 185$).

Conclusions: Pulmonary vessel volume can identify CHP patients at risk of aggressive disease and a poor IPF-like prognosis.

Keywords: Chronic hypersensitivity pneumonitis, Pulmonary vessel volume, Idiopathic pulmonary fibrosis, Quantitative CT analysis

Background

The majority of patients with hypersensitivity pneumonitis who present to specialist centres have the chronic fibrotic form of the disease [1–3]. Within the population of chronic hypersensitivity pneumonitis (CHP) patients, it has been observed that some patients may show an accelerated rate of progression, comparable to the trajectory of idiopathic pulmonary fibrosis (IPF) [2, 4, 5]. The overlap with IPF is also evident in the often-challenging differentiation of CHP from IPF in a multi-disciplinary team (MDT) setting [5–7]. The early identification of a rapidly progressive fibrosing lung disease is increasingly relevant in an era of anti-fibrotic therapies, in which treatment guidelines are likely to increasingly broaden the spectrum of diagnoses for which anti-fibrotic treatment is indicated.

Given the varied outcome and unpredictable prognosis in CHP, the American National Heart, Lung and Blood Institute, in collaboration with the Office of Rare Diseases, convened a workshop in 2005 to discuss future research priorities in HP [8]. Amongst the various recommendations was a need to improve the characterisation of different HP phenotypes. The workshop also emphasized the desirability of exploring quantitative CT analysis in longitudinal studies of HP patients [8].

Automated computer-based quantitative imaging has advanced rapidly in recent years, with quantitatively scored CT variables shown to be superior to visual CT

* Correspondence: joseph.jacob@nhs.net
[1]Department of Radiology, Royal Brompton Hospital, Royal Brompton and Harefield NHS Foundation Trust, London, UK
Full list of author information is available at the end of the article

scores in predicting mortality in IPF. [9] To date however, quantitative CT tools have not been applied to the study of outcome in patients with CHP. Our study specifically set out to identify whether, in patients without end-stage lung disease, there are visual or quantitative CT features that characterize CHP patients who have a poor IPF-like outcome.

Methods

Study population and clinical information

All new consecutive patients with an MDT diagnosis of CHP and IPF according to published guidelines [10–12], over a four and a half year period (January 2007–July 2011) were identified from the Interstital Lung Disease Unit database. Patients with a non-contrast, supine, volumetric thin-section CT were captured. Individuals with no overt CT signs of fibrosis (the absence of honeycombing/reticular pattern/traction bronchiectasis on visual scoring by both radiologist scorers, RE and ALB) were excluded from analysis (Fig. 1).

Approval for this retrospective study of clinically indicated CT and pulmonary function test (PFT) data was obtained from the Institutional Ethics Committee and informed patient consent was not required.

CT scanning, echocardiography, PFT protocols were as previously described [9, 13] and are included in the online appendices. CALIPER CT data processing steps [9, 13] are also detailed in the online appendices.

CALIPER CT pattern quantitation

CALIPER evaluation of CT data involved algorithmic identification and volumetric quantification of 15x15x15 voxel volume units into one of six radiological parenchymal features: ground glass opacity (GGO), reticular pattern, honeycombing, emphysema, pulmonary vessel volume (PVV), and normal lung (Figs. 2 and 3).

A *fibrosis score* represented the sum of reticular pattern and honeycombing whilst the *ILD extent* additionally summed GGO extent. PVV represented the sum of the volumes of the pulmonary arteries and veins, excluding vessels at the lung hilum. All parenchymal pattern volumes were divided by the total lung volume, also derived by CALIPER, to generate percentages for each pattern.

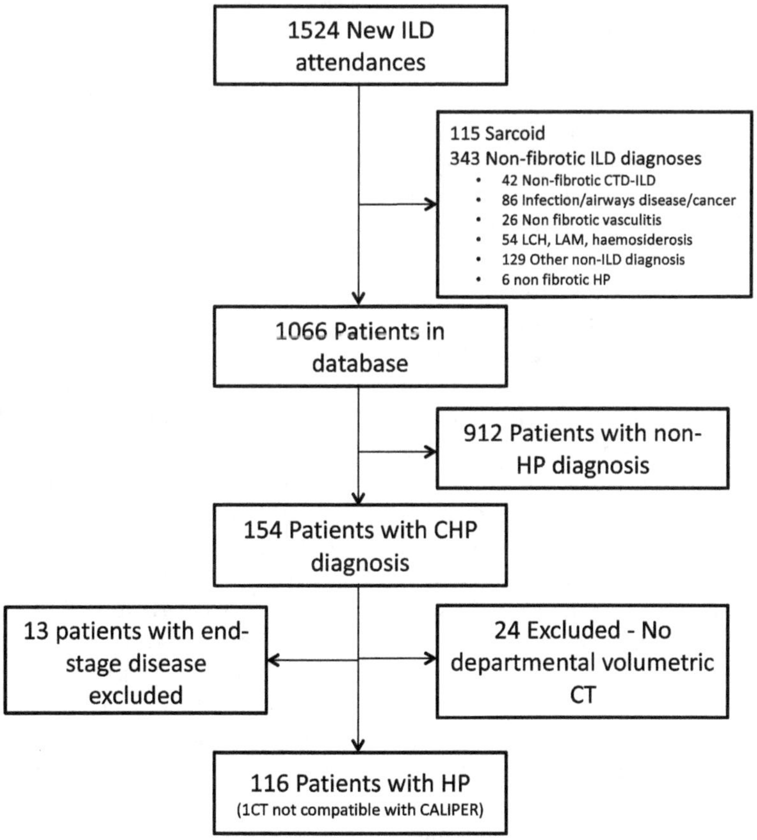

Fig. 1 Flowchart illustrating the selection of patients for the final chronic hypersensitivity pneumonitis study population. ILD = interstitial lung disease, CTD = connective tissue disease, CHP = chronic hypersensitivity pneumonitis, LCH = Langerhans cell histiocytosis, LAM = lymphangioleiomyomatosis, CT = computed tomography

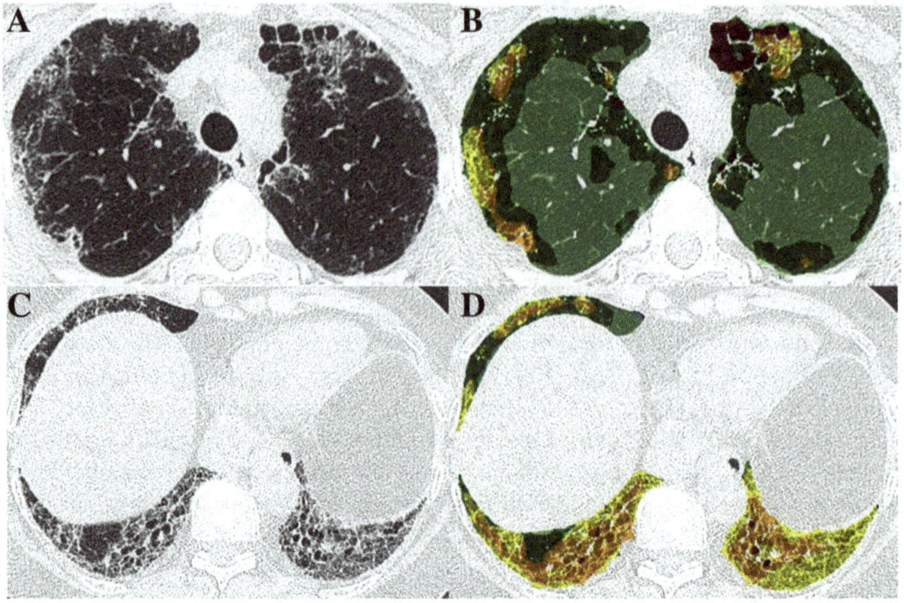

Fig. 2 Axial CT image in a 46-year-old female never smoker (**a**), diagnosed with chronic hypersensitivity pneumonitis following surgical lung biopsy. An upper lobe predominant fibrosing lung disease associated with honeycomb cysts is demonstrated. On the CALIPER colour overlay image (**b**), ground glass opacities (yellow) are interspaced with reticular pattern (orange) in the lung periphery. In the anterior left upper lobe, there are honeycomb cysts visible (brown). Light and dark green areas represent normal lung parenchyma. Axial CT image in a 55-year-old female 2-pack-year ex-smoker (**c**), diagnosed with chronic hypersensitivity pneumonitis following surgical lung biopsy with more extensive fibrosis involving the lower lobes. CALIPER colour overlay images show minor misclassification of traction bronchiectasis as honeycomb cysts in the left lower lobe (**d**), but extensive ground glass opacities (yellow) and interspaced reticular pattern (orange)

CT visual quantitation

Each CHP CT was evaluated independently by two radiologists (ALB, RE with 5 and 7 years thoracic imaging experience respectively), blinded to all clinical information. Methods by which discordant CT scores were consensed are given in the Additional file 1.

Additional visually quantified CT features included consolidation, mosaicism (decreased attenuation component), and traction bronchiectasis (no comparable CALIPER score) [details in Additional file 1]. There was no analogous visual score of PVV. A CT index of pulmonary hypertension (main pulmonary artery:ascending aorta ratio) was recorded by a single scorer using electronic caliper measurements of the ascending aorta and pulmonary artery diameters at the level of the pulmonary artery bifurcation [14, 15]. A CT UIP pattern was evaluated by one radiologist (JJ, with 5 years thoracic imaging experience) who was blinded to all clinical information.

Identification of CHP patients with end-stage disease

The study aim was to identify characteristics of the subset of CHP patients who do not have end-stage disease yet progress to death rapidly with an IPF-like trajectory. Two methods were used to identify CHP with end stage disease:

1. Contained within the consecutive CHP cases were individuals with respiratory failure secondary to end-stage fibrosing lung disease, which in itself predicates a poor outcome. PaO_2 values were examined to separate out patients who would have an inevitably rapid decline because of end-stage disease at baseline. 102/129 (79%) patients had a measured PaO_2. Patients were identified as having end-stage disease if they had a $PaO_2 < 7 \cdot 5$kPa ($n = 13$). In the 27 patients without a measured PaO_2, the use of supplementary oxygen therapy (recommended at a threshold of $<7 \cdot 3$kPaO_2 [10]) was used to identify patients with respiratory failure and therefore end-stage disease ($n = 3$). The first study group consisted of 116 CHP patients.
2. A threshold of FVC ≥ 50% predicted was also used to separate CHP patients into those with and without end-stage disease at baseline. 98/123 (80%) patients had a FVC ≥ 50% predicted. In 6 patients without a measured FVC, only one patient required supplemental home oxygen and was therefore excluded. The second study group consisted of 103 CHP patients. Analysis of this second population of non end-stage CHP patients is provided in Additional files 1, Additional file 2 and 3.

Statistical analysis

Data are given as medians, means with standard deviations, or numbers of patients with percentages where

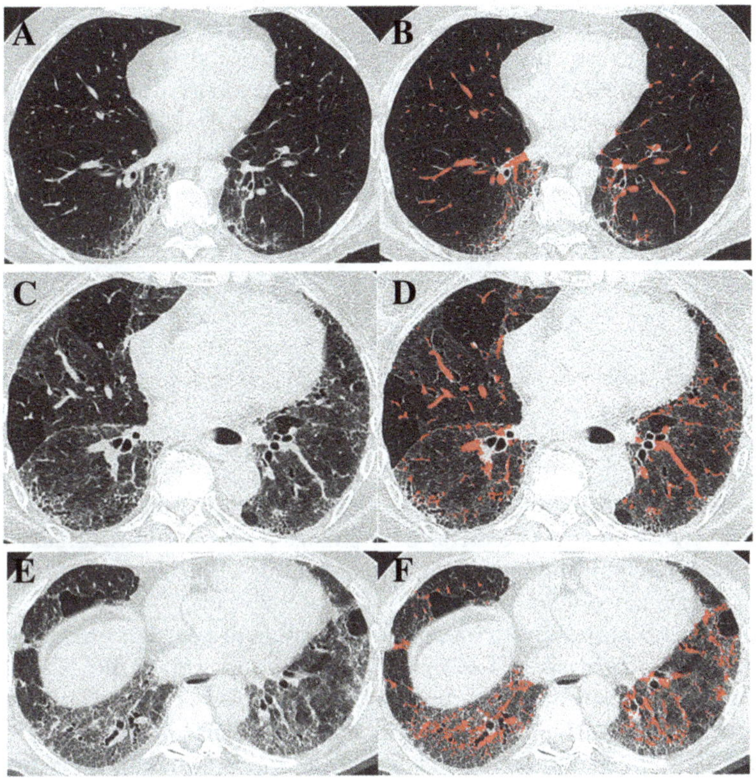

Fig. 3 Corresponding axial CT images and colour overlay maps of CALIPER quantitation of pulmonary vessel volume (red), a volumetric measure of pulmonary arteries and veins within the lung, excluding vessels at the lung hilum in three chronic hypersensitivity pneumonitis patients with mild (**a** + **b**), moderate (**c** + **d**) and severe (**e** + **f**) extents of fibrosis. Note there is misclassification of small regions of the reticular pattern in the paravertebral regions (**b**) and right lower lobe (**f**) as vessels

appropriate. Interobserver variation for visual scores was assessed using the single determination standard deviation. Univariate and multivariate Cox regression analyses of the CHP cohort were used to investigate relationships within and between the three data sets: CALIPER CT evaluation, visual CT evaluation and PFTs. To evaluate group differences, the *T*-test and Mann Whitney *U* test were used for mean and median continuous variables and the Chi-squared tests was used for categorical variables.

Cox regression analyses of CALIPER and PFT variables were used to compare the CHP and IPF cohorts. The robustness of the results was confirmed using bootstrapping and resampling of the dataset up to 1000 times. Survival curves were created using Kaplan Meier analyses and statistically significant differences between curves evaluated using the Log-Rank test. In all study analyses, a p-value of <0.05 was considered significant. Assumptions of linearity and proportional hazards were tested by visual inspection of Martingale residuals and scaled Schoenfeld residuals. Statistical analyses were performed with STATA (version 12, StatCorp, College Station, TX, USA).

Results

Demographic data

The initial study population, which has not been previously described, comprised 129 consecutive patients newly presenting with an MDT diagnosis of CHP based on a compatible clinical history and review of the following data: antigen exposure history (positive in 53/129 [41%] patients), precipitating antibodies (positive in 50/129 [39%] patients), bronchoalveolar lavage (BAL) findings (performed in 73/129 [57%] patients), CT imaging (129/129 [100%] of patients), and histopathology (60/129 [46%] of patients).

The median age at presentation was 60 years. Patient status and mean follow up time (58.0 ± 17 · 5 months) were obtained by contacting the patient's primary care giver on a given date. 50/129 patients (39%) died during the study period. Data on vital status was completed on 98% of cases with 3 patients censored. 41/73 (56%) patients undergoing BAL had a lymphocytosis ≥20% and 25/73 (34%) had a lymphocytosis ≥30%. A right ventricular systolic pressure (RVSP) >50 mmHg measured on transthoracic echocardiography was considered representative of pulmonary hypertension [16], and was found in 10/69 (14%) of the CHP cohort.

When separating the CHP population into those with and without end-stage disease using a PaO_2 threshold of $7 \cdot 5kPa0_2$, using Kaplan Meier curves, the $7 \cdot 5kPa0_2$ threshold was shown to clearly distinguish groups with a good and bad outcome (Log rank $p < 0.0001$) (Fig. 4). The primary study group consisted of 116 CHP patients. Demographic data and average visual score, CALIPER score and PFT data are provided in Table 1. Interobserver variation values for the visual scores are provided in Additional file 1 (Table 1).

CHP mortality analyses

Strong univariate CALIPER and visually-scored CT predictors of mortality in the CHP cohort included reticular pattern, honeycombing, visual traction bronchiectasis, PVV and the fibrosis score (Table 2). CALIPER and visually scored emphysema were not predictive of survival.

On bivariate analyses, PVV was a stronger predictor of mortality than FVC, DLco, and CPI (Additional file 1 [Table 2]). The results were maintained following adjustment for patient age and gender with no PFTs retaining significance in the model. In a subanalysis of CHP patients with either histopathological confirmation or antibody positivity to precipitating antigens, after adjusting for patient age and gender, PVV ($p = 0 \cdot 005$) remained a stronger predictor of mortality than FVC ($p = 0 \cdot 10$), DLco ($p = 0 \cdot 009$) and CPI ($p = 0 \cdot 01$).

Benchmarking of an IPF outcome in patients with CHP

A consecutive population of IPF patients ($n = 283$), presenting to our institution over the same period as the CHP study population was analyzed to establish a mortality profile of IPF. The IPF population has been previously evaluated in two studies [9, 13]. To identify and exclude patients with respiratory failure and end-stage disease, in a similar way to the CHP cohort, all IPF patients without a measured $Pa0_2$ ($n = 70$), as well as those patients with a $Pa0_2 < 7 \cdot 5kPa$ ($n = 28$) were excluded. 185 IPF patients were subsequently evaluated with Kaplan Meier analysis which identified the mean survival to be $38 \cdot 4 \pm 2 \cdot 2$ months (Fig. 5). Of the final population of 185 IPF patients, 74/185 (40%) patients demonstrated a definite UIP pattern on CT and 102/185 (55%) patients demonstrated a possible UIP pattern on CT. 9/185 (5%) patients had a CT pattern that was inconsistent with a UIP pattern, but which was characterised as UIP on open lung biopsy, and confirmed as IPF following MDT discussion with no support for a diagnosis of CHP or connective tissue disease related-ILD (alternative explanations of UIP).

Derivation of poor-outcome using PVV thresholds

CHP patients with an IPF-like outcome were identified by separating the CHP population into two age and gender-matched cohorts comprising 58 patients (Additional file 1 [Table 3]). No significant differences were identified for PFTs or CT parenchymal pattern scores between groups. Various PVV thresholds predictive of mortality were investigated. A PVV threshold $>6 \cdot 5\%$ of the lung showed a mean survival most comparable to IPF patients in both CHP groups: Group 1 mean survival $= 39 \cdot 7 \pm 7 \cdot 8$ months ($n = 11$; 19%); Group 2 mean survival $= 28 \cdot 2 \pm 8 \cdot 1$ months ($n = 9$; 16%).

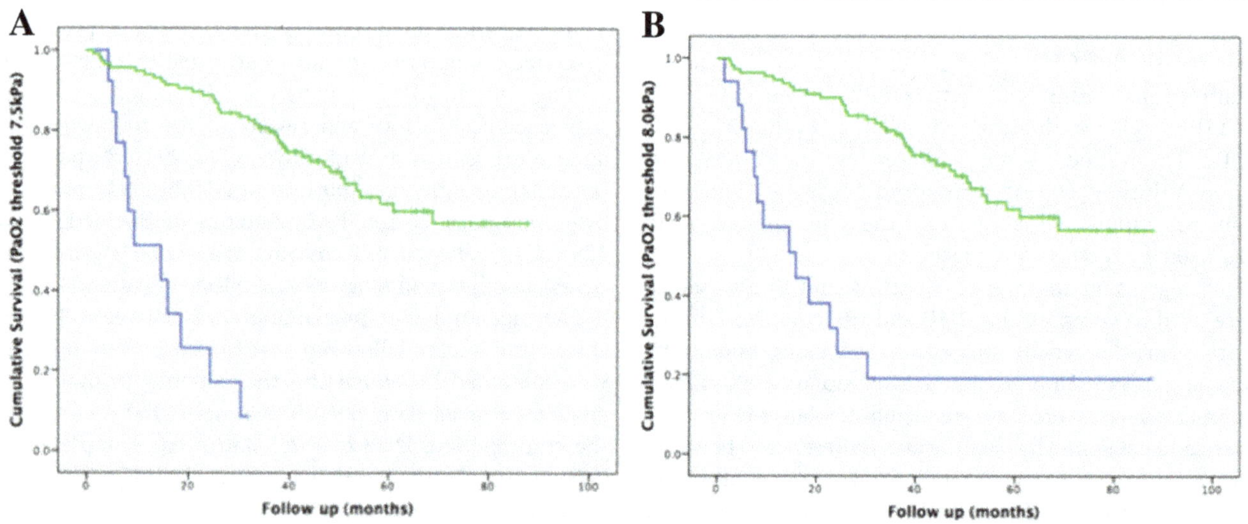

Fig. 4 Survival curves demonstrating differences in survival between chronic hypersensitivity pneumonitis patients with differing PaO2 thresholds. **a** Differences between patients with a PaO2 $>7 \cdot 5kPa$ (green)($n = 116$; mean survival $= 65 \cdot 6 \pm 2 \cdot 9$ months) and patients with a PaO2 $< 7 \cdot 5kPa$ (blue)($n = 13$; mean survival $= 14 \cdot 9 \pm 2 \cdot 7$ months). Log rank test $p = <0 \cdot 0001$. **b** Differences in survival between patients with a PaO2 $> 8kPa$ (green)($n = 112$; mean survival $= 66 \cdot 0 \pm 2 \cdot 9$ months) and patients with a PaO2 $< 8kPa$ (blue)($n = 17$; mean survival $= 27 \cdot 4 \pm 7 \cdot 6$ months). Log rank test $p = <0 \cdot 0001$

Table 1 Patient age, gender and mean and standard deviations of pulmonary function indices, CALIPER and visually scored CT parameters, and echocardiography data in patients with chronic hypersensitivity pneumonitis. Data represent mean values with standard deviations. CT computed tomography, FEV1 forced expiratory volume in one second, FVC forced vital capacity, DLco diffusing capacity for carbon monoxide, Kco carbon monoxide transfer coefficient, TLC total lung capacity, CPI composite physiological index, ILD interstitial lung disease, RVSP right ventricular systolic pressure, TxBx = traction bronchiectasis. Baseline variables in patients with hypersensitivity pneumonitis

Variable (n = 116 unless stated) Units are percentage unless stated	Value
Median Age (years)	58·5
Male/female	39/77
Survival (alive/dead)	77/39
Never smokers/ever/current-smokers (n = 128)	71/42/2
Pack years	17.5 ± 16.2
Follow up time (months)	58.0 ± 17·5
FEV1 % predicted (n = 112)	68·6 ± 19·7
FVC % predicted (n = 112)	72·2 ± 22·8
DLco % predicted (n = 109)	42·9 ± 15·8
Kco % predicted (n = 109)	70·1 ± 16·3
TLC% predicted (n = 103)	72·0 ± 16·8
CPI (n = 108)	47·9 ± 15·2
Echocardiography RVSP (mmHg) (n = 58)	35·0 ± 14·9
CALIPER ILD extent	24·3 ± 22·5
CALIPER Fibrosis extent	4·8 ± 4·1
CALIPER Ground glass opacity	19·6 ± 20·9
CALIPER Reticular pattern	4·4 ± 3·9
CALIPER Honeycombing	0·3 ± 0·6
CALIPER Emphysema	0·5 ± 1·7
CALIPER Pulmonary vessel volume	4·5 ± 1·9
CALIPER Normal lung	70·7 ± 23·8
Visual ILD extent	62·1 ± 24·6
Visual fibrosis extent	27·4 ± 19·0
Visual Ground glass opacity	33·4 ± 24·0
Visual Reticular pattern	26·4 ± 18·2
Visual Honeycombing	0·9 ± 4·1
Visual Consolidation	0·8 ± 3·3
Visual Mosaicism	5.0 ± 7·1
Visual Emphysema	3·0 ± 8v4
Visual TxBx severity (max score 18)	5·9 ± 4·7
Main pulmonary artery diameter (mm)	29·6 ± 4·9
Ascending aorta diameter (mm)	33·1 ± 3·9
Pulmonary artery:ascending aorta ratio	0.9 ± 0·1

The two CHP groups were combined and PVV thresholds were reanalyzed and compared to outcomes in the IPF population (Fig. 5). No statistically significant difference between Kaplan Meier survival curves was identified on comparison of the IPF and poor-outcome CHP groups when using a PVV threshold of 6·5% (Log rank test $p = 0·89$).

Percent-predicted DLco and CPI thresholds indicative of an IPF-equivalent outcome were examined in the CHP population ($n = 116$) and compared to the 6·5% PVV threshold. A DLco of <25% predicted was associated with a mean survival of 41·8 ± 8·1 months and a CPI threshold >65 was associated with a mean survival of 38·1 ± 6·1 months. The PVV threshold was a stronger predictor of mortality than either PFT threshold.

Combined analysis of IPF and poor-outcome CHP cases

The 20 CHP cases with an IPF-like outcome were combined with the 185 IPF cases and evaluated together using Cox proportional hazards analyses. An MDT diagnosis of CHP was not associated with an improved outcome over patients diagnosed with IPF on univariate analysis. Results were confirmed following correction for age, gender and disease severity (as estimated by the CPI) and bootstrapping of 1000 samples at a confidence interval level of 95%. Results did not change when the 70 IPF patients without a measured PaO_2 were included in the IPF cohort.

When patients were categorized as non end-stage disease using an FVC ≥ 50% predicted threshold the results were essentially unchanged (see Additional files 1, Additional file 2 and 3).

Subanalysis of the poor outcome CHP population

No difference in patient age, gender or smoking history was identified between good and bad outcome CHP patients. 13/20 (65%) of poor outcome CHP patients had histopathological or antibody-positive confirmation of a CHP diagnosis and more ILD measured visually ($p = 0·008$) and by CALIPER ($p < 0·0001$) than good outcome patients (Table 3). Overall, CALIPER variables were better able to identify differences between CHP outcome groups than visual CT scores. The mean FVC, DLco and CPI between groups were significantly different ($p < 0·0001$). However no difference was identified in either the mean RVSP ($p = 0·96$), or an RVSP value indicative of pulmonary hypertension [>50 mm Hg] [16] between outcome groups. The lack of a vasculopathic signal was reinforced by the lack of an appreciable difference in Kco values between groups ($p = 0·88$).

Discussion

Our study is the first to our knowledge to evaluate the prognostic value of quantitatively derived CT variables in

Table 2 Univariate Cox regression analysis of chronic hypersensitivity pneumonitis patients demonstrating mortality according to CALIPER indices (top white), visually derived CT indices (light grey), pulmonary function tests (dark grey), echocardiography, and clinical indices (lower white). ILD = Interstitial lung disease, DA = decreased attenuation, TxBx = traction bronchiectasis, PA = pulmonary artery, Ao = Aorta, PVV = pulmonary vessel volume, FEV_1 = forced expiratory volume in one second, FVC = forced vital capacity, TLC = total lung capacity, DLco = diffusing capacity for carbon monoxide, Kco = Carbon monoxide transfer coefficient, CPI = composite physiologic index, RVSP = right ventricular systolic pressure, NS = not significant

	Number of patients	Hazard ratio	*P* value	95.0% Confidence interval	
				Lower	Upper
Caliper indices					
Total ILD extent	116	1·02	0·001	1·01	1·03
Total fibrosis extent	116	1·32	<0·0001	1·22	1·43
Ground glass opacity	116	1·02	0·02	1·00	1·03
Reticular pattern	116	1·33	<0·0001	1·22	1·44
Honeycombing	116	2·71	0·001	1·54	4·76
Emphysema	116		NS		
Normal lung	116	0·98	0·001	0·97	0·99
PVV	116	1·56	<0·0001	1·31	1·84
Visual indices					
ILD extent	116		NS		
Fibrosis extent	116	1·06	<0·0001	1·04	1·08
Ground glass opacity	116	0·98	0·02	0·97	1·00
Reticular pattern	116	1·05	<0·0001	1·03	1·07
Honeycombing	116	1·19	0·001	1·07	1·31
Consolidation	116		NS		
Total emphysema	116		NS		
Mosaicism	116		NS		
TxBx severity	116	1·16	<0·0001	1·09	1·23
Main PA	116	1·09	0·002	1·03	1·15
Aorta	116		NS		
PA:Ao ratio	116	1·03	0·02	1·01	1·05
Pulmonary function indices					
FEV_1	112	0·98	0·02	0·96	1·00
FVC	112	0·98	0·006	0·97	0·99
TLC	103	0·96	0·0001	0·93	0·98
DLco	109	0·96	0·001	0·93	0·98
Kco	109		NS		
CPI	108	1·04	0·001	1·02	1·07
Other indices					
ECHOCARDIOGRAPHY RVSP	58		NS		
Age	116		NS		
Gender	116		NS		
Smoking history	115		NS		

patients with chronic hypersensitivity pneumonitis. Importantly, we have shown that the pulmonary vessel volume (PVV) provides a robust prognostic signal, independent of PFTs and thresholding of the PVV allowed clear prognostic distinctions to be made in CHP patients. 17% of the CHP study population had a PVV above 6·5% of the total lung volume, and these patients demonstrated a rate of disease progression, nearly identical to that of IPF.

Previous studies have reported that a proportion of CHP patients exhibit rapid decline and progression to

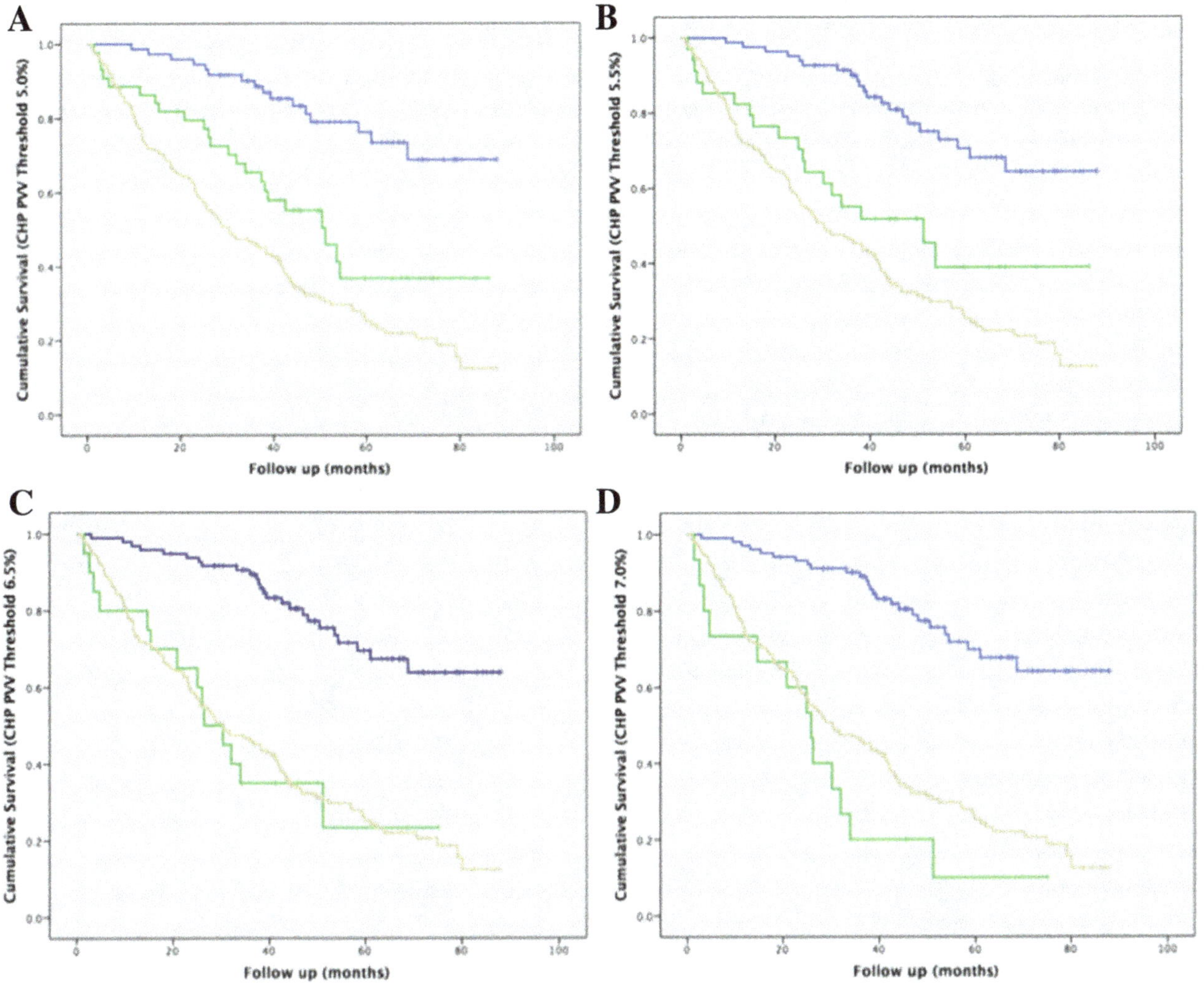

Fig. 5 Survival curves for patients with idiopathic pulmonary fibrosis (IPF) (yellow) and chronic hypersensitivity pneumonitis (CHP) (green and blue). CHP cases with end stage disease (denoted by a PaO2 < 7 · 5kPa) were excluded. IPF cases without a measured PaO2 or with end stage disease (denoted by a PaO2 < 7 · 5kPa) were excluded. IPF patients ($n = 185$) were compared to CHP cases at pulmonary vessel volume (PVV) thresholds above (green) and below (blue) 5%, 5 · 5%, 6 · 5% and 7% (**a–d**). The IPF and poor-outcome CHP curves were most comparable at a CHP PVV threshold of 6 · 5% where the mean survival in the IPF population (38 · 4 ± 2 · 2 months; $n = 185$) was found to be similar to the poor-outcome CHP population (35 · 3 ± 6 · 1 months; $n = 20$) and distinct from the good-outcome CHP population (71 · 3 ± 2 · 8 months; $n = 96$). The PVV > 6% threshold contained only two patients more than the PVV > 6 · 5% threshold which did not significantly alter the results and accordingly was not been formally plotted

death, similar to patients with IPF [4, 5]. A study of 47 histologically-confirmed UIP patients performed by Pérez-Padilla et al [4] showed that after correcting for CT disease extent, patients exposed to avian antigens had similar outcomes to patients unexposed to avian antigens [4]. A study by Mooney et al [17] demonstrated that the quartile of CHP patients with the most extensive fibrosis (the sum of visual CT reticulation and honeycomb extent scores), had an outcome comparable to IPF at 4 years. However the study by Mooney et al included CHP patients with respiratory failure and end-stage disease who would be expected to have a poor, IPF-like outcome. In our study our specific aim was to demonstrate that even with the exclusion of patients with end-stage disease, a proportion of CHP patients progress to death with an IPF-like disease course.

A prior study in CHP patients with interspaced CT imaging demonstrated that computer-derived CT variables were strongly predictive of mortality [18]. However the interspaced nature of the dataset precluded certain variables such as the pulmonary vessel volume form being adequately examined as a predictor of mortality. Given that a previous report in patients with IPF demonstrated the PVV to be the strongest CT variable for predicting mortality [9], it was a logical step to examine this key variable in a separate CHP population with volumetric CT imaging. The similar severity-adjusted survival between a subgroup of CHP patients and IPF

Table 3 Patient demographics, pulmonary function indices, CALIPER and visually scored CT parameters and echocardiography data in 2 groups of chronic hypersensitivity pneumonitis patients. Group 1 had an IPF-like outcome ($n = 20$) and group 2 had a good outcome ($n = 96$). Differences between groups were assessed using the *T*-test for continuous variables, the Mann Whitney *U* test for differences in continuous median values and the Chi-Squared test for categorical variables. CT = computed tomography, FEV1 = forced expiratory volume in one second, FVC = forced vital capacity, DLco = diffusing capacity for carbon monoxide, Kco = carbon monoxide transfer coefficient, TLC = total lung capacity, CPI = composite physiological index, ILD = interstitial lung disease, RVSP = right ventricular systolic pressure TxBx = traction bronchiectasis, PA = pulmonary artery. Comparison of hypersensitivity pneumonitis patients groups: IPF-like versus non-IPF-like outcome

Variable Units are percentage unless stated	Group 1 (*n* = 20 unless stated in brackets)	Group 2 (*n* = 96 unless stated in brackets)	Group Differences
Median Age (years)	56·5	59	NS
Male/female	7/13	32/64	NS
Survival (alive/dead)	6/14	71/25	<0·0001
Never/ever/current smokers	15/4/0 (19)	56/38/2	NS
Pack years	28·5 ± 26·5	16·4 ± 14·9	NS
FEV1 % predicted	48·1 ± 12·1 (18)	72·5 ± 18·4 (94)	<0·0001
FVC % predicted	45·6± 10·8 (18)	77·3 ± 20·9 (94)	<0·0001
DLco % predicted	28·1 ± 8·4 (16)	45·5 ± 15·4 (93)	<0·0001
Kco % predicted	70·4± 16·4 (16)	70·1 ± 16·3 (93)	NS
TLC% predicted	50·9± 7·2 (14)	75·3 ± 15·4 (89)	<0·0001
CPI	64·6± 6·5 (16)	45·0 ± 14·3 (92)	<0·0001
Echocardiography RVSP (mmHg)	33·0± 6·5 (8)	35·4 ± 15·9 (50)	NS
CALIPER ILD extent	58·6± 17·2	17·2 ± 15·9	<0·0001
CALIPER Ground glass opacity	48·7± 21·1	13·5 ± 14·9	<0·0001
CALIPER Reticular pattern	9·4 ± 5·1	3·4 ± 2·5	<0·0001
CALIPER Honeycombing	0·5 ± 1·1	0·3 ± 0·4	NS
CALIPER Emphysema	0·2 ± 0·4	0·5 ± 1·8	NS
CALIPER Pulmonary vessel volume	7·7 ± 0v8	3·8 ± 1·3	<0·0001
Visual ILD extent	74·9± 17·4	59·5 ± 25·1	=0·002
Visual Ground glass opacity	24·1 ± 13·5	35·3 ± 25·3	=0.006
Visual Reticular pattern	44·4± 14·7	22·7 ± 16·6	<0·0001
Visual Honeycombing	3·6 ± 9·5	0·4 ± 1·1	NS
Visual Emphysema	0·3 ± 0·5	3·5 ± 9·2	=0·001
Visual TxBx severity (max score 18)	9·2 ± 4·9	5·2 ± 4·4	=0·0004
Main PA diameter (mm)	31·5 ± 4·5	29·2 ± 4·9	NS
Ascending aorta diameter (mm)	32·2 ± 4·3	33·3 ± 3·9	NS
PA:ascending aorta ratio	1.0 ± 0.2	0.9 ± 0.1	=0.006

patients identified in the current study corroborates previous observations that a subset of CHP patients have an outcome nearly identical to IPF. [2, 4, 5] Whilst our findings do not identify the mechanism for this difference, three potential contributing factors could be considered.

Firstly, the PVV threshold may identify CHP patients that have more aggressive lung disease. Alternatively PVV may be providing added information regarding pulmonary vasculopathy, though the similarities in RVSP and Kco between good and bad outcome CHP groups makes this unlikely. Lastly vessel size may be a better marker of interstitial severity than functional indices. The high negative intrathoracic pressures generated during respiration in patients with fibrosing lung disease may increase as fibrosis worsens, drawing extra blood into the lungs as well as concomitantly exerting a pull on pulmonary vessel walls. The mortality signal associated with a high PVV may therefore reflect worsening pulmonary fibrosis.

Intriguingly, a study evaluating pulmonary angiogenesis in patients with CHP has identified elevated levels of vascular endothelial growth factor in the lungs of CHP patients when compared to control subjects [19]. Angiogenesis represents a physiological, hypoxia-induced response within the tissues to facilitate improvements in gas exchange. Therefore an increase in the PVV may represent a response to the progressive impairment in gas exchange that results as the interstitial damage progresses.

The PVV threshold of >6·5% of the lung demonstrated a stronger distinction between groups than any individual PFT and has the additional benefit of avoiding the issue of observer disagreement associated with subjective visual CT scoring. Furthermore, given recent evidence suggesting variability between MDTs in making a CHP diagnosis [7], we were able to confirm the PVV signal strength in patients with either a histopathological CHP diagnosis or antibody positivity.

Significant univariate predictors of mortality in the current study are in line with previous reports that have identified CT markers of fibrosis including reticulation [17], honeycombing [20, 21], traction bronchiectasis [3] and a fibrosis score (sum of reticulation and honeycombing) [1, 17, 22] as predictors of a poor prognosis in CHP. A mosaic attenuation pattern (scored as the decreased attenuation component), however, was not predictive of mortality in contrast to the findings in histopathologically proven CHP cases of Lima et al. [1] Emphysema extent scored on CT had no bearing on prognosis, a result which could arguably be reconciled with the relatively limited extent of emphysema in our CHP cohort.

In the CHP group with an IPF-like outcome, the majority (79%) of patients were never smokers and unlike previous reports in CHP, smoking was not associated with a worse outcome [23]. Similarly, the presence of pulmonary hypertension was not associated with a worsened prognosis in contrast to the study by Koschel et al. [24] However the study by Koschel et al [24] did not correct for baseline disease extent when analyzing outcome in CHP patients with pulmonary hypertension which could have negated the study findings.

Of the PFTs, the total lung capacity (TLC) was the strongest predictor of mortality on univariate analysis, echoing the findings of Mooney et al [17]. However, the same association of TLC with mortality was not replicated in a study by Vourlekis et al [2]. On multivariate analysis, CT variables, particularly CALIPER PVV, were stronger predictors of mortality than FVC, DLco, and CPI. The findings mirror the results of the study by Walsh et al which reported the superiority of visual CT variables over any PFTs in predicting mortality in CHP [3].

In our analysis, we deliberately excluded patients with end-stage fibrosing lung disease to allow the identification of patients at risk of a poor outcome, but in whom, targeted intervention might reasonably be expected to modify disease progression. Patients with end-stage disease, characterized by the requirement of oxygen therapy at rest, more usually enter palliative care pathways rather than aggressive medical treatment. The poor outcome of such end-stage CHP cases was highlighted in the study by Mooney et al in which, unsurprisingly, oxygen therapy was shown to be predictive of mortality on multivariate analysis [17]. In our study, with the exclusion of end-stage patients, a significant proportion of CHP patients (17%) had an outcome comparable to IPF.

There are limitations to the current study. In an era in which the MDT diagnosis is the accepted diagnostic standard, the number of patients undergoing surgical biopsy for tissue diagnosis is inevitably reduced. Though only 46% of patients in the final study had a surgical biopsy, the diagnosis of CHP on a histopathological examination alone may not be definitive, as studies have shown that the majority of biopsy samples do not show all of the classical pathological features [1, 6]. The PVV variable was found to be liable to minor contamination as areas of reticular pattern, predominantly in the lung periphery, were captured and classified as vessels. The noise associated with the PVV signal when improved in future iterations of similar software would likely strengthen our observations. Though the median age of our CHP population was slightly higher than several prior CHP studies [2, 25, 26], it was similar to the study by Mooney et al [17] whilst the median age of the poor-outcome CHP group was similar to the HP population in the study by Lacasse et al [25]. We do not believe that these limitations diminish the applicability of our results to patients with an MDT diagnosis of CHP.

Conclusions

In conclusion, we have demonstrated that a significant proportion of CHP patients have an IPF-like outcome and that this can be predicted from the PVV derived from CALIPER software. This novel finding may have a role in identifying the subgroup of CHP patients who may benefit from close monitoring and intervention to control disease progression.

Additional files

Additional file 1: Brief description of data: Methodological information regarding: pulmonary function test, echocardiography and CT scanning protocols and details regarding CALIPER CT scoring and visual CT scoring and consensus formulation of visual CT scores. A further analysis of end-stage patients defined using an FVC threshold <50% predicted is also included. Two tables highlighting the single determination standard deviation values for the two radiologist scores and a comparison of age and gender matched hypersensitivity pneumonitis groups are also included.

Additional file 2: Figure S1. Brief description of data: Survival curves demonstrating outcomes in non end-stage (defined using an FVC threshold >50% predicted) hypersensitivity pneumonitis patients.

Additional file 3: Figure S2. Brief description of data: Survival curves comparing poor-outcome (defined using an FVC threshold >50% predicted) chronic hypersensitivity pneumonitis patients and idiopathic pulmonary fibrosis patients using Kaplan Meier curve analysis.

Abbreviations

Ao: Aorta; BAL: Broncho-alveolar lavage; CALIPER: Computer-aided lung informatics for pathology evaluation and rating; CHP: Chronic hypersensitivity pneumonitis; CI: Confidence interval; CPI: Composite physiologic index; CT: Computed tomography; DA: Decreased attenuation; DLco: Diffusing capacity for carbon monoxide; FEV1: Forced expiratory volume in one second; FVC: Forced vital capacity; GGO: Ground glass opacity; HR: Hazard ratio; ILD: Interstitial lung disease; IPF: Idiopathic pulmonary fibrosis; Kco: Carbon monoxide transfer coefficient; MDT: Multi-disciplinary team; PA: Pulmonary artery; PaO_2: Partial pressure of oxygen; PFT: Pulmonary function test; PVV: Pulmonary vessel volume; RVSP: Right ventricular systolic pressure; TLC: Total lung capacity; TxBx: Traction bronchiectasis; UIP: Usual interstitial pneumonia

Acknowledgements

The manuscript was supported by the National Institute of Health Research Respiratory Disease Biomedical Research Unit at the Royal Brompton and Harefield NHS Foundation Trust and Imperial College London.

We would also like to thank Professor David Hansell without whom the bulk of this work would not have been possible.

Funding

There is no funding source for the current study. Joseph Jacob had full access to all the data in the study and had final responsibility for the decision to submit for publication.

Authors' contributions

JJ, MK, RE, ALB, AUW, DMH were involved in either the acquisition, or analysis or interpretation of data for the study. JJ, AUW and DMH were also involved in the conception and design of the study. BJB, RK and SR invented and developed CALIPER. They were involved in processing the raw CT scans and in generation of figures but were not involved with the analysis or interpretation of the data in the study. All authors revised the work for important intellectual content and gave final approval for the version to be published. All authors agree to be accountable for the all aspects of the work in ensuring that questions related to the accuracy or integrity of any part of the work are appropriately investigated and resolved.

Competing interests

JJ reports personal fees from Boehringer Ingelheim unrelated to the work in the current manuscript. BJB, RK, SR report a grant from the Royal Brompton Hospital during the conduct of the study; another from Imbio, LLC, was outside the submitted work; and all have a patent: SYSTEMS AND METHODS FOR ANALYZING IN VIVO TISSUE VOLUMES USING MEDICAL IMAGING DATA licensed to Imbio, LLC. AUW receives personal fees for participating in advisory boards and speaking at symposia from Boehringer Ingelheim, Intermune, Roche and Bayer, and for participating in advisory boards from Gilead, MSD and speaker fees from Chiesi. DMH has received a grant from Intermune for creating an educational website and consultancy and receives personal consultancy fees from AstraZeneca, Boehringer Ingelheim, Intermune, Roche, Sanofi, Glaxo Smith Kline. DMH is the recipient of a National Institute of Health Research Senior Investigator Award.

Consent for publication

Not applicable.

Author details

[1]Department of Radiology, Royal Brompton Hospital, Royal Brompton and Harefield NHS Foundation Trust, London, UK. [2]Division of Radiology, Mayo Clinic Rochester, Rochester, MN, USA. [3]Department of Radiology, Faculty of Medicine, Saga University, 5-1-1 Nabeshima, Saga-City, Japan. [4]Department of Physiology and Biomedical Engineering, Mayo Clinic Rochester, Rochester, MN, USA. [5]Interstitial Lung Disease Unit, Royal Brompton Hospital, Royal Brompton and Harefield NHS Foundation Trust, London, UK.

References

1. Lima MS, Coletta ENAM, Ferreira RG, et al. Subacute and chronic hypersensitivity pneumonitis: Histopathological patterns and survival. Respir Med. 2009;103(4): 508–15.
2. Vourlekis JS, Schwarz MI, Cherniack RM, et al. The effect of pulmonary fibrosis on survival in patients with hypersensitivity pneumonitis. Am J Med. 2004;116:662–8.
3. Walsh SL, Sverzellati N, Devaraj A, et al. Chronic hypersensitivity pneumonitis: high resolution computed tomography patterns and pulmonary function indices as prognostic determinants. Eur Radiol. 2012;22(8):1672–9.
4. Perez-Padilla R, Salas J, Chapel R, et al. Mortality in Mexican patients with chronic pigeon breeder's lung compared to those with usual interstitial pneumonia. Am Rev Respir Dis. 1993;148:49–53.
5. Churg A, Sin DD, Everett D, et al. Pathologic patterns and survival in chronic hypersensitivity pneumonitis. Am J Surg Pathol. 2009;33(12):1765–70.
6. Morell F, Villar A, Montero M-I, et al. Chronic hypersensitivity pneumonitis in patients diagnosed with idiopathic pulmonary fibrosis: a prospective case-cohort study. Lancet Respir Med. 2013;1(9):685–94.
7. Walsh SLF, Wells AU, Desai SR, et al. Multicentre evaluation of multidisciplinary team meeting agreement on diagnosis in diffuse parenchymal lung disease: a case-cohort study. Lancet Respir Med. 2016;4(7):557–65.
8. Fink JN, Ortega HG, Reynolds HY, et al. Needs and opportunities for research in hypersensitivity pneumonitis. Am J Respir Crit Care Med. 2005;171(7):792–8.
9. Jacob J, Bartholmai B, Rajagopalan S, et al. Mortality prediction in idiopathic pulmonary fibrosis: evaluation of automated computer tomographic analysis with conventional severity measures. Eur Respir J. 2016; doi: 10.1183/13993003.01011-2016.
10. Wells AU, Hirani N. Interstitial lung disease guideline. Thorax. 2008;63 Suppl 5:v1–v58.
11. Travis WD, Costabel U, Hansell DM, et al. An official American thoracic society/European respiratory society statement: update of the international multidisciplinary classification of the idiopathic interstitial pneumonias. Am J Respir Crit Care Med. 2013;188(6):733–48.
12. Raghu G, Collard HR, Egan JJ, et al. An official ATS/ERS/JRS/ALAT statement: idiopathic pulmonary fibrosis: evidence-based guidelines for diagnosis and management. Am J Respir Crit Care Med. 2011;183(6):788–824.
13. Jacob J, Bartholmai B, Rajagopalan S, et al. Automated quantitative CT versus visual CT scoring in idiopathic pulmonary fibrosis: validation against pulmonary function. J Thorac Imaging. 2016;31:304–11.
14. Ng CS, Wells AU, Padley SP. A CT sign of chronic pulmonary arterial hypertension: the ratio of main pulmonary artery to aortic diameter. J Thorac Imaging. 1999; 14(4):270–8.
15. Edwards PD, Bull RK, Coulden R. CT measurement of main pulmonary artery diameter. Br J Radiol. 1998;71:1018–20.
16. Bossone E, D'Andrea A, D'Alto M, et al. Echocardiography in pulmonary arterial hypertension: from diagnosis to prognosis. J Am Soc Echocardiogr. 2013;26(1):1–14.
17. Mooney JJ, Elicker BM, Urbania TH, et al. Radiographic fibrosis score predicts survival in hypersensitivity pneumonitis. Chest. 2013;144(2):586–92.
18. Jacob J, Bartholmai B, Rajagopalan S, et al. Automated computer-based CT stratification as a predictor of outcome in hypersensitivity pneumonitis. Eur Radiol. 2016;Accepted for publication.
19. Navarro C, Ruiz V, Gaxiola M, et al. Angiogenesis in hypersensitivity pneumonitis. Arch Physiol Biochem. 2003;111(4):365–8.

20. Gaxiola M, Buendía-Roldán I, Mejía M, et al. Morphologic diversity of chronic pigeon breeders disease: clinical features and survival. Respir Med. 2011; 105(4):608–14.
21. Tateishi T, Ohtani Y, Takemura T, et al. Serial high-resolution computed tomography findings of acute and chronic hypersensitivity pneumonitis induced by avian antigen. J Comput Assist Tomogr. 2011;35(2):272–9.
22. Hanak V, Golbin JM, Hartman TE, et al. High-resolution CT findings of parenchymal fibrosis correlate with prognosis in hypersensitivity pneumonitis. Chest. 2008;134(1):133–8.
23. Ohtsuka Y, Munakata M, Tanimura K, et al. Smoking promotes insidious and chronic farmer's lung disease, and deteriorates the clinical outcome. Intern Med. 1995;34(10):966–71.
24. Koschel DS, Cardoso C, Weidemann B, Hoffken G, Halank M. Pulmonary hypertension in chronic hypersensitivity pneumonitis. Lung. 2012;190:295–302.
25. Lacasse Y, Selman M, Costabel U, et al. Clinical diagnosis of hypersensitivity pneumonitis. Am J Respir Crit Care Med. 2003;168(8):952–8.
26. Hanak V, Golbin JM, Ryu JH. Causes and presenting features in 85 consecutive patients with hypersensitivity pneumonitis. Mayo Clin Proc. 2007;82(7):812–6.

16

Single use and conventional bronchoscopes for Broncho alveolar lavage (BAL) in research: a comparative study (NCT 02515591)

Seher Raza Zaidi[1,2*†], Andrea M. Collins[1,2*†], Elena Mitsi[1], Jesús Reiné[1], Kayleigh Davies[2], Angela D Wright[1,2,3], Jessica Owugha[1], Richard Fitzgerald[2], Amitava Ganguli[2], Stephen B Gordon[4], Daniela Mulari Ferreira[1] and Jamie Rylance[1,2]

Abstract

Background: Broncho alveolar lavage (BAL) is widely used for investigative research to study innate, cellular and humoral immune responses, and in early phase drug trials. Conventional (multiple use) flexible bronchoscopes have time and monetary costs associated with cleaning, and carries a small risk of cross infection. Single use bronchoscopes may provide an alternative, but have not been evaluated in this context.

Methods: Healthy volunteers underwent bronchoscopy at a day-case clinical research unit using the Ambu® aScope™ single-use flexible intubation bronchoscope. Broncho alveolar lavage was performed from a sub segmental bronchus within the right middle lobe; a total of 200 ml of warmed normal saline was instilled then aspirated using handheld suction. BAL volume yield, cell yield and viability were recorded.

Results: Ten volunteers, (mean age 23 years, six male) participated. Bronchoscopies were carried out by one of two senior bronchoscopists, experienced in the technique of obtaining BAL for research purposes. The results were compared to 50 (mean age 23, 14 male) procedures performed using the conventional scope by the same two bronchoscopists. The total volume yield was significantly higher in the disposable group median 152 ml (IQR 141–166 ml) as compared to conventional 124 ml (110–135 ml), $p = <0.01$. The total cell yield and viability were similar in both groups, with no significant differences.

Conclusions: With single use bronchoscopes, we achieved a larger BAL volume yield than conventional bronchoscopes, with comparable cell yield and viability. Better volume yields can potentially reduce post procedure side effects such as pleuritic chest pain and cough. The risk of cross infection can be eliminated, providing reassurance to researchers and participants. Reduced maintenance requirements can be cost effective. These could potentially be used for early phase drug development studies.

Keywords: Research Bronchoscopy, Bronchoalveolar Lavage, Single use bronchoscopes, Bronchoscopy, Bronchoalveolar lavage fluid, Lung diseases

* Correspondence: seher.zaidi@lstmed.ac.uk; andrea.collins@liverpool.ac.uk
†Equal contributors
[1]Respiratory Infection Group, Liverpool School of Tropical Medicine, Pembroke Place, Liverpool L3 5QA, UK
Full list of author information is available at the end of the article

Background

Flexible bronchoscopy is widely performed in adults and children for investigation of pulmonary pathology [1, 2]. Broncho alveolar lavage (BAL) sampling is used to study innate, cellular and humoral immune responses, determining the cell population profiles that can facilitate the diagnosis of various diffuse lung diseases [3–7]. It is used in early phase drug development studies and has a well-proven safety record in both research and in clinical applications. BAL is easily performed and well-tolerated with rare complications [8–10].

Typically, conventional flexible bronchoscopes are used but they are associated with significant costs related to initial purchase, ongoing maintenance, and sterilisation [11, 12]. Single use bronchoscopes offer an alternative [11] and are currently used in many UK NHS trusts for both emergency and elective airway intubations [13]. Single use scopes are more portable, and might also improve working efficiency [12]. Their efficacy for research studies has not yet been demonstrated, notably in research BAL the cell number and viability, and the returned volume of epithelial lining fluid is critical. Maximising the volume of BAL fluid returned has potential advantages to both researchers and participants: procedures that return less than 100 mL are more frequently associated with side effects such as cough, pleuritic chest pain and fever. Larger total instilled volumes of a minimum of 100 mL and a recommended standard 240 mL using standard 4×60 mL aliquots have therefore been recommended by the European Respiratory Society (ERS) to improve standardization when more efficient alveolar sampling and accurate quantitative measurements are required [14]. For cellular studies, function and viability are important, and may be maximised by the use of manual suction which minimises cellular shear forces [8]. Rapid processing by designated laboratory staff highly trained in handling of BALF (BAL fluid) samples is ideal. However, it should be noted that there is no strong relationship between the volumes returned and cell numbers obtained (unpublished data from our group).

This study presents a comparison of single use disposable bronchoscopes and conventional bronchoscopes with regards to BAL volumes, cell yields and viability using each method.

Methods

The aim of the study was to compare the BAL volume yield, total cell yield and viability between samples obtained using single use and conventional bronchoscopes. Table 1 compares different features of the single use and flexible bronchoscopes.

Recruitment

We enrolled healthy volunteers aged 18–55 years old, to undergo bronchoscopy using the Ambu® aScope™ Regular 5.0/2.2 single-use flexible intubation bronchoscope. The study was carried out in the Clinical Research Unit (CRU) at the Royal Liverpool University Hospital (RLUH). The primary aim was to compare the BAL volume yield (mL), cell yield (total cell number) and proportion of viable cells (alveolar macrophages [AM] and lymphocytes), with recent data from procedures using conventional bronchoscopes. Conventional procedures were performed on 50 healthy volunteers recruited at the same site with identical inclusion and exclusion criteria. The demographics are described in Table 2.

A physical examination including vital signs was performed. A detailed history of complications associated with other procedures or trauma was obtained, and risks for bleeding sought according to guidelines [7], specifically medications (e.g. clopidogrel, aspirin, Coumadin, heparin), and relevant medical conditions (e.g. uremia). Exclusion criteria were: a history of allergic reaction to benzodiazepines, or any anaesthetic agent; smoking history of > 10 pack years; any tobacco smoking in the preceding 3 months; pregnancy; abnormalities of screening blood tests (haemoglobin, white cell count, platelets, liver transaminases, bilirubin, renal and clotting profile).

Table 1 Features of Single-use and Multiple Use Bronchoscopes

		Multiple Use Bronchoscope	Single-use Bronchoscope
Optical Systems	Field of View	120°	85°
	Direction of View	Forward Viewing	Forward Viewing
	Depth of field	2–100 mm	8–19 mm
Insertion section	Distal end outer diameter	4.8 mm	5.4 mm
	Insertion tube outer diameter	4.9 mm	5.0 mm
	Working length	600 mm	600 mm
Instrument Channel		2.0 mm	2.0 mm
Risk of cross infection		Yes	No
Potential delay due to cleaning		Yes	No
Cost		Sterilisation Servicing Initial equipment cost	Repeated purchase cost
Portability		Depends on location of image processing unit	Can be hand held

Table 2 Demographics

	Single-use ($n = 10$)	Conventional ($n = 50$)
Age (yr) mean ± SD [a]	23.4 ± 1.8	25.9 ± 4.2
Males (%)	6 (60%)	19 (37.2%)

[a] Un-paired T-test

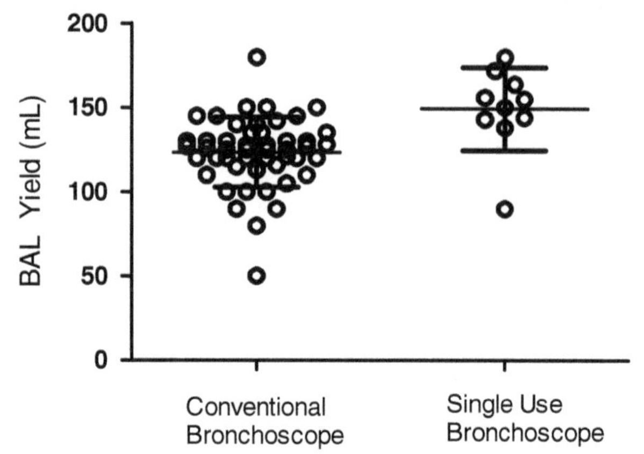

Fig. 1 BAL Fluid Volume Yield (mL) from Conventional vs Single-use Bronchoscopes

Bronchoscopy and Broncho alveolar lavage

Bronchoscopy was carried out as a day case according to previously published protocol [8]. Briefly, local anaesthesia was attained using topical lidocaine gel and spray, with further 4% lidocaine administered to the larynx and 2% lidocaine to the bronchial tree via the scope. Warmed 0.9% saline was instilled to the right middle lobe in sequential aliquots (60, 50 and 40 mL), with aspiration into a sterile syringe using gentle manual suction. BAL yields were recorded, and fluid transported immediately to the laboratory on melting ice [8]. We used continuous monitoring of heart rate, blood pressure and oxygen saturations during the procedure, with supplemental oxygen given by nasal cannula.

All procedures were carried out by one of two senior bronchoscopists, experienced in obtaining BAL for research purposes. Hospital procedures required that conventional bronchoscopy was performed in the surgical theatres, whereas flexible bronchoscopy was performed in the research ward: this was the only difference between the groups.

Sample processing

BAL fluid (BALF) was filtered through double layered gauze to remove mucus plugs. Cells were pelleted by centrifugation (1500 rpm for 10 min at 4 °C), and washed with 50 mL cold RPMI medium (Gibco™ RPMI 1640 Medium) containing antibiotics (Penicillin, Neomycin and Streptomycin, Sigma-Aldrich, Sigma Chemical Co. St. Louis, MO, USA). The centrifugation step was repeated once, and the cell pellet was re-suspended in culture medium, with the addition of 10% FBS Gibco-Invitrogen (Life Technologies GmbH, Eggenstein, Germany). Cell suspensions were examined as five times diluted in trypan blue for counting and viability assessment using a haemocytometer.

Statistical analysis

Primary outcome measures were compared with values from the preceding 50 conventional procedures using the Mann Whitney U Test. Statistical analyses were performed with Graph Pad Prism version 5.0, Graph Pad Software, La Jolla, CA, USA).

Results

Ten participants (6 male), mean age of 23.4 years (range 20–26 years) were enrolled. All participants were intubated nasally, and only one requested sedation (midazolam 3 mg used). The median BAL volume yield from the single-use bronchoscopes was 152 mL (IQR 141–166 mL) as compared to conventional 124 mL (110–135 mL), $p < 0.01$ (Fig. 1). The median total cell yield from single-use bronchoscopes was 7.33×10^6 (5.13×10^6–9.80×10^6) compared with 7.0×10^6 (4.53×10^6–1.64×10^7) for conventional procedures, $p = 0.61$ (Fig. 2). The median cell viability for samples from single use bronchoscopes was 98.5% (93.8–100) compared to 98.2% (93.7–100%), $p = 0.75$ (Fig. 3). The comparison for the demographics is described in Table 2.

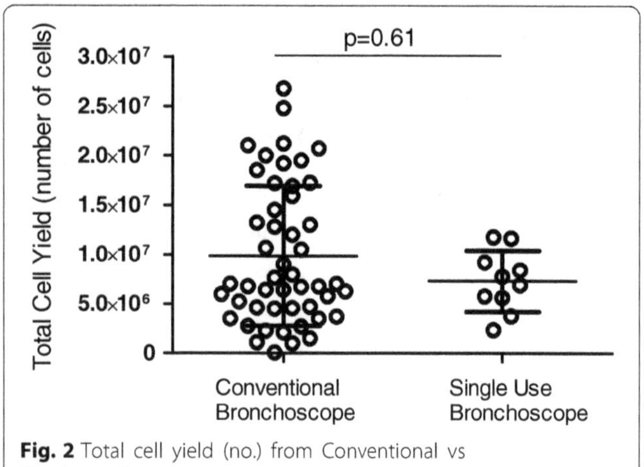

Fig. 2 Total cell yield (no.) from Conventional vs Single-use Bronchoscopes

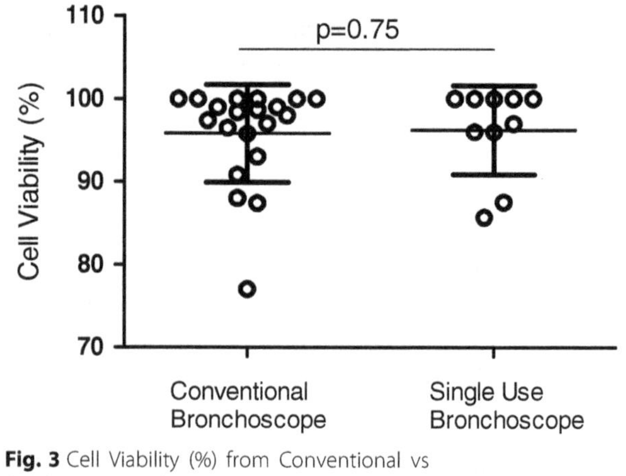

Fig. 3 Cell Viability (%) from Conventional vs Single-use Bronchoscopes

Discussion

Broncho alveolar lavage with single-use flexible bronchoscope achieved greater BAL volume yields than with conventional bronchoscopes. There was no significant difference between the cell yield and viability between the methods.

Single-use bronchoscopes have been evaluated in the critical care setting with favourable evaluation for bronchoscopy, tracheostomy, intubation and suction [11]. Our group has experience of over 1500 research BALs, and the procedures in this study were performed by senior bronchoscopists with extensive experience of BAL for research purposes; allowing good comparison with the use of conventional bronchoscopes. BAL volume yields were similar in male and female participants in our study, as seen in other studies [15].

The greater BAL volume return achieved with single-use bronchoscopes could lead to reduced risk of post-procedural side effects such as cough, pleuritic chest pain and fever, which may improve tolerability and participant comfort. However, we have not systematically collected these data.

Single use flexible bronchoscopes have the potential for use in pharmaceutical preclinical and clinical studies for medicine development.

Conclusion

Single-use flexible bronchoscopes can be used to obtain BAL for research purposes to study immune responses and in early phase drug development studies.

Abbreviations

BAL: Broncho alveolar Lavage; RML: Right Middle Lobe bronchus

Acknowledgements

We would like to thank all the volunteers for their participation, the staff on the RLUH clinical research unit and in the LSTM laboratory for help and support during the study and also Ambu® for supporting this study, by providing single use flexible bronchoscopes.

Funding

Data for this study was collected with grant support from Bill and Melinda Gates Foundation and the Medical Research Council. Personnel and estates costs were also provided by the clinical research unit at the Royal Liverpool University Hospital and the Liverpool School of Tropical Medicine.

Authors' contributions

SZ Manuscript writing and drafting, data analysis and interpretation. AC Manuscript writing and drafting, writing study protocol, performing procedures and recruitment. EM Manuscript writing and drafting, sample processing, obtaining data, data analysis and interpretation. KD Manuscript writing and drafting, study protocol, recruitment and assisting in procedures. AW Manuscript writing and drafting, study protocol, recruitment and assisting in procedures. JO Manuscript writing and drafting, sample processing, obtaining data. JR Manuscript writing and drafting, sample processing, obtaining data. RF Manuscript writing and drafting, study protocol, recruitment. AG Manuscript writing and drafting, study protocol, recruitment. SG Manuscript writing and drafting, study protocol. DF Manuscript writing and drafting, study protocol, sample processing, obtaining data, data analysis and interpretation. JR Manuscript writing and drafting, performed procedures, study protocol, recruitment, sample processing, obtaining data, data analysis and interpretation. All authors read and approved the final manuscript.

Competing interests

Authors do not have any competing interests related to this study. The single use, flexible bronchoscopes were provided free of charge for use by Ambu®, with no input in the study design, analysis or manuscript drafting.

Consent for publication

Not applicable.

Author details

[1]Respiratory Infection Group, Liverpool School of Tropical Medicine, Pembroke Place, Liverpool L3 5QA, UK. [2]Respiratory Research Group, Royal Liverpool and Broadgreen University Hospital NHS Trust, Liverpool L7 8XP, UK. [3]Clinical Research Network, Northwest Coast, Liverpool, UK. [4]Malawi-Liverpool-Wellcome Trust Clinical Research Programme, Blantyre, Malawi.

References

1. Rose AS, Knox KS. Bronchoalveolar lavage as a research tool. Semin Respir Crit Care Med. 2007;28(5):561–73.
2. Davies J, Payne D. Research applications of bronchoscopy. Paediatr Respir Rev. 2003;4(3):230–6.
3. Gordon SB, Irving GR, Lawson RA, Lee ME, Read RC. Intracellular trafficking and killing of Streptococcus pneumoniae by human alveolar macrophages are influenced by opsonins. Infect Immun. 2000;68(4):2286–93.
4. Gordon SB, Miller DE, Day RB, Ferry T, Wilkes DS, Schnizlein-Bick CT, et al. Pulmonary Immunoglobulin Responses to Streptococcus pneumoniae Are Altered but Not Reduced in Human Immunodeficiency Virus–Infected Malawian Adults. J Infect Dis. 2003;188(5):666–70.
5. Jambo KC, Sepako E, Fullerton DG, Mzinza D, Glennie S, Wright AK, et al. Bronchoalveolar CD4+ T cell responses to respiratory antigens are impaired in HIV-infected adults. Thorax. 2011;66(5):375–82.
6. Eagan R, Twigg HL, French N, Musaya J, Day RB, Zijlstra EE, et al. Lung Fluid Immunoglobulin from HIV-Infected Subjects Has Impaired Opsonic Function against Pneumococci. Clin Infect Dis. 2007;44(12):1632–8.
7. Meyer KC, Raghu G, Baughman RP, Brown KK, Costabel U, du Bois RM, et al. An Official American Thoracic Society Clinical Practice Guideline: The Clinical Utility of Bronchoalveolar Lavage Cellular Analysis in Interstitial Lung Disease. Am J Respir Crit Care Med. 2012;185(9):1004–14.
8. Collins AM, Rylance J, Wootton DG, Wright AD, Wright AKA, Fullerton DG, et al. Bronchoalveolar Lavage (BAL) for Research; Obtaining Adequate Sample Yield. Journal of Visualised Experiments. 2014;(85):e4345. doi:10.3791/4345.
9. Strumpf IJ, Feld MK, Cornelius MJ, Keogh BA, Crystal RG. Safety of Fiberoptic Bronchoalveolar Lavage in Evaluation of Interstitial Lung Disease. Chest. 1981;80(3):268–71.
10. Begara I, Luján L, McLaren L, Collie DDS, Miller HRP, Watt NJ. Quantitation of transforming growth factor-β in plasma and pulmonary epithelial lining fluid of sheep experimentally infected with maedi-visna virus. Vet Immunol Immunopathol. 1995;48(3):261–73.
11. Mankikian J, Ehrmann S, Guilleminault L, Le Fol T, Barc C, Ferrandiere M, et al. An evaluation of a new single-use flexible bronchoscope with a large suction channel: reliability of bronchoalveolar lavage in ventilated piglets and initial clinical experience. Anaesthesia. 2014;69(7):701–6.

12. Colt HG, Beamis JJ, Harrell JH, Mathur PM. Novel flexible bronchoscope and single-use disposable-sheath endoscope system. A preliminary technology evaluation. Chest. 2000;118(1):183–7.
13. Pujol E, López AM, Valero R. Use of the Ambu® aScope™ in 10 patients with predicted difficult intubation. Anaesthesia. 2010;65(10):1037–40.
14. Haslam PL, Baughman RP. Report of ERS Task Force: guidelines for measurement of acellular components and standardization of BAL. Eur Respir J. 1999;14(2):245–8.
15. Olsen HH, Grunewald J, Tornling G, Sköld CM, Eklund A. Bronchoalveolar Lavage Results Are Independent of Season, Age, Gender and Collection Site. PLoS ONE. 2012;7(8):e43644.

17

Diagnostic value of medical thoracoscopy in malignant pleural effusion

Yan-Bing Wu†, Li-Li Xu†, Xiao-Juan Wang, Zhen Wang, Jun Zhang, Zhao-Hui Tong and Huan-Zhong Shi*

Abstract

Background: Medical thoracoscopy has been shown to be an efficacious procedure in diagnosing unexplained exudative pleural effusions with excellent safety. This study aimed to assess the diagnostic significance of thoracoscopy in the management of patients with malignant pleural effusion (MPE).

Methods: Consecutive patients with malignant pleural effusion were retrospectively reviewed, and their demographic, radiographic, thoracoscopic and histological data were collected.

Results: Between July 2005 and June 2014, 342 of 833 patients undergoing thoracoscopy were finally confirmed to suffer from MPE. The top three frequent causes of MPE were metastatic carcinoma (79.5%), malignant mesothelioma (10.2%), and lymphoma (2.9%). Among metastatic malignancies, the most common cancer was lung cancer (85.2%), followed by breast cancer (4.4%), ovarian cancer (2.2%), pancreatic cancer (1.8%), etc. No serious adverse events associated with thoracoscopy were recorded.

Conclusions: Medical thoracoscopy is a valuable and safe tool in diagnosing malignant pleural effusion with minimal complication rates.

Keywords: Diagnosis, Malignant pleural effusion, Pleural biopsy, Sensitivity and specificity, Thoracoscopy

Background

The identification of malignant cells in a pleural lavage in patients without pleural effusion suggests micrometastatic disease, and our previous meta-analysis [1] showed that positive pleural lavage cytological findings are associated with a higher recurrence rate and significant poorer survival, with the overall hazard ratio for patients having malignant cells in pleural lavage was 5.61 (95% confidence interval 3.98–7.90). In non-small-cell lung cancer patients, the evidence of even a minimal pleural effusion at diagnosis is an independent prognostic factor for worse survival [2]. Malignant pleural effusion (MPE) is frequently observed in multiple malignancies, and lung cancer is the most common cause [3]. The existence of MPE in patients indicates systemic dissemination of cancer and declining in life expectancy and quality [4, 5].

The current guideline recommended that thoracentesis and/or closed pleural biopsy can be used as the first diagnostic steps in the diagnosis of MPE [6]. However, these procedures usually do not work when pleural effusion with thickness less than 10 mm on chest computed tomography (CT) scans. Instead, the more invasive approaches, such as medical thoracoscopy (MT), can be considered to identify whether pleural biopsy contains malignant cells [3, 7]. As a matter of fact, MT is a highly sensitive and safe method for diagnosing exudative pleural effusions [8–10]. The recent developed semi-rigid MT is easy to use and can gain popularity among respiratory physicians who are accustomed to flexible bronchoscope [11, 12].

In the present retrospective study of patients with MPE having undergone at least one semi-rigid MT over a 9-year period in a Chinese 1600-bed general hospital, we analyzed the diagnostic efficiency and safety of MT in the diagnosis of MPE.

* Correspondence: shihuanzhong@sina.com
†Equal contributors
Department of Respiratory and Critical Care Medicine, Beijing Institute of Respiratory Medicine and Beijing Chaoyang Hospital, Capital Medical University, Beijing, China

Methods

The study protocol and ethical approval was approved by the Institutional Review Board for human studies of Beijing Chao-Yang Hospital, China. Informed consents were not required as this was considered a review of clinical practice.

Information including medical history, clinical presentation, laboratory examination results, and image data of unexplained exudative pleural effusions patients who underwent MT in our hospital between July 2005 and June 2014 were gathered, and only MPE patients were finally included in the current study. Unexplained exudative pleural effusions were defined as the patients underwent the initial diagnostic approaches including thoracentesis and/or closed pleural biopsy, and their diseases remain undiagnosed. The characteristics of the study population are listed in Table 1.

MT procedures have been described in our previous publications [13, 14]. The diagnosis of MPE was established by the presence of the positive findings for malignancy in pleural biopsy.

Table 1 Characteristics of the study population (n = 342)

Variables	Values
Age, yr., mean ± SD	62.8 ± 9.7
Sex, male/female, n (%)	183/159 (53.5/46.5)
Smoking status, n (%)	
Current or previous smoker	127 (37.1)
Non-smoker	149 (43.6)
Not clear	66 (19.3)
History of malignancy	32 (9.4)
CT imaging	
Mediastinal and hilum lymphadenopathy	196 (57.3)
Pleural thickening	159 (46.5)
Pulmonary consolidation or infiltration	158 (46.2)
Pulmonary mass or nodules	134 (39.2)
Pulmonary atelectasis	126 (36.8)
Pleural nodularity	51 (14.9)
Side of effusion, n (%)	
Right	149 (43.6)
Left	133 (38.9)
Bilateral	60 (17.5)
Size of effusion, n (%)	
Small	57 (16.7)
Moderate	44 (12.9)
Large	241 (70.4)
Effusion appearance, n (%)	
Blood- tinged	191 (55.9)
Yellow	151 (44.1)

Descriptive statistical methods were used in the data analysis (mean ± standard deviation [SD] or/and range).

Results

Between July 2005 and June 2014, 833 patients with undiagnosed pleural effusions successfully underwent medical thoracoscopy [15]. Eventually, 342 patients with lymphocytic exudates were finally diagnosed with MPE; the mean age was 62.8 ± 9.7 years.

For 149 MPE patients, pleural fluid occurred only in the right side, for 133 only in the left, and for the rest 60 both sides were involved (Table 1). The size of a pleural effusion was clarified as small, moderate, or large based on CT imaging according to the methods described by Moy and colleagues [16]. In both unilateral and bilateral effusion, the proportions of small, moderate, and large size of pleural effusions were 16.7, 12.9, and 70.4%, respectively. The appearance of pleural effusion was blood-stained in 55.9% of patients, and in 44.1% was yellow.

In addition to pleural effusion, CT imaging revealed mediastinal and hilum lymphadenopathy, pleural thickening, pulmonary consolidation or infiltration, pulmonary mass or nodules, pulmonary atelectasis, and pleural nodularity (Table 1).

In all patients studied, we observed one or more abnormalities on the surface of parietal or/and visceral pleura under medical thoracoscopy. As shown in Table 2, pleural nodules, hyperemia, pleural adhesion, pleural plaques, ulcer, and the other pleural pathological changes were observed.

The most common etiological causes of MPE were metastatic carcinomas (n = 272), pleural malignant mesothelioma (n = 35), lymphoma (n = 10). It should be mentioned that we could not identify the original malignancies in 25 patients with MPE (Table 3). Among metastatic malignancies that resulted in MPE, the most common cancer included lung cancer, followed by breast cancer, ovarian cancer, pancreatic cancer (Table 4).

No serious adverse events were observed, and transient chest pain (43.9%) induced by the indwelling chest tube was the most frequent minor complication. Subcutaneous

Table 2 Procedural details (n = 342)

Procedural details	Value
Pleural fluid removed, mL	1306.7 ± 753.0
Parietal pleura biopsies, n	10 ± 2
Thoracoscopic findings, n (%)	
Pleural nodules	243 (71.1)
Hyperemia	159 (46.5)
Pleural adhesion	125 (36.6)
Pleural plaques	69 (20.2)
Ulcer	10 (2.9)
Other pleural pathological changes	97 (28.4)

Table 3 Diagnoses established by thoracoscopy in patients with MPE (n = 342)

Diagnoses	n (%)
Non-small cell lung cancer	221 (64.6)
Adenocarcinoma	215 (97.3)
Squamous cell carcinoma	6 (2.7)
Small cell lung cancer	11 (3.2)
Other metastatic carcinoma	40 (11.7)
Malignant mesothelioma	35 (10.2)
Epithelioid	
Sarcomatoid	
Biphasic	
Undifferentiated	
Lymphoma	10 (2.9)
Undetermined	25 (7.3)

emphysema was found in 8.5% of patients who recovered after chest-tube drainage. Minor bleeding was recorded in 6.4% of patients. And 5.6% of patients appeared with transient self-limited fever (38 °C or more).

Discussion

Because the prognosis for patients with MPE is poor, an efficacious procedure that can establish a definite diagnosis as early as possible with a minimum of risk and discomfort would be highly desirable. If a patient with undiagnosed pleural effusion is suspected as malignant, cytologic examination of pleural fluid is the first recommendation [6]. Although repeated thoracenteses can enhance the sensitivity of cytology, it is usually only 50 to 70% [17]. When cytology fails, closed percutaneous needle biopsy was traditionally performed blindly by an Abrams or Ramel needle [18–20]. Nevertheless, its role in diagnosing MPE has been challenged, as the positive diagnostic rate of closed pleural biopsy was only about 50% [21, 22]. More recently, the real time image-guided pleural biopsy has been shown to be a promising procedure for sampling the pleura, since it can increase the sensitivity for diagnosing MPE to about 80% [21, 23–25].

Table 4 Types of metastatic cancers (n = 272)

Metastatic cancers	n (%)
Lung cancer	232 (85.2)
Breast cancer	12 (4.4)
Ovarian cancer	6 (2.2)
Pancreatic cancer	5 (1.8)
Hepatic carcinoma	3 (1.1)
Esophageal carcinoma	2 (0.7)
Renal carcinoma	2 (0.7)
Thymic carcinoma	2 (0.7)
Gastric carcinoma	1 (0.4)
Myeloma	1 (0.4)
Sinuethmoid cancer	1 (0.4)
Malignant hemangioendothelioma	1 (0.4)
Base tongue carcinoma	1 (0.4)
Malignant melanoma	1 (0.4)
Cervical cancer	1 (0.4)
Endometrial cancer	1 (0.4)

Numerous tumor markers have been intensively examined for improving the diagnosis of MPE, however, seeking for a highly accurate pleural fluid tumor marker that reliably diagnoses MPE has been in vain so far [26]. Using one tumor marker alone for diagnosing MPE is not recommend according to the recent evidences, however, when combined two or more tumor markers together, the diagnostic sensitivity seems to be improved [27, 28]. The diagnostic performance of tumor markers for MPE seems to be similar with conventional tests including cytological examination–high specificity and low sensitivity. Tumor markers are less important in practice, since they do not complement the properties of conventional tests.

CT- or ultrasound-guided pleural biopsies are quite sensitive and safe, with the only reported complications being local hematoma and minor hemoptysis [21, 29]. The limitation of the image-guided pleural biopsy is the blindness of the procedure. MT overcomes this problem by allowing for the visualization of abnormal areas and for a direct biopsy, and thus improves the diagnostic accuracy of pleural effusions [8, 9]. Since June 2005, our institution started using MT as a routine method for patients with undiagnosed exudative pleural effusion in cases when either clinical, radiologic, laboratory, or cytologic investigation was failed. During a period of 9 years, 833 patients with unexplained pleural effusions underwent MT successfully, and among them, 342 were eventually diagnosed with MPE [15].

One or more abnormalities on the surface of parietal or/and visceral pleura were observed in the whole population in this study, including pleural nodules, hyperemia, pleural adhesion, pleural plaques, ulcer, and the other pleural pathological changes. Pathological examination revealed the presence of the positive findings for malignancy in pleural biopsy in 342 patients. The data in detail presented in the current study derived from our whole MT study population [15]. As reported in the previous publication [15], after a complete work-up including MT biopsies, the definite diagnoses of 92.6% (771/833) of patients with pleural effusions can be established definitely by MT followed by histopathological study.

It was noted that no etiological causes of pleural effusions can be identified in 7.4% (62/833) of patients even after MT [15]. All of these patients were followed up for at least 12 months, and did not complain about a new pleural effusion. No diagnosis other than benign pleural effusion was found in these 62 patients. Several studies suggest that among the patients with histological diagnosis of non-specific pleurisy made after MT, 8.3–18% of them were eventually diagnosed with MPE, usually pleural mesothelioma, during long term follow-up [30–32]. Therefore, we cannot exclude the possibility that a few patients with MPE-negative MT results would be finally diagnosed with MPE if we prolong the follow-up.

It has been reported that carcinoma from any organ can metastasize to the pleura, but lung, and breast carcinomas and lymphomas are the most common causes, digestive and ovary carcinomas are less frequent [33]. Our recent unpublished data indicated that during the past 3 years, 23.7% (365/1541) of pleural effusion patients admitted to our hospital were diagnosed with MPE. In the present study, our data showed that the most common etiological causes of MPE confirmed by MT were metastatic carcinomas, and followed by pleural malignant mesothelioma, lymphoma, and the other malignancies. Among metastatic malignancies that resulted in MPE, the most common cancer was lung cancer, followed by breast cancer, ovarian cancer, and pancreatic cancer.

MT has an excellent safety profile when performed by a trained physician, and a mortality rate associated with MT is always ≤0.8% [34]. A recent meta-analysis further suggested that mortality associated with MT was not observed, and that the major complication rate of MT was 1.5% and the minor complication rate was 10.5% [10]. In our 9-year study, MT procedures were well tolerated with a low rate of complications without serious adverse events, and transient chest pain caused by the indwelling chest tube was the most frequent minor complication. Large volumes of pleural fluid could be safely aspirated, although some patients suffered from coughing and chest discomfort after lung re-expansion with a chest tube.

The strengthen of this study was that study population was in a large size, in which 342 MPE patients were included. At the same time, our study also had limitations. First, as a retrospective study, it's impossible to collect and analyze the required data in a prospective way. Second, we could only retrospectively reviewed the data from patients with MPE, and no data from the other control group, such as the patients with tuberculous pleurisy, were available, it was therefore not possible to calculate the sensitivity and specificity of MT in diagnosing MPE. Third, blind needle biopsies or image-assisted biopsies were performed only in a few patients before undergoing MT in our series. This partially explained why there were so many pleural effusion patients (833 cases) receiving MT examination in our institution during 9 years.

Conclusions

In summary, MT is simple and safe with a high positive rate in the diagnosis of MPE. Due to its convenience and compatibility with existing bronchoscopy, MT appears to be a more widely performed procedure. Thus MT should be performed actively for proper patients with suspected MPE.

Abbreviations

CT: Computed tomography; MPE: Malignant pleural effusion; MT: Medical thoracoscopy; SD: Standard deviation

Acknowledgements

The authors feel thankful to Department of Pathology in Beijing Chao-Yang Hospital, Capital Medical University, Beijing, China and in particular Dr. Mu-Lan Jin and Dr. Xiao-Li Diao for their effort in evaluating and validating of the histological abnormalities in pleural biopsy specimen of this study.

Funding

This work was funded in part by grants from National Natural Science Foundation of China (No. 91442109, No. 31470883, and No. 81270149), and in part by key project of the department of science and technology, Beijing, China (D141107005214003). The funding source play no role in study design, data collection, data analysis, data interpretation, writing of the report, or in the decision to submit the report for publication.

Authors' contributions

HZS designed the study, had full access to all of the data in the study, was the guarantor for this manuscript, and took responsibility for the integrity of the data and the accuracy of the data analysis. YBW, LLX, XJW, ZW, JZ, and ZHT performed medical thoracoscopy and collected data. YBW, LLX, and HZS contributed to writing manuscript. No writing assistance was involved in this manuscript. All authors have read the manuscript and approve its submission.

Consent for publication

Not applicable.

Competing interests

No part of the research presented has been funded by tobacco industry sources. And all the authors have declared that competing interest exists.

References

1. Li YN, Shi HZ, Liang QL, Yang HB, Huang GM. Prognostic significance of pleural lavage cytology in patients with lung cancer: a meta-analysis. Lung Cancer. 2008;60(2):183–92.
2. Ryu JS, Ryu HJ, Lee SN, Memon A, Lee SK, Nam HS, Kim HJ, Lee KH, Cho JH, Hwang SS. Prognostic impact of minimal pleural effusion in non-small-cell lung cancer. J Clin Oncol. 2014;32(9):960–7.
3. Light RW. Clinical practice. Pleural effusion. N Engl J Med. 2002;346(25):1971–7.
4. Sugiura S, Ando Y, Minami H, Ando M, Sakai S, Shimokata K. Prognostic value of pleural effusion in patients with non-small cell lung cancer. Clin Cancer Res. 1997;3(1):47–50.
5. Goldstraw P, Crowley J, Chansky K, Giroux DJ, Groome PA, Rami-Porta R, Postmus PE, Rusch V, Sobin L. The IASLC lung cancer staging project: proposals for the revision of the TNM stage groupings in the forthcoming

(seventh) edition of the TNM classification of malignant tumours. J Thorac Oncol. 2007;2(8):706–14.
6. Roberts ME, Neville E, Berrisford RG, Antunes G, Ali NJ. Management of a malignant pleural effusion: British Thoracic Society pleural disease guideline 2010. Thorax. 2010;65(Suppl 2):ii32–40.
7. Heffner JE. Diagnosis and management of malignant pleural effusions. Respirology. 2008;13(1):5–20.
8. Loddenkemper R. Thoracoscopy–state of the art. Eur Respir J. 1998;11(1):213–21.
9. Rodriguez-Panadero F. Medical thoracoscopy. Respiration. 2008;76(4):363–72.
10. Agarwal R, Aggarwal AN, Gupta D. Diagnostic accuracy and safety of semirigid thoracoscopy in exudative pleural effusions: a meta-analysis. Chest. 2013;144(6):1857–67.
11. Ernst A, Hersh CP, Herth F, Thurer R, LoCicero J 3rd, Beamis J, Mathur P. A novel instrument for the evaluation of the pleural space: an experience in 34 patients. Chest. 2002;122(5):1530–4.
12. Munavvar M, Khan MA, Edwards J, Waqaruddin Z, Mills J. The autoclavable semirigid thoracoscope: the way forward in pleural disease? Eur Respir J. 2007;29(3):571–4.
13. Wang Z, Tong ZH, Li HJ, Zhao TT, Li XY, Xu LL, Luo J, Jin ML, Li RS, Wang C. Semi-rigid thoracoscopy for undiagnosed exudative pleural effusions: a comparative study. Chin Med J. 2008;121(15):1384–9.
14. Wang Z, Xu LL, Wu YB, Wang XJ, Yang Y, Zhang J, Tong ZH, Shi HZ. Diagnostic value and safety of medical thoracoscopy in tuberculous pleural effusion. Respir Med. 2015;109(9):1188–92.
15. Wang XJ, Yang Y, Wang Z, Xu LL, Wu YB, Zhang J, Tong ZH, Shi HZ. Efficacy and safety of diagnostic thoracoscopy in undiagnosed pleural effusions. Respiration. 2015;90(3):251–5.
16. Moy MP, Levsky JM, Berko NS, Godelman A, Jain VR, Haramati LB. A new, simple method for estimating pleural effusion size on CT scans. Chest. 2013;143(4):1054–9.
17. Bennett R, Maskell N. Management of malignant pleural effusions. Curr Opin Pulm Med. 2005;11(4):296–300.
18. Abrams LD. A pleural-biopsy punch. Lancet. 1958;1(7010):30–1.
19. Prakash UB, Reiman HM. Comparison of needle biopsy with cytologic analysis for the evaluation of pleural effusion: analysis of 414 cases. Mayo Clin Proc. 1985;60(3):158–64.
20. Renshaw AA, Dean BR, Antman KH, Sugarbaker DJ, Cibas ES. The role of cytologic evaluation of pleural fluid in the diagnosis of malignant mesothelioma. Chest. 1997;111(1):106–9.
21. Maskell NA, Gleeson FV, Davies RJ. Standard pleural biopsy versus CT-guided cutting-needle biopsy for diagnosis of malignant disease in pleural effusions: a randomised controlled trial. Lancet. 2003;361(9366):1326–30.
22. Chakrabarti B, Ryland I, Sheard J, Warburton CJ, Earis JE. The role of Abrams percutaneous pleural biopsy in the investigation of exudative pleural effusions. Chest. 2006;129(6):1549–55.
23. Adams RF, Gray W, Davies RJ, Gleeson FV. Percutaneous image-guided cutting needle biopsy of the pleura in the diagnosis of malignant mesothelioma. Chest. 2001;120(6):1798–802.
24. Benamore RE, Scott K, Richards CJ, Entwisle JJ. Image-guided pleural biopsy: diagnostic yield and complications. Clin Radiol. 2006;61(8):700–5.
25. Metintas M, Ak G, Dundar E, Yildirim H, Ozkan R, Kurt E, Erginel S, Alatas F, Metintas S. Medical thoracoscopy vs CT scan-guided Abrams pleural needle biopsy for diagnosis of patients with pleural effusions: a randomized, controlled trial. Chest. 2010;137(6):1362–8.
26. Light RW. Tumor markers in undiagnosed pleural effusions. Chest. 2004;126(6):1721–2.
27. Shi HZ, Liang QL, Jiang J, Qin XJ, Yang HB. Diagnostic value of carcinoembryonic antigen in malignant pleural effusion: a meta-analysis. Respirology (Carlton, Vic). 2008;13(4):518–27.
28. Liang QL, Shi HZ, Qin XJ, Liang XD, Jiang J, Yang HB. Diagnostic accuracy of tumour markers for malignant pleural effusion: a meta-analysis. Thorax. 2008;63(1):35–41.
29. Koegelenberg CF, Bolliger CT, Theron J, Walzl G, Wright CA, Louw M, Diacon AH. Direct comparison of the diagnostic yield of ultrasound-assisted Abrams and Tru-cut needle biopsies for pleural tuberculosis. Thorax. 2010;65(10): 857–62.
30. Venekamp LN, Velkeniers B, Noppen M. Does 'idiopathic pleuritis' exist? Natural history of non-specific pleuritis diagnosed after thoracoscopy. Respiration. 2005;72(1):74–8.
31. Davies HE, Nicholson JE, Rahman NM, Wilkinson EM, Davies RJ, Lee YC. Outcome of patients with nonspecific pleuritis/fibrosis on thoracoscopic pleural biopsies. Eur J Cardiothorac Surg. 2010;38(4):472–7.
32. Metintas M, Ak G, Cadirci O, Yildirim H, Dundar E, Metintas S. Outcome of patients diagnosed with fibrinous pleuritis after medical thoracoscopy. Respir Med. 2012;106(8):1177–83.
33. Marel M, Stastny B, Melinova L, Svandova E, Light RW. Diagnosis of pleural effusions. Experience with clinical studies, 1986 to 1990. Chest. 1995;107(6): 1598–603.
34. Michaud G, Berkowitz DM, Ernst A. Pleuroscopy for diagnosis and therapy for pleural effusions. Chest. 2010;138(5):1242–6.

Serum concentrations of Krebs von den Lungen-6, surfactant protein D, and matrix metalloproteinase-2 as diagnostic biomarkers in patients with asbestosis and silicosis

Changjiang Xue[1], Na Wu[1], Xue Li[2], Meihua Qiu[1], Xuqin Du[1] and Qiao Ye[1*]

Abstract

Background: Asbestosis and silicosis are progressive pneumoconioses characterized by interstitial fibrosis following exposure to asbestos or silica dust. We evaluated the potential diagnostic biomarkers for these diseases.

Methods: The serum concentrations of Krebs von den Lungen-6 (KL-6), surfactant protein D (SP-D), and matrix metalloproteinase-2 (MMP-2), MMP-7, and MMP-9 were measured in 43 patients with asbestosis, 45 patients with silicosis, 40 dust-exposed workers (DEWs) without pneumoconiosis, and 45 healthy controls (HCs). Chest high-resolution computed tomography (HRCT) images were reviewed by experts blinded to the clinical data. According to the receiver operating characteristic (ROC) curve, the ideal level of each biomarker and its diagnostic sensitivity were obtained.

Results: The serum KL-6 and MMP-2 concentrations were highest in patients with asbestosis, particularly in comparison with those in DEWs and HCs ($P<0.05$). The serum SP-D concentration was significantly higher in patients with asbestosis than in patients with silicosis, DEWs, and HCs ($P<0.01$), whereas no significant difference was noted among patients with silicosis, DEWs, and HCs. No significant difference in the serum MMP-7 or -9 concentration was found among patients with asbestosis, patients with silicosis, DEWs, or HCs. Among patients with asbestosis, the serum KL-6 concentration was significantly correlated with the lung fibrosis scores on HRCT and negatively correlated with the forced vital capacity (FVC) % predicted and diffusing capacity of the lung for carbon monoxide (DL_{CO}) % predicted. The serum SP-D and MMP-2 concentrations were negatively correlated with the DL_{CO} % predicted (all $P<0.05$). The order of diagnostic accuracy according to the ROC curve was KL-6, SP-D, and MMP-2 in patients with asbestosis alone and in the combination of both patients with asbestosis and those with silicosis. The combination of all three biomarkers may increase the possibility of diagnosing asbestosis (sensitivity, 93%; specificity, 57%) and both asbestosis and silicosis (sensitivity, 83%; specificity, 62%).

Conclusions: KL-6, SP-D, and MMP-2 are available biomarkers for the adjuvant diagnosis of asbestosis and silicosis. The combination of all three biomarkers may improve the diagnostic sensitivity for asbestosis and silicosis.

Keywords: Asbestosis, Silicosis, Biomarker, Krebs von den Lungen-6, Surfactant protein D, Matrix metalloproteinase, Pulmonary function

* Correspondence: yeqiao_chaoyang@sina.com
[1]Department of Occupational Medicine and Toxicology, Clinical Center for Interstitial Lung Diseases, Beijing Chao-Yang Hospital, Capital Medical University, 8 Gongren Tiyuchang Nanlu, Chao-Yang District, Beijing 100020, China
Full list of author information is available at the end of the article

Background

Asbestosis and silicosis are progressive pneumoconioses characterized by interstitial fibrosis following exposure to asbestos or silica dust. Disease progression usually leads to irreversible complications and death. Clinical detection and diagnosis of asbestosis and silicosis mainly relies on a history of occupational exposure and radiological abnormalities [1, 2]. China, where the asbestos and silica exposure industries have not been greatly limited, has invariably exhibited a sustained epidemic of asbestosis and silicosis [3, 4]. Biomarkers with which to detect these pneumoconioses other than imaging and lung function testing are warranted [5]. Krebs von den Lungen 6 (KL-6), surfactant protein D (SP-D), and matrix metalloproteinases (MMPs) are potential biomarkers for diagnosing and monitoring progression of various fibrotic lung diseases.

KL-6, classified in humans as mucin, is a circulating high-molecular-weight glycoprotein [6]. KL-6 has served as a useful biomarker in the differential diagnosis of various chronic lung fibroses and pulmonary alveolar proteinosis, evaluation of disease activity, and prediction of disease outcome [6–10]. The regenerating type II pneumocytes can be positively stained by the KL-6 monoclonal antibody in the lung tissue of patients with lung fibrosis [6, 7]. KL-6 is detectable in both the serum and bronchoalveolar lavage fluid of patients with lung fibrosis [6].

SP-D, which belongs to the collecting subgroup of the C-type lectin superfamily, is produced by two types of nonciliated epithelial cells in the peripheral airway (alveolar type II cells and Clara cells) and is secreted into the alveolar space [11]. It functions at the air–liquid interface to reduce surface tension and thereby prevent alveolar collapse and atelectasis; it also plays important roles in the innate immune system of the lungs [12]. The serum concentration of SP-D can reflect the pathological changes of lungs affected by idiopathic pulmonary fibrosis (IPF) by migration from the air space into the bloodstream [11].

In addition to type II pneumocyte-derived biomarkers, MMPs can degrade extracellular matrix components and numerous nonmatrix proteins [13]. MMPs and their inhibitors, tissue inhibitors of MMPs, have been implicated in the pathogenesis of pulmonary fibrosis based upon the results of clinical studies that showed elevated levels of MMPs in both blood and/or lung samples, indicating that they can serve as potential diagnostic and prognostic markers of chronic lung fibrosis [14–17].

Several biomarkers, such as interleukin-1β, type IV collagen, tumor necrosis factor-α, neopterin, and proteomic profiling, have shown potential significance in patients with lung fibrosis [18–21]. However, no previous investigations have evaluated the diagnostic values of pneumocyte-derived biomarkers in various pneumoconioses. To clarify the potential diagnostic biomarkers for asbestosis and silicosis, we measured the serum concentrations of KL-6, SP-D, and MMP-2, -7, and -9 in discriminating patients with asbestosis and silicosis from dust-exposed workers (DEWs) without pneumoconiosis and healthy controls (HCs).

Methods

A case–control study of patients with asbestosis, patients with silicosis, DEWs without pneumoconiosis, and HCs was conducted using a sandwich-type electrochemiluminescence immunoassay (ECLIA) or commercially available enzyme-linked immunosorbent assay (ELISA) to detect the serum concentrations of KL-6, SP-D, and MMP-2, -7, and -9. All participants underwent chest X-ray and/or chest high-resolution computed tomography (HRCT) and pulmonary function testing. The study was approved by the Institutional Ethics Committee for Human Research, Beijing Chao-Yang Hospital. Informed consent was obtained from all participants before blood sample collection.

Patients' characteristics

In total, 43 outpatients with newly diagnosed asbestosis, 45 with silicosis and 40 dust-exposed workers (DEWs) without pneumoconiosis were sequentially recruited from the Department of Occupational Medicine and Toxicology, Beijing Chao-Yang Hospital, during a 2-year period (January 2015 to December 2016). All patients were diagnosed according to the diagnostic criteria of pneumoconiosis based on the 2011 International Labour Organization classification [22]. Patients with bronchial asthma, tuberculosis, autoimmune disease, severe liver and kidney dysfunction, and malignant tumors were excluded.

Forty DEWs, including 19 coal mine workers, 7 sand moulding workers, 5 jade polishers, 4 asbestos textile workers, and 5 boiler maintenance workers, had occupational exposure to silica or asbestos dust. They underwent all examinations without showing evidence of a pneumoconiosis.

The HCs comprised 45 age-, sex-, and smoking status-matched healthy volunteers from the health examination center of Beijing Chao-yang Hospital during the same period of time.

All participants' smoking status was carefully determined, and they were categorized as non-smokers, ex-smokers (had quit smoking ≥12 months previously), and smokers (currently smoking or had quit smoking <12 months previously). Cigarette smoking is shown by pack-years.

Occupational dust exposure

All participants completed a standardized questionnaire to collect information on their work history. All jobs within the participant's working life were taken into account. The 43 patients with asbestosis were local residents who had been exposed to chrysotile dust or fibers, including 36 (83.7%) involved in the manufacture of asbestos textiles or asbestos-based products and 7 (16.3%) exposed to asbestos products in a working atmosphere (e.g., heat insulation workers and boiler maintenance workers). The 45 patients with silicosis were local residents who had been exposed to silica dust in the processing of jade. The asbestos product plants were open from the 1950s to 1970s, and the jade-processing factories were open from the 1970s to 1990s. Our hospital is the largest center for evaluation of occupational diseases in the city and is located 20 to 30 km away from the plants.

Because of the absence of atmospheric measurements and the lack of detailed information on the frequency of exposure for each job suspected to be associated with asbestos exposure, the duration of asbestos exposure (number of years) was determined.

Measurements of KL-6, SP-D, and MMP-2, -7, and -9 concentrations

The serum samples were collected from each participant and stored at −80°C until serum analysis. All samples were measured within two weeks of the storage. The serum KL-6 concentration was measured by ECLIA using a Lumipulse G1200 Analyzer (Rebio, Fuji, Japan). The serum SP-D and MMP-2, -7, and -9 concentrations were measured by commercially available ELISA kits (RayBiotech, Norcross, GA, USA).

Pulmonary function tests

Pulmonary function tests were performed according to the guidelines of the hospital physiology laboratory. Parameters used for analysis of the flow–volume curve were the forced vital capacity (FVC), forced expired volume in the first second (FEV_1), and FEV_1/FVC ratio. Each participant also underwent evaluation of their total lung capacity and diffusing capacity of the lung for carbon monoxide (DL_{CO} SB) (single-breath method, with the values corrected for the present hemoglobin concentration). The results are expressed as percentages of predicted values on the basis of age, height, and sex using equations established by the European Respiratory Society [23]. The forced expiratory maneuvers were repeated until three sequential measurements were obtained. The indices were obtained from the best curve, which was associated with the highest value of FEV_1 plus FVC.

Lung fibrosis scores on HRCT

HRCT scans in the patients with asbestosis were performed with 0.625-mm sections, a 1-second scan time, and a 10-mm interval in the apex base scans with inclusion of both lungs in the field of view. The HRCT images were reviewed by two experts blinded to the patients' clinical data. Two experts scored the HRCT images, which comprised three images taken at the level of the aortic arch, carina, and 1 cm above the diaphragm. Each lung lobe was scored on a scale of 0 to 5 for interstitial abnormalities according to a previously described protocol [24]. The HRCT score for each patient was the sum of the five lung lobes and ranged from 1 to 25. The final score was the mean of the scores from the two experts. The interobserver correlation was good. The kappa coefficient for the correlation between the patterns was 0.742 (P=0.006).

Conventional chest radiographs were performed in each patient with silicosis and independently evaluated by two occupational medicine experts according to the International Labour Organization classification [22]. Briefly, the lung fields were divided into six zones on the posterior chest radiograph. When the highest density of small opacities was ≥1/0 and the distribution affected two or more zones, the patients were classified into Stage I. When the highest density of small opacities was ≥2/1 and the distribution affected more than four zones, or the highest density of small opacities was ≥3/2 and the distribution affected four or more zones, the patients were classified into Stage II. When the highest density of small opacities was ≥3/2 and the distribution affected four or more zones with aggregation of small or large opacities, or the diameter of the largest opacity was ≥20 × 10 mm, the patients were classified into Stage III. The interobserver correlation was good. The kappa coefficient for the correlation between the patterns was 0.653 (P=0.009).

Statistical analysis

The results are expressed as mean ± standard deviation, and the differences among the four groups were tested using the Kruskal–Wallis test or one-way analysis of variance. Counting data were analyzed using the chi-square test. Correlations between parameters were assessed by Pearson's correlation coefficient. The levels of serum biomarkers were further analyzed by a receiver operating characteristic (ROC) curve to determine the cut-off levels that resulted in the optimal diagnostic accuracy for each marker between the patients and controls. The use of these cut-off levels allowed for calculation of the sensitivity, specificity, and likelihood ratio of the biomarkers for separating the patients from the controls. Statistical analyses were performed using SPSS version 17.0 for Windows (SPSS Inc., Chicago, IL, USA). A P value of <0.05 was considered statistically significant.

Results

Demographics of the participants

The demographics of each participant group are summarized in Table 1. There was no significant difference in sex, age, or smoking status among the groups. However, the pulmonary function values, including the FEV_1/FVC

Table 1 Demographics of the study participants

	Asbestosis	Silicosis	DEWs	HCs	*P* value
n	43	45	40	45	
Male: Female	19:24	23:22	21:19	22:23	0.879
Age, years	68.2 ± 8.6	65.1 ± 11.3	63.1 ± 8.7	65.6 ± 11.4	0.152
Smokers: nonsmokers	17:26	20:25	22:18	18:27	0.460
Current smoker: Exsmoker	6:11	8:12	13:9	11:7	0.275
Duration of exposure, years	7.4 ± 2.6	9.3 ± 3.1	7.8 ± 3.0	NA	0.107
FVC, predicted %	77.7 ± 23.4	79.2 ± 20.9	82.8 ± 18.2	83.3 ± 17.4	0.484
FEV_1, predicted %	71.2 ± 12.5	77.1 ± 12.1	80.3 ± 11.5	80.8 ± 11.4	**0.002**
FEV_1/FVC, %	75.5 ± 9.2	81.2 ± 8.0	81.7 ± 7.8	83.9 ± 11.7	**<0.001**
DL_{CO}, predicted %	65.9 ± 14.1	74.3 ± 11.6	80.8 ± 7.8	80.6 ± 8.9	**<0.001**
Lung fibrosis scores	10.1 ± 6.4	NA	NA	NA	

P values were computed by chi-square test for sex and smoking status, and the one-way analysis of variance for age, duration of exposure and pulmonary function parameters. Significant results are highlighted in bold. *NA* not available

ratio, the predicted percentages of FEV_1 and DL_{CO}, showed significant differences among the groups.

Serum concentrations of KL-6, SP-D, and MMP-2, -7, and -9

As shown in Fig. 1, the serum KL-6 and MMP-2 concentrations were highest in patients with asbestosis and second highest in patients with silicosis; these concentrations were significantly different from those in DEWs and HCs ($P<0.05$). The serum SP-D concentration was significantly higher in patients with asbestosis than in patients with silicosis, DEWs, or HCs ($P<0.01$), whereas no significant difference was found among patients with silicosis, DEWs, and HCs. No significant differences were found in the serum MMP-7 or -9 concentration among patients with asbestosis, patients with silicosis, DEWs, and HCs. The serum concentrations of KL-6, SP-D, and MMP-2 were not significantly different among the various stages of silicosis (Table 2).

Correlations between the KL-6, SP-D, and MMP-2 concentrations and clinical parameters in patients with asbestosis

As shown in Fig. 2, the serum KL-6 concentration was positively correlated with the lung fibrosis scores on HRCT in the patients with asbestosis while negatively correlated with the FVC % predicted and DL_{CO} % predicted ($P<0.05$). The serum SP-D and MMP-2 concentration was also negatively correlated with the DL_{CO} % predicted ($P<0.05$).

ROC curve analysis for identification of asbestosis or asbestosis and silicosis

ROC curve analysis was used to evaluate the ability of the serum KL-6, SP-D, and MMP-2 concentrations to differentiate patients with asbestosis from patients with silicosis, DEWs and HCs or asbestosis and silicosis from DEWs and HCs (Table 3). The area under the curve (AUC) for KL-6 was larger than that for SP-D and MMP-2 (Fig. 3), indicating that the order of diagnostic accuracy by the ROC curve was KL-6, SP-D, and MMP-2 in patients with asbestosis alone or in both patients with asbestosis and those with silicosis. The sensitivity and specificity of the combination of all three biomarkers for the diagnosis of asbestosis were 93% and 57%, respectively; however, they were 83% and 62% for the diagnosis of both asbestosis and silicosis.

Discussion

In the present study, we showed that the diagnostic value of the serum biomarkers KL-6, SP-D, and MMP-2 was higher in patients with asbestosis or patients with silicosis than in DEWs and HCs. In patients with asbestosis, the serum KL-6 concentration was significantly correlated with the lung fibrosis scores on HRCT while negatively correlated with the FVC % predicted and DL_{CO} % predicted. In addition, the serum SP-D and MMP-2 concentrations were negatively correlated with the DL_{CO} % predicted in patients with asbestosis. The order of diagnostic accuracy according to the ROC curve was KL-6, SP-D, and MMP-2 in patients with asbestosis alone and in patients with asbestosis plus those with silicosis. The combination of KL-6, SP-D, and MMP-2 may improve the diagnostic sensitivity for asbestosis and silicosis.

KL-6 is mainly localized in the cytoplasm and membrane of alveolar type II epithelial cells and bronchial epithelial cells [7]. KL-6 is also expressed in the cytoplasm of Clara cells and in bronchial glands [7]. KL-6 can promote the proliferation and migration of fibroblasts, inhibit cell apoptosis, and increase the development of pulmonary fibrosis [25]. The proliferation of type II alveolar epithelial cells in dust-related lung fibroses such as asbestosis or silicosis may release KL-6 into

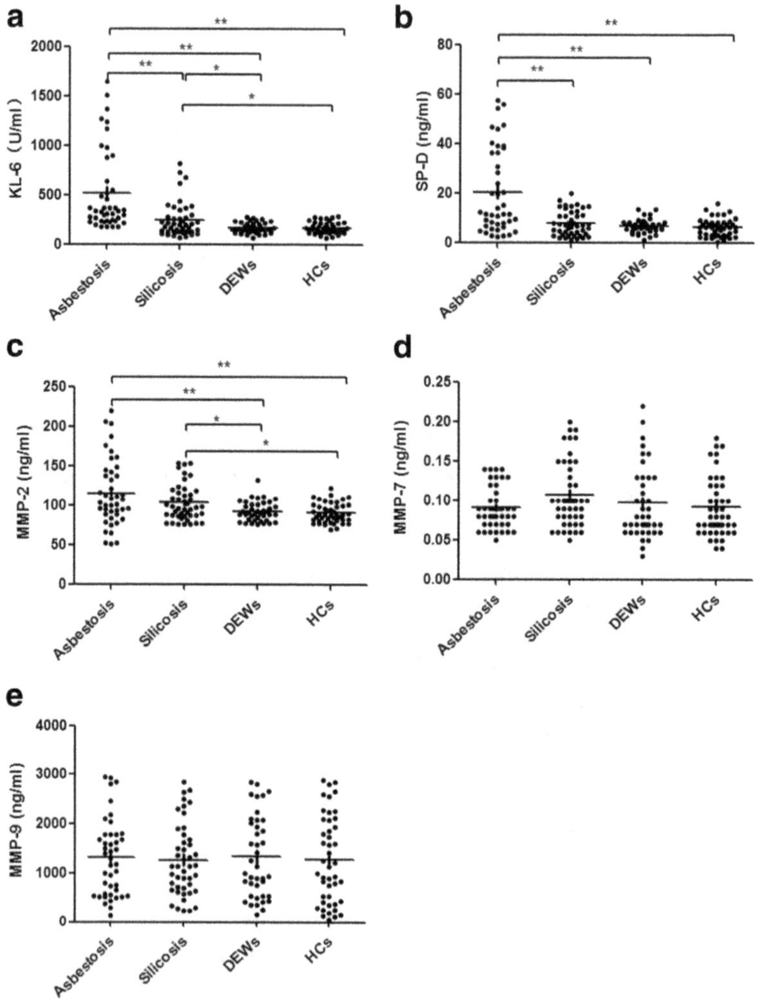

Fig. 1 Comparison of serum concentrations of KL-6, SP-D, and MMP-2, -7, and -9 among the study groups using the Kruskal–Wallis test. **a**. KL-6. **b**. SP-D. **c**. MMP-2. **d**. MMP-7. **e**. MMP-9. **P*<0.05; ***P*<0.01

the peripheral blood, resulting in a significantly elevated serum KL-6 concentration. An increased concentration of KL-6 in the epithelial lining fluid may stimulate fibrotic processes in patients with interstitial lung diseases and raise the possibility of the need for treatment with anti-KL-6 antibodies [26]. The serum KL-6 concentration in patients with interstitial lung diseases reflects the overall extent of interstitial lesions and serves as a powerful predictor of acute exacerbations of IPF [27, 28]. In the present study, KL-6 was higher with diagnostic value in both patients with asbestosis and patients with silicosis than in DEWs and HCs.

Table 2 Serum concentrations of of KL-6, SP-D and MMP-2 in the patients with various stages of silicosis

	Stage I	stage II	Stage III	*P* value
n	21	8	16	
KL-6, U/ml	200.2 ± 101.6	206.0 ± 127.8	314.6 ± 248.2	0.122
SP-D, ng/ml	7.0 ± 4.2	10.5 ± 7.0	7.3 ± 4.7	0.235
MMP-2, ng/ml	105.0 ± 27.4	100.9 ± 18.4	101.5 ± 19.3	0.869

P value were computed by Kruskal–Wallis test

SP-D is also a type II pneumocyte-derived biomarker. SP-D plays an important role in lung innate immunity [29], and its serum concentration reflects the severity and prognosis of interstitial lung diseases [30, 31]. SP-A and SP-D are very similar in terms of structure and function. However, evaluation of their hydrophilicity suggests that SP-D migrates into the blood more easily than does SP-A in patients with IPF [11]. SP-D may more easily leak into the bloodstream, whereas SP-A remains bound to surfactant lipids in the alveolar space. Previous data have suggested that the serum SP-D concentration may more accurately reflect pathological changes in IPF-affected lungs than the serum SP-A concentration [11]. The present data show that the SP-D

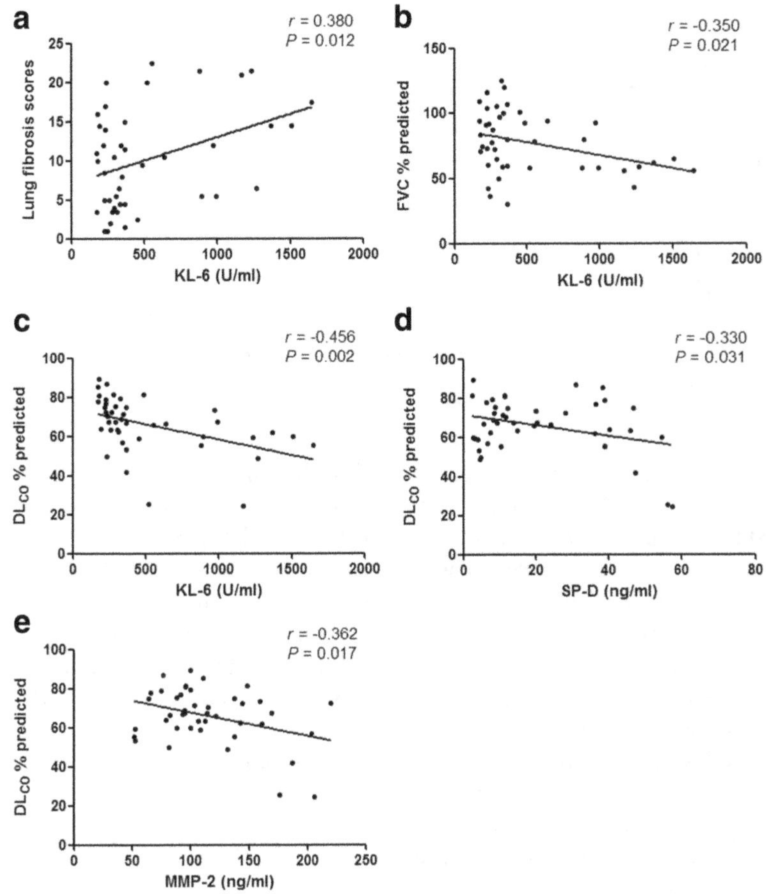

Fig. 2 Correlation between KL-6, SP-D, and MMP-2 and clinical parameters in patients with asbestosis. **a**. KL-6 and lung fibrosis scores. **b**. KL-6 and FVC % predicted. **c**. KL-6 and DL_{CO} % predicted. **d**. SP-D and DL_{CO} % predicted. **e**. MMP-2 and DL_{CO} % predicted

concentrations in patients with asbestosis were significantly higher than those in patients with silicosis, DEWs, or HCs. Our results indicate that the serum SP-D concentration might be an effective biomarker of asbestosis.

MMPs are a family of endopeptidases that can degrade several components of the extracellular matrix and control the activity of several proteins that function in immunity; damage, repair, and remodeling of collagen; and fibrosis [13]. The levels of MMP-7 and MMP-9 in both serum and bronchoalveolar lavage fluid are significantly higher in patients with IPF than in healthy controls [32]. MMP-2, -7, and -9 have also been shown to be upregulated in the lungs in patients with IPF, particularly in alveolar macrophages, hyperplastic epithelial cells, and myofibroblasts [14, 32, 33]. Elevated serum MMP-7 concentrations are correlated with severe lung fibrosis and poorer survival in patients with IPF [34]. Our data failed to show the diagnostic value of the serum MMP-7 and -9 concentrations in patients with asbestosis and in those with silicosis compared with DEWs and HCs, but our data

Table 3 Cut-off values and the identifying ability of KL-6, SP-D and MMP-2 by ROC curve analysis

	Identifying asbestosis			Identifying asbestosis and silicosis		
	KL-6	SP-D	MMP-2	KL-6	SP-D	MMP-2
AUC	0.874	0.757	0.641	0.751	0.657	0.655
95% CI	0.815-0.919	0.686-0.818	0.564-0.712	0.679-0.813	0.581-0.728	0.579-0.725
Cut-off value	216 U/ml	8.82 ng/ml	110.6 ng/ml	222 U/ml	9.9 ng/ml	110.6 ng/ml
Sensitivity, %	88.4	65.1	44.2	62.5	46.6	37.5
Specificity, %	73.1	76.9	86.2	81.2	88.2	95.3
Likelihood ratio	3.28	2.82	3.19	3.32	3.96	7.97

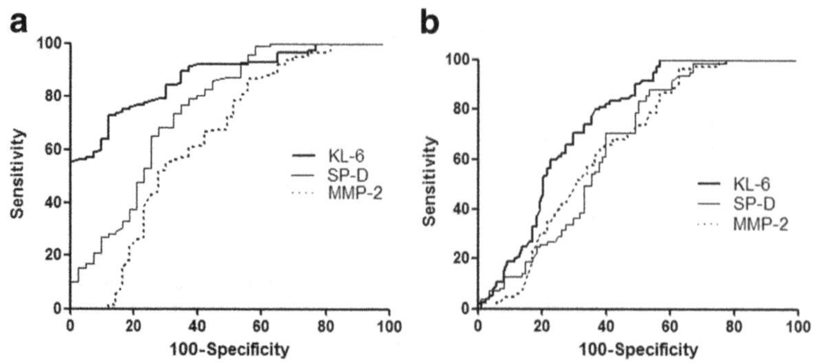

Fig. 3 a. ROC curve analysis to differentiate patients with asbestosis from patients with silicosis, DEWs and HCs. **b**. ROC curve analysis to differentiate patients with asbestosis and silicosis from DEWs and HCs

did show the diagnostic value of the MMP-2 concentration. This finding may suggest that MMPs have different roles between dust-related fibrotic lung diseases and IPF.

The typical radiological abnormalities associated with asbestosis are pulmonary fibrosis and pleural plaques [35]. Like other pulmonary fibrotic diseases, asbestosis can be evaluated by the lung fibrosis scores on HRCT to describe the degree of pulmonary fibrosis [36]. As in patients with IPF, our data showed that the serum KL-6 concentration was correlated with the extent of diffuse fibrosis in patients with asbestosis; however, it was not correlated with the density in patients with nodular fibrosis. The serum KL-6 concentration was significantly correlated with lung fibrosis scores on HRCT, indicating the use of KL-6 in the evaluation of pulmonary fibrosis. In the analysis of the KL-6, SP-D, and MMP-2 concentrations and pulmonary function in patients with asbestosis, a higher serum KL-6 concentration was significantly negatively correlated with the FVC % predicted and DL_{CO} % predicted, suggesting that high expression of KL-6 is associated with decreased pulmonary ventilation function and diffusion function in patients with asbestosis. The serum SP-D and MMP-2 concentrations were negatively correlated with DL_{CO} % predicted, indicating impairment of pulmonary diffusion function [37, 38]. The ROC curve analysis showed that the area under the curve of KL-6 was the largest, indicating that it is more effective than SP-D and MMP-2 in the diagnosis of asbestosis or silicosis. The sensitivity of the combination of all three biomarkers was higher than that of any single serum marker. Therefore, the combination of KL-6, SP-D, and MMP-2 can improve the sensitivity of diagnosis of asbestosis and silicosis.

Some limitations of this study should be mentioned. First, we could not continuously monitor the biomarker concentrations in every patient to evaluate the dynamic changes in the progression of asbestosis and silicosis. In addition, other biomarkers may be effective for monitoring and evaluating disease progression and prognosis.

Conclusions

This study showed that KL-6, SP-D, and MMP-2 are readily available biomarkers for the adjuvant diagnosis of asbestosis and silicosis. The combination of all three biomarkers may improve the sensitivity of differentiating patients with asbestosis or silicosis from DEWs or HCs. Further study is warranted to justify KL-6, SP-D and MMP-2 as confirmation of early occupational lung fibrosis in the workers exposure to dusts for the possibility of intervention or prevention of the diseases.

Abbreviations

AUC: The area under the curve; DEWs: Dust-exposed workers; DL_{CO}: Diffusing capacity of the lung for carbon monoxide; ECLIA: Electrochemiluminescence immunoassay; ELISA: Enzyme-linked immunosorbent assay; FEV_1: Forced expired volume in the first second; FVC: Forced vital capacity; HCs: Healthy controls; HRCT: High-resolution computed tomography; IPF: Idiopathic pulmonary fibrosis; KL-6: Krebs von den Lungen-6; MMP: Matrix metalloproteinase; ROC: Receiver operating characteristic; SP-D: Surfactant protein D

Acknowledgements

We thank all patients and investigators who were involved in these studies. We express our thanks to our colleagues Yan Yongji and Ma Jing.

Funding

The work was supported by National Major Scientific and Technological Special Project for Significant New Drugs Development (2014ZX09J15104, 2014ZX09303302) and National Natural Science Foundation of China (81370159).

Authors' contributions

XC performed all data collection, collected and processed samples, analyzing the data and wrote the manuscript. WN, LX and QM were responsible for recruiting the patients. DX was responsible for analyzing the data. YQ contributed as primary investigator and was responsible for designing the study, recruiting the patients and writing the manuscript. All authors read and approved the final manuscript.

Consent for publication

Not applicable.

Competing interests

The authors declare that they have no competing interests.

Author details

[1]Department of Occupational Medicine and Toxicology, Clinical Center for Interstitial Lung Diseases, Beijing Chao-Yang Hospital, Capital Medical University, 8 Gongren Tiyuchang Nanlu, Chao-Yang District, Beijing 100020, China. [2]Department of Pathology, Beijing Chao-Yang Hospital, Capital Medical University, 8 Gongren Tiyuchang Nanlu, Chao-Yang District, Beijing 100020, China.

References

1. Leong SL, Zainudin R, Kazan-Allen L, Robinson BW. Asbestos in Asia. Respirology. 2015;20(4):548–55.
2. Castranova V, Vallyathan V. Silicosis and coal workers' pneumoconiosis. Environ Health Perspect. 2000;108(Suppl 4):675–84.
3. Courtice MN, Lin S, Wang X. An updated review on asbestos and related diseases in China. Int J Occup Environ Health. 2012;18(3):247–53.
4. Zhang M, Wang D, Zheng YD, XY DU, Chen SY. Analyses on the characteristics and the trends of pneumoconiosis notified between 1997 and 2009 in China. Zhonghua Lao Dong Wei Sheng Zhi Ye Bing Za Zhi. 2013;31(5):321–34.
5. Pandey JK, Agarwal D. Biomarkers. A potential prognostic tool for silicosis. Indian J Occup Environ Med. 2012;16:101–7.
6. Takahashi T, Munakata M, Suzuki I, Kawakami Y. Serum and bronchoalveolar fluid KL-6 levels in patients with pulmonary alveolar proteinosis. *Am J Respir Crit Care Med*. 1998;158, 1294:–8.
7. Ohnishi H, Yokoyama A, Kondo K, Hamada H, Abe M, Nishimura K, Hiwada K, Kohno N. Comparative study of KL-6, surfactant protein-A, surfactant protein-D, and monocyte chemoattractant protein-1 as serum markers for interstitial lung diseases. Am J Respir Crit Care Med. 2002;165:378–81.
8. Yokoyama A, Kohno N, Hamada H, Sakatani M, Ueda E, Kondo K, Hirasawa Y, Hiwada K. Circulating KL-6 predicts the outcome of rapidly progressive idiopathic pulmonary fibrosis. Am J Respir Crit Care Med. 1998;158:1680–4.
9. Satoh H, Kurishima K, Ishikawa H, Ohtsuka M. Increased levels of KL-6 and subsequent mortality in patients with interstitial lung diseases. J Intern Med. 2006;260:429–34.
10. Yamakawa H, Hagiwara E, Kitamura H, Yamanaka Y, Ikeda S, Sekine A, Baba T, Okudela K, Iwasawa T, Takemura T, Kuwano K, Ogura T. Serum KL-6 and surfactant protein-D as monitoring and predictive markers of interstitial lung disease in patients with systemic sclerosis and mixed connective tissue disease. J Thorac Dis. 2017;9(2):362–71.
11. Nishikiori H, Chiba H, Ariki S, Kuronuma K, Otsuka M, Shiratori M, Ikeda K, Watanabe A, Kuroki Y, Takahashi H. Distinct compartmentalization of SP-A and SP-D in the vasculature and lungs of patients with idiopathic pulmonary fibrosis. BMC Pulm Med. 2014;14:196.
12. Takahashi H, Sano H, Chiba H, Kuroki Y. Pulmonary surfactant proteins A and D: innate immune functions and biomarkers for lung diseases. Curr Pharm Des. 2006;12(5):589–98.
13. Craig VJ, Zhang L, Hagood JS, Owen CA. Matrix metalloproteinases as therapeutic targets for idiopathic pulmonary fibrosis. Am J Respir Cell Mol Biol. 2015;53(5):585–600.
14. Selman M, Ruiz V, Cabrera S, Segura L, Ramirez R, Barrios R, Pardo A. TIMP-1, -2, -3, and -4 in idiopathic pulmonary fibrosis: a prevailing nondegradative lung microenvironment? Am J Physiol Lung Cell Mol Physiol. 2000;279:L562–74.
15. Morais A, Beltrão M, Sokhatska O, Costa D, Melo N, Mota P, Marques A, Delgado L. Serum metalloproteinases 1 and 7 in the diagnosis of idiopathic pulmonary fibrosis and other interstitial pneumonias. Respir Med. 2015;109:1063–8.
16. Zuo F, Kaminski N, Eugui E, Allard J, Yakhini Z, Ben-Dor A, Lollini L, Morris D, Kim Y, DeLustro B, et al. Gene expression analysis reveals matrilysin as a key regulator of pulmonary fibrosis in mice and humans. Proc Natl Acad Sci USA. 2002;99:6292–7.
17. Henry MT, McMahon K, Mackarel AJ, Prikk K, Sorsa T, Maisi P, Sepper R, Fitzgerald MX, O'Connor CM. Matrix metalloproteinases and tissue inhibitor of metalloproteinase-1 in sarcoidosis and IPF. Eur Respir J. 2002;20:1220–7.
18. Prince P, Boulay ME, Pagé N, Desmeules M, Boulet LP. Induced sputum markers of fibrosis and decline in pulmonary function in asbestosis and silicosis: a pilot study. Int J Tuberc Lung Dis. 2008;12:813–9.
19. Jiang PR, Cao Z, Qiu ZL, Pan JW, Zhang N, Wu YF. Plasma levels of TNF-α and MMP-9 in patients with silicosis. Eur Rev Med Pharmacol Sci. 2015;19:1716–20.
20. Pingle SK, Tumane RG, Jawade AA. Neopterin: Biomarker of cell-mediated immunity and potent usage as biomarker in silicosis and other occupational diseases. Indian J Occup Environ Med. 2008;12:107–11.
21. Miao R, Ding B, Zhang Y, Xia Q, Li Y, Zhu B. Proteomic profiling change during the early development of silicosis disease. J Thorac Dis. 2016;8:329–41.
22. International Labour Office. International Classification of Radiographs of Pneumoconiosis, revised. Occupational Safety and Health Series. 2011; 22:Rev 2011.
23. Cotes JE, Chinn DJ, Quanjer PH, Roca J, Yernault JC. Standardization of the measurement of transfer factor (diffusing capacity), report working party standardization of lung function tests, European Community for steel and coal: official statement of the European Respiratory Society. Eur Respir J. 1993;6:41–53.
24. Kazerooni EA, Martinez FJ, Flint A, Jamadar DA, Gross BH, Spizarny DL, Cascade PN, Whyte RI, Lynch JP 3rd, Toews G. Thin-section CT obtained at 10-mm increments versus limited three-level thin-section CT for idiopathic pulmonary fibrosis: correlation with pathologic scoring. AJR Am J Roentgenol. 1997;169:977–83.
25. Ohshimo S, Yokoyama A, Hattori N, Ishikawa N, Hirasawa Y, Kohno N. KL-6, a human MUC1 mucin, promotes proliferation and survival of lung fibroblasts. Biochem Biophys Res Commun. 2005;338:1845–52.
26. Wakamatsu K, Nagata N, Kumazoe H, Oda K, Ishimoto H, Yoshimi M, Takata S, Hamada M, Koreeda Y, Takakura K, Ishizu M, Hara M, Ise S, Izumi M, Akasaki T, Maki S, Kawabata M, Mukae H, Kawasaki M. Prognostic value of serial serum KL-6 measurements in patients with idiopathic pulmonary fibrosis. Respir Investig. 2017;55:16–23.
27. Hu Y, Wang LS, Jin YP, Du SS, Du YK, He X, Weng D, Zhou Y, Li QH, Shen L, Zhang F, Su YL, Sun XL, Ding JJ, Zhang WH, Cai HR, Dai HP, Dai JH, Li HP. Serum Krebs von den Lungen-6 level as a diagnostic biomarker for interstitial lung disease in Chinese patients. Clin Respir J. 2017;11(3):337–45.
28. Kishaba T, Shimaoka Y, Fukuyama H, Yoshida K, Tanaka M, Yamashiro S, Tamaki H. A cohort study of mortality predictors and characteristics of patients with combined pulmonary fibrosis and emphysema. BMJ Open. 2012;15:2(3).
29. Ariki S, Nishitani C, Kuroki Y. Diverse functions of pulmonary collectins in host defense of the lung. J Biomed Biotechnol. 2012;2012:532071.
30. Takahashi H, Fujishima T, Koba H, Murakami S, Kurokawa K, Shibuya Y, Hiratori M, Kuroki Y, Abe S. Serum surfactant proteins A and D as prognostic factors in idiopathic pulmonary fibrosis and their relationshipto disease extent. Am J Respir Crit Care Med. 2000;162(3 Pt 1):1109–14.
31. Greene KE, King TE Jr, Kuroki Y, Bucher-Bartelson B, Hunninghake GW, Newman LS, Nagae H, Mason RJ. Serum surfactant proteins-A and -D as biomarkers in idiopathic pulmonary fibrosis. Eur Respir J. 2002;19(3):439–46.
32. Rosas IO, Richards TJ, Konishi K, Zhang Y, Gibson K, Lokshin AE, Lindell KO, Cisneros J, Macdonald SD, Pardo A, et al. MMP1 and MMP7 as potential peripheral blood biomarkers in idiopathic pulmonary fibrosis. PLoS Med. 2008;5:e93.
33. Craig VJ, Polverino F, Laucho-Contreras ME, Shi Y, Liu Y, Osorio JC, Tesfaigzi Y, Pinto-Plata V, Gochuico BR, Rosas IO, et al. Mononuclear phagocytes and airway epithelial cells: novel sources of matrix metalloproteinase-8 (MMP-8) in patients with idiopathic pulmonary fibrosis. PLoS One. 2014;9:e97485.
34. Song JW, Do KH, Jang SJ, Colby TV, Han S, Kim DS. Blood biomarkers MMP-7 and SP-A: predictors of outcome in idiopathic pulmonary fibrosis. Chest. 2013;143(5):1422–9.
35. Akira M, Morinaga K. The comparison of high-resolution computed tomography findings in asbestosis and idiopathic pulmonary fibrosis. Am J Ind Med. 2016;59:301–6.
36. Arakawa H, Kishimoto T, Ashizawa K, Kato K, Okamoto K, Honma K, Hayashi S, Akira M. Asbestosis and other pulmonary fibrosis in asbestos-exposed workers: high-resolution CT features with pathological correlations. Eur Radiol. 2016;26:1485–92.
37. Yang XL, Zhu XL, Li A, Du XQ, Song YG, Ye Q. Characteristics of lung function in patients with asbestosis of different stages. Zhonghua Lao Dong Wei Sheng Zhi Ye Bing Za Zhi. 2016;34:687–90.
38. Gothi D, Gahlot T, Sah RB, Saxena M, Ojha UC, Verma AK, Spalgais S. Asbestos-induced lung disease in small-scale clutch manufacturing workers. Indian J Occup Environ Med. 2016;20:95–102.

19

Pleural plaques in lung cancer screening by low-dose computed tomography: prevalence, association with lung cancer and mortality

Mario Silva[1,2*], Nicola Sverzellati[1,2], Davide Colombi[1], Gianluca Milanese[1,2], Carlo La Vecchia[3], Carlotta Galeone[3], Alfonso Marchianò[4] and Ugo Pastorino[2]

Abstract

Background: To report the prevalence of pleural plaques in a lung cancer screening trial by low-dose computed tomography (LDCT) and to test the association with incidence of lung cancer and mortality.

Methods: The LDCT of 2303 screenees were retrospectively reviewed with the specific aim of describing the prevalence and features of pleural plaques. Self-administered questionnaire was used to assess asbestos exposure. Frequency of lung cancer, lung cancer mortality, and overall mortality were detailed according to presence of pleural findings. Statistical analyses included comparison of mean or median, contingency tables, and Cox model for calculation of hazard ratio (HR) and its 95% confidence interval (CI).

Results: Among male screenees, 31/1570 (2%) showed pleural abnormalities, 128/1570 (8.2%) disclosed asbestos exposure, 23/31 (74.2%) subjects with pleural plaques consistently denied exposure to asbestos. There was a trend for higher frequency of lung cancer among subjects with pleural plaques (9.7% vs 4.2%). Lung cancer in subjects with pleural plaques was always diagnosed in advanced stage. Subjects with pleural plaques showed HR 5.48 (95% CI 1.61–18.70) for mortality from lung cancer.

Conclusions: Pleural plaques are a risk factor for lung cancer mortality that can be detected in lung cancer screening by LDCT, also in subjects that are not aware of asbestos exposure.

Keywords: Lung cancer screening, Pleural abnormalities, Asbestos exposure, Pleural plaques, Self-disclosure of asbestos exposure, Post-test refinement of individual risk

* Correspondence: mario.silva@unipr.it
[1]Department of Medicine and Surgery (DiMeC), Section of Radiology, Unit of Surgical Sciences, University of Parma, Padiglione Barbieri, Via Gramsci 14, 43126 Parma, Italy
[2]Department of Thoracic Surgery, Fondazione IRCCS Istituto Nazionale dei Tumori, Milan, Italy
Full list of author information is available at the end of the article

Background

Lung cancer screening by low-dose computed tomography (LDCT) has the main purpose of reducing lung cancer mortality in subjects that have several risk factors contributing to increased risk of lung cancer [1]. Asbestos exposure is a well-known risk factor for thoracic malignancies and non-malignant respiratory diseases [2–5], hence, the majority of lung cancer risk models include exposure to asbestos for pre-test calculation of lung cancer risk [3, 6, 7]. However, there is limited reliability on reference methods for the assessment of life-time exposure from occupational and, notably, non-occupational inhalation.

Signs of asbestos exposure can be detected by LDCT, with variable degrees of accuracy. Pleural plaques are among the chest abnormalities significantly related with exposure to asbestos [8, 9]. In the setting of professional exposure to asbestos, several studies reported the association between reduced survival and asbestos-related LDCT signs, including pleural plaques [4, 10]. The detection of pleural plaques and their prognostic value in non-occupational setting has not been investigated, yet. Lung cancer screening trials by LDCT provide the unique opportunity of investigating pleural plaques out of the specific setting of professional surveillance.

The aim of this study was to describe the prevalence of pleural plaques in a population of lung cancer screening participants, and to test their relation with incidence of lung cancer and mortality.

Methods

The Institutional Review Board approved the Multicenter Italian Lung Detection (MILD) protocol, and written informed consent was obtained from all participants. Informed consent included retrospective evaluation of MILD data, as performed in this study. Therefore, specific consent was waived for this study. Eligibility criteria were as follows: age 50–75 years, current or former (having quit <10 years before enrollment) smokers with a tobacco burden ≥20 pack-years, and no history of cancer in the 5 years before enrollment. Details on screening strategy and lung cancer specific mortality rates of the MILD trial are published elsewhere [11]. In brief, the MILD trial enrolled a total of 4099 participants from September 2005 to January 2011. These subjects were randomly assigned to two groups: the early detection group (2376 participants) received a LDCT either every 12 months (1190 participants) or every 24 months (1186 participants), and the control group (1723 participants) received only primary prevention program with pulmonary function test and blood sample collection.

This investigation aimed to evaluate pleural abnormalities on baseline LDCT, and was thus based on the early detection group only. Baseline LDCT was available for 2303 out of 2376 participants (1570 men and 733 women; median age 60 years, interquartile range - IQR - 55 to 65 years). These subjects were evaluated for pleural abnormalities. The MILD protocol included self-administered questionnaire about medical history (i.e. oncologic history, cardio-vascular and respiratory anamnesis, metabolic diseases, and family history of lung cancer), smoking history (i.e. cigarette smokers were differentiated from other smokers, duration of smoking, amount of daily cigarette, pack-years, and Fagerstrom test) [12], exposure to asbestos, respiratory symptoms, subjective awareness of lung cancer risk related to smoking, and willing to quitting smoking [13]. Also, height and weight were recorded and body mass index (BMI) was calculated.

Visual assessment of pleural plaques on LDCT

LDCT technique

LDCT was performed with a 16-detector CT scanner (Somatom Sensation; Siemens Healthcare, Forchheim, Germany) without contrast agent, and with standardized low dose acquisition protocol: potential 120 kVp, current 30 effective mAs, collimation 0.75 mm, rotation time 0.5 s, and pitch 1.5. For each LDCT examination, the reconstruction protocol was as follows: slice thickness 1 mm, slice increment 1 mm, and kernel b50. For this study, the reconstructed images were stored to a dedicated workstation for diagnostic work-up (Osirix, Pixmeo SARL, Bernex, Switzerland); window width (WW) and window level (WL) were optimized for assessment of pleura (soft tissue setting: WW 350 HU and WL 50 HU) and lung parenchyma (lung setting: WW 1600 and WL -600 HU).

Pleural findings

LDCTs were reviewed by two radiologists for the detection of pleural abnormalities (both radiologists had three-year experience in lung cancer screening LDCT: 1201 LDCTs read by MS and 1102 LDCTs read by DC). A senior radiologist (NS, with 10-year experience in lung cancer screening LDCT) reviewed LDCT of all subjects with pleural abnormalities and selected those evocative of asbestos exposure, as described thereafter. Pleural plaques and diffuse pleural thickening were deemed findings evocative of asbestos exposure [8, 9]. In particular, pleural plaques were described as solid thickening of pleural surface with clear-cut edges, with or without calcification [14, 15] (Fig. 1). Diffuse pleural thickening was described as single continuous pleural thickening thicker than 3 mm, larger than 5 cm on axial plane, and longer than 8 cm in z-axis [8, 14]. From now on, all pleural abnormalities evocative of asbestos exposure will be referred as pleural plaques. All pleural plaques were visually scored according to a pre-formatted score sheet, adapted from the literature [14–17], namely: *a) distribution* according to

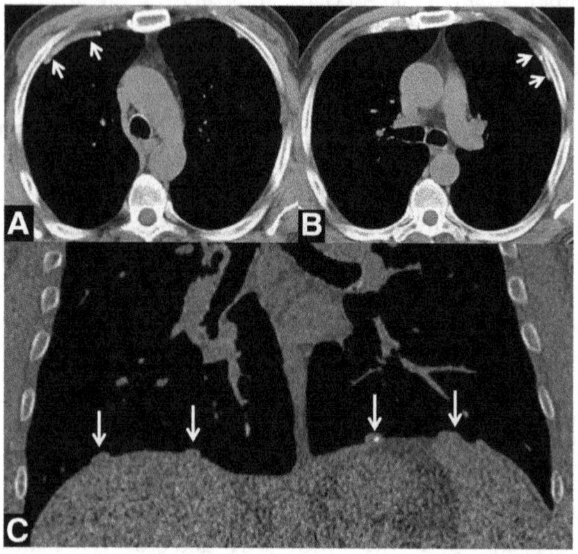

Fig. 1 a-c Pleural plaques. **a-b** - Transverse CT image of the chest shows smooth solid thickening of pleural surface with clear-cut edge. **c** – Coronal reconstruction of the chest shows smooth solid thickening of pleural surface above the diaphragm, with scant calcification

side (unilateral or bilateral) and pleural anatomical compartment (subcostal, para-mediastinal, diaphragmatic, and fissural); *b)* presence of *calcifications*; *c) aspect* was described as smooth or nodular; *d) cumulative extent* was classified into 4 groups: smaller than 1 cm, between 1 cm and 25% of pleural surface, 25%–50% of pleural surface, and > 50% of pleural surface; *e) thickness* was classified into 4 groups: < 2 mm, 2–5 mm, 5–10 mm, and > 10 mm.

Self-reported asbestos exposure

The self-administered questionnaire included disclosure of asbestos exposure. It was administered at the recruitment appointment and at any following LDCT appointment. Subjects with consistent positive disclosure about asbestos exposure over the consecutive questionnaires were deemed *exposed*. Conversely, *non-exposed* subjects were those with consistent negative disclosure or inconsistent disclosures along the consecutive questionnaires (e.g. positive disclosure at baseline questionnaire and negative disclosure at follow-up, or vice versa). The self-reported asbestos exposure was compared with the presence of pleural plaques to investigate awareness of exposure.

Frequency of lung cancer and assessment of cause of mortality

Lung cancers were recorded from the surgical registry, in particular, histology and stage were reported [18]. Mortality from lung cancer and mortality from any cause were retrieved from the National Registry Office database. Data were updated to April 2016.

Statistical analysis

Statistical analysis was selectively performed on male population to avoid multivariate model bias from gender-related variables (e.g. height, weight, and BMI) related to the odd distribution of pleural plaques between genders. The continuous variables were given as median with their interquartile range (IQR) and were analyzed using a two-sided Student's t-test, if data were normally distributed (based on the Shapiro-Wilk statistic), or a two-sided Wilcoxon rank-sum test, if otherwise. The categorical variables were given as numbers and percentages and were analyzed using the contingency table analysis with the Chi-square or Fisher's test, as appropriate.

The Cox model adjusted for age, BMI, pack-years, and self-disclosure of asbestos exposure was used to calculate the hazard ratio (HR) and the corresponding 95% confidence intervals (CI) for lung cancer incidence, lung cancer mortality, mortality from causes different from lung cancer, and overall mortality. All tests were two-sided and a p-value < 0.05 was considered as statistically significant. All statistical analyses were performed with MedCalc 12 (MedCalc Software, Belgium).

Results

Visual assessment of pleural plaques on LDCT

Pleural plaques were reported in 33/2303 subjects (1.4%), in particular 31/1570 men (2.0%) and 2/733 women (0.3%) ($p < 0.001$). Demographics, biometrics, smoking history, and self-disclosure of asbestos exposure of male screenees were reported in Table 1, according to presence of pleural plaques. Men with pleural plaques were older ($p = 0.005$), with similar biometrics and smoking history compared to men without pleural plaques. The geographic area of screenee provenance was summarized in Fig. 2 and the distribution of pleural plaques was detailed as the ratio of screenees from each area of provenance. LDCT features of pleural plaques were summarized in Table 2, notably pleural effusion was reported in 1/31 men (3.2%) and it was not associated with lung cancer or mesothelioma.

Self-reported asbestos exposure

Asbestos exposure was consistently self-reported by 128/1570 men (8.2%), whereas 68/1570 (4.3%) provided inconsistent disclosure, and 1374/1570 (87.5%) consistently denied asbestos exposure. The consistent self-reported exposure to asbestos was significantly related to presence of pleural plaques ($p = 0.003$; Table 1), however the majority of men with pleural plaques consistently denied exposure to asbestos (23/31, 74.2%).

Frequency of lung cancer and cause of mortality

Sixty-eight lung cancers were diagnosed in 1570 men over 14,533.3 person-years (467/100,000 person-years),

Table 1 Demographics, biometrics, smoking history, and self-disclosure of asbestos exposure in the overall male population and according to the presence of pleural plaques

	All men ($n = 1570$)	Men with pleural plaques ($n = 31$)	Men without pleural plaques ($n = 1539$)	p^a
Age [years]	58 [54–62]	62 [57–66]	58 [54–62]	0.0054
Height [cm]	174 [170–178]	177 [170–180]	174 [170–178]	0.2536
Weight [kg]	80 [73–88]	83 [75–92]	80 [73–88]	0.101
BMI [kg/m^2]	26.4 [24.4–28.7]	27.2 [24.8–30.2]	26.4 [24.4–28.7]	0.1949
Smoking history				
Current smoker	1007 (64.1%)	19 (61.3%)	988 (64.2%)	0.7103[b]
Former smoker	563 (35.9%)	12 (38.7%)	551(35.8%)	
Duration [years]	39 [34–43]	40 [36–45]	39 [34–43]	0.2501
Pack years	40.0 [32.0–54.0]	41.0 [35.0–61.5]	40.0 [32.0–54.0]	0.6378
Self-disclosure of asbestos exposure	128 (8.2%)	8 (25.8%)	120 (7.8%)	0.0025[b]

[a]Wilcoxon test
[b]Fisher exact test

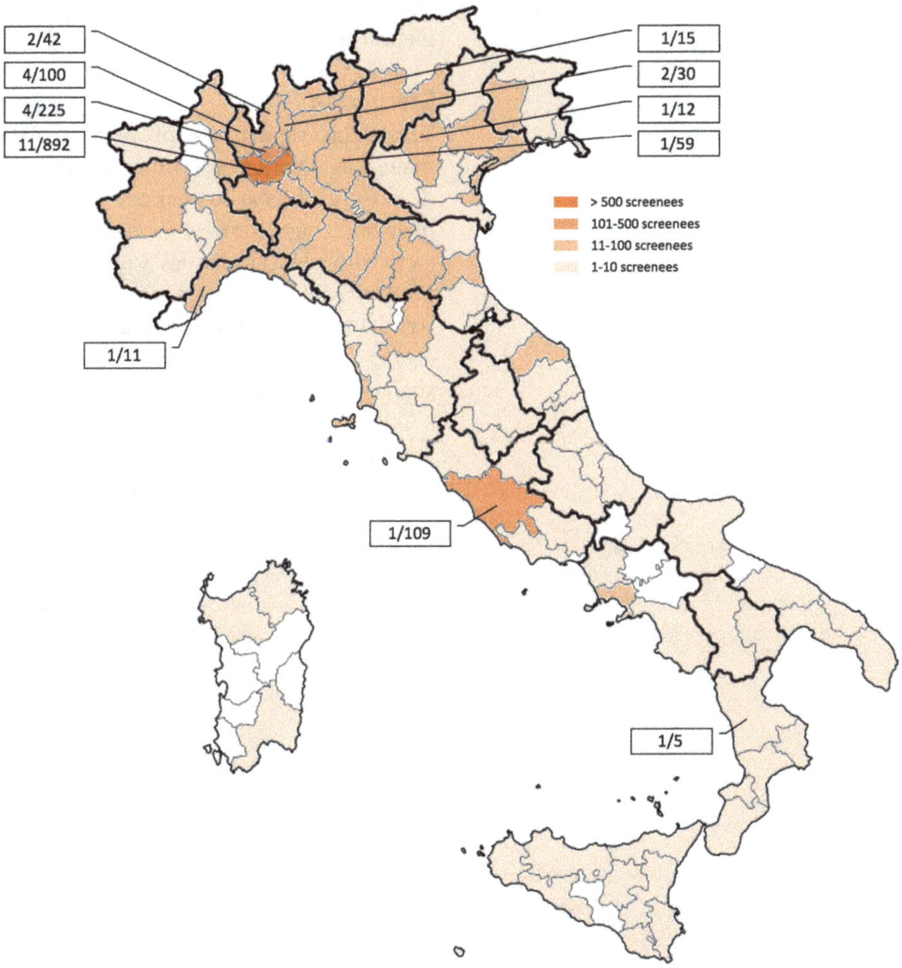

Fig. 2 Geographic area of provenance of screenees are summarized according to numeric categories: 1–10 screenees, 11–100 screenees, 101–500 screenees, and > 500 screenees. The geographic distribution of pleural plaques is reported as the ratio between the number of screenees with pleural plaques and specific number of screenees from each geographic area (adapted from https://commons.m.wikimedia.org)

Table 2 LDCT features of pleural plaques detected by LDCT in 31/1570 men

LDCT features of pleural plaques	*N (%)* 31 (100%)
Distribution by side:	
Bilateral	28 (90%)
Unilateral	3 (10%)
Distribution by anatomical compartment:	
More than one pleural compartment	21 (68%)
Subcostal only	9 (29%)
Para-mediastinal only	1 (3%)
Extent:	
< 1 cm	1 (3%)
1 cm to 25%	25 (81%)
25 to 50%	4 (13%)
> 50%	1 (3%)
Thickness:	
< 2 mm	1 (3%)
2–5 mm	7 (23%)
5–10 mm	19 (61%)
> 10 mm	4 (13%)
Calcification:	
Calcified	21 (68%)
Non-calcified	10 (32%)
Aspect morphology:	
Nodular aspect	19 (61%)
Smooth aspect	12 (39%)
Pleural effusion	1 (3%)

until April 2016 (Table 3). In particular, the frequency of lung cancer was 3/31 in men with pleural plaques (1079/100,000 person-years) and 65/1539 in men without pleural plaques (456/100,000 person-years), with a non-statistically significant difference between the groups ($p = 0.148$). In particular, all men with pleural plaques showed stage 4 lung cancer. The mortality from lung cancer in men with pleural plaques was statistically higher compared to those without pleural plaques ($p = 0.015$), whereas the mortality from causes other than lung cancer was similar between the two groups.

A single mesothelioma was diagnosed in a subject who did not have pleural plaques nor disclosed asbestos exposure.

Table 4 details the HR for overall or specific mortality and for incidence of lung cancer in subjects with pleural plaques. The HR for overall mortality was higher in men with pleural plaques (HR 2.02), allegedly conditioned by the exceptionally high HR for mortality from lung cancer (HR 5.48). Of note, the HR for lung cancer incidence was slightly but not significantly higher in men with pleural plaques (HR 1.84).

Discussion

This study reports 2% prevalence of pleural plaques in male participants of a lung cancer screening trial. Self-disclosure of asbestos exposure was recorded in 8.2% of male screenees, however a significant proportion of subjects with pleural plaques were not aware of asbestos exposure. Male screenees with pleural plaques showed a trend for higher risk of lung cancer and significant increase of lung cancer mortality compared to male screenees without pleural plaques.

The relationship between asbestos exposure and lung cancer has been investigated in several studies based on occupational surveillance programs for asbestos workers

Table 3 Comparison of lung cancer frequency, stage, and cause of mortality according to presence pleural plaques. The table includes events from the entire period of lung cancer screening (median follow-up 9.5 years). Notably, pleural plaques were searched on baseline LDCT, therefore detection of pleural plaques either preceded (e.g. event at incidence rounds) or was synchronous (e.g. event at baseline round) to each detailed event

	All patients (*n* = 1570)	Men with pleural plaques (*n* = 31)	Men without pleural plaques (*n* = 1539)	*p*[a]
Total person-years follow-up	14,533.3	278.0	14,255.3	
Median person-years follow-up	9.5	9.4	9.5	
Patients with lung cancer	68 (4.3%)	3 (9.7%)	65 (4.2%)	0.148
Lung cancer stage				
I or II	39 (57.4%)	0	39 (60%)	0.073
III or IV	29 (42.6%)	3 (100%)	26 (40.0)	
Total deaths	87 (5.5%)	4 (12.9%)	83 (5.4%)	0.088
Lung cancer deaths	27 (1.7%)	3 (9.7%)	24 (1.6%)	0.015
Deaths from causes other than lung cancer	60 (3.8%)	1 (3.2%)	59 (3.8%)	1.0

[a]Fisher exact test

Table 4 Hazard ratios (HR)[a] of overall mortality, lung cancer mortality and lung cancer occurrence among 1570 men according to pleural findings

	Pleural findings HR[a] (95% CI)
Overall mortality ($N = 87$)	2.02 (0.73–5.56)
Mortality from lung cancer ($N = 27$)	5.48 (1.61–18.70)
Mortality from other causes than lung cancer ($N = 60$)	0.70 (0.10–5.10)
Lung cancer incidence ($N = 68$)	1.84 (0.57–5.93)

[a]Estimated from Cox model adjusted for age, BMI, pack-years, self-disclosure of asbestos exposure

[19–22]. Current or recent occupational exposure to asbestos is a known risk factor for lung cancer with a reported two-fold increase of lung cancer risk among smokers [7]. Mastrangelo et al. reported progressive decrease of relative risk of lung cancer after 15–20 years since last exposure to asbestos [22], comparable to smoking cessation. Nevertheless, increased risk of thoracic malignancy has been demonstrated also for extremely low exposure, such as non-occupational and environmental exposure [23, 24]. Accordingly, several lung cancer risk models for selection of lung cancer screening population include asbestos exposure among risk factors, even in case of non-occupational exposure [3, 7]. Non-occupational exposure is likely to become more relevant in industrialized countries were asbestos ban was issued more than 20 years ago [10]. The assessment of non-occupational exposure to asbestos is extremely challenging, indeed more controversial that the assessment of occupational exposure [25]. Self-administered questionnaires have been employed to collect data on asbestos exposure in participants of lung cancer screening trials, despite this assessment demands specialized operators for thorough investigation of potential pollutant [26]. Our data showed that signs of asbestos exposure such pleural plaques were associated with increased risk of lung cancer mortality, including subjects who were not aware of occupational exposure. The increased risk was independent from tobacco burden. We encourage specific investigation of asbestos exposure (both occupational and non-occupational) for selection of subjects for lung cancer screening, even when tobacco burden does not meet the reference level for recruitment in such screening.

Previous lung cancer screening trials reported prevalence of asbestos-exposure ranging 5.6–7.3% [27, 28]. In our study, similar results were obtained by self-disclosure of asbestos exposure (overall self-disclosed exposure 6.5% - data not reported in results), however almost 75% of male screenees with pleural plaques did not disclose the exposure. This observation confirms that self-disclosure of asbestos exposure is not reliable, as it was reported in the literature [29]. Ledda et al. reported a significant increase of pleural plaques prevalence among subjects in an area with high environmental concentration of fibrous amphibole [30]. Of note, the CT features of pleural plaques reported by Ledda in environmentally exposed subjects were similar to those reported in our lung cancer screening population, in particular the majority of subjects showed plaque extent between 1 cm and 25% of pleural surface. Pleural plaques in subjects that are not aware of exposure to asbestos could be associated with non-occupational and environmental exposure, and this should be particularly emphasized in high-risk subjects that undergo lung cancer screening by LDCT.

Bach et al. showed increase of lung cancer risk in association to asbestos exposure in participants of lung cancer screening trials [31]. In our study, screenees with pleural plaques showed higher risk of lung cancer mortality compared to the remainder screenees. We underline that screenees with pleural plaques were diagnosed with advanced stage lung cancer. Hence, we suggest that increased mortality could have been driven by a more aggressive pattern of lung cancer in this group of screenees. Again, it is apparent that assessment of pleural plaques in lung cancer screening participant contributes to the detection of subjects with minor or unknown exposure. For this purpose, the objective assessment of pleural abnormalities could be regarded as potential marker of increased risk of lung cancer associated to asbestos exposure, and should be investigated for post-test refinement of subjective risk of lung cancer. Furthermore, from a demographic point of view, detection of pleural plaques in screenees that are not aware of the exposure should prompt active investigation of environmental exposure to asbestos in specific areas.

Among occupationally exposed subjects, the correlation between pleural plaques and lung cancer appears to be lower compared to the relative risk associated with asbestosis [10]. Both asbestosis and pleural plaques can be seen on LDCT, however pleural plaques are more specific than asbestosis findings in the absence of known exposure to asbestos. Vehmas et al. reported significant increase of lung cancer death in asbestos workers with pleural plaques [4]. This report in workers exposed to asbestos is confirmed by our data in the setting of lung cancer screening trial. Screenees with pleural plaques showed a trend for increased incidence of lung cancer, noteworthy the clinical evolution of lung cancer in these subjects was extremely aggressive. Lung cancer in subjects with pleural plaques were all diagnosed in stage 4 and, thus, lung cancer mortality was significantly higher compared to screenees with cancer diagnosis but without pleural plaques, suggesting that mortality from lung cancer in subjects with pleural plaques could be influenced by more factors rather than the simple incidence of lung cancer (e.g. aggressive biology). Risk models for post-test risk refinement are mostly based on the presence and characteristics of nodule and have been validated [32–34]. Looking forward to screening implementation, post-test risk model enrichment is fostered including other non-nodular LDCT findings such as emphysema and other interstitial lung abnormalities. Pleural plaques should be considered as additional non-nodular finding for post-test risk model.

This study has some limitations. Asbestos exposure was investigated by prospectively self-administered questionnaire, which is known to be inconsistent for assessment of asbestos exposure. However, self-administered questionnaire is the affordable option for implementation in lung cancer screening by LDCT. Moreover, asbestos exposure was not further investigated in subjects with pleural plaques and unaware of asbestos exposure. This could be regarded as a limitation because the specific description of exposure hazard in this subgroup could have provided information to improve anamnestic collection of this specific pollutant. Moreover, the asbestos exposure was investigated with a binary question (e.g. yes or no), without specific description of exposure duration and intensity. This limitation was driven by the management and financial plan within lung cancer screening trial with a large population of screenees. We foster future studies testing the correlation between detailed descriptors of asbestos exposure and lung cancer outcomes within lung cancer screening programs. Finally, parenchymal signs of asbestos exposure were not investigated, despite they are associated with risk of lung cancer. Notably, parenchymal signs were not scored because they are not specific for asbestos exposure when the exposure is not formally confirmed. It would be ideal that reliable information about asbestos exposure in lung cancer screening allow specific investigation of interstitial lung abnormalities related with the exposure, since they are significantly related with the risk of lung cancer [10].

Conclusions

In conclusion, pleural plaques can be detected in a sizeable proportion of subjects undergoing lung cancer screening by LDCT. Screenees with pleural plaques show increased risk of lung cancer mortality, therefore pleural plaques could be considered in risk models for post-test refinement of subjective risk.

Abbreviations

BMI: Body mass index; CI: Confidence interval; HR: Hazard ratio; IQR: Interquartile range; LDCT: Low-dose computed tomography; WL: Window level; WW: Window width

Acknowledgements

The authors would like to thank all the MILD participants and their families. Moreover, the authors wish to thank Claudio Jacomelli and Claudio Citterio for data management and the MILD staff (Elena Bertocchi, Annamaria Calanca, Carolina Ninni, Stefano Sestini, Paola Suatoni). The Authors thank Dr. Francesca Marezza (University of Parma) for her contribution in the field of medico-legal implication of asbestos exposure.

Funding

The MILD project was supported by grants from the Italian Ministry of Health (RF 2004), the Italian Association for Cancer Research (AIRC 2004 IG 1227 and AIRC 5xmille IG 12162), and the Fondazione Cariplo (2004–1560).

Authors' contributions

Study concepts and design: NS, MS, DC, UP, CLV. Literature research: MS, NS, DC, GM, AM. Data collection: MS, DC, NS, GM, CG. Data Analysis: MS, NS, UP, CLV, CG. Statistical analysis: CG, CLV. Manuscript preparation: MS, NS, UP. Manuscript editing: DC, GM, CLV, CG, AM. All authors have read and approved the final version of this manuscript.

Consent for publication

Not applicable

Competing interests

The authors declare that they have no competing interests..

Author details

[1]Department of Medicine and Surgery (DiMeC), Section of Radiology, Unit of Surgical Sciences, University of Parma, Padiglione Barbieri, Via Gramsci 14, 43126 Parma, Italy. [2]Department of Thoracic Surgery, Fondazione IRCCS Istituto Nazionale dei Tumori, Milan, Italy. [3]Department of Clinical Sciences and Community Health, University of Milan, Milan, Italy. [4]Department of Radiology and Radiotherapy, Fondazione IRCCS Istituto Nazionale dei Tumori, Milan, Italy.

References

1. Field JK, Devaraj A, Duffy SW, Baldwin DR. CT screening for lung cancer: is the evidence strong enough? Lung Cancer. 2016;91:29–35.
2. Hammond EC, Selikoff IJ, Seidman H. Asbestos exposure, cigarette smoking and death rates. Ann N Y Acad Sci. 1979;330:473–90.
3. Cassidy A, Myles JP, van Tongeren M, Page RD, Liloglou T, Duffy SW, Field JK. The LLP risk model: an individual risk prediction model for lung cancer. Br J Cancer. 2008;98(2):270–6.
4. Vehmas T, Oksa P, Kivisaari L. Lung and pleural CT signs predict deaths: 10-year follow-up after lung cancer screening of asbestos-exposed workers. Int Arch Occup Environ Health. 2012;85(2):207–13.
5. Lopatin S, Tsay JC, Addrizzo-Harris D, Munger JS, Pass H, Rom WN. Reduced lung function in smokers in a lung cancer screening cohort with asbestos exposure and pleural plaques. Am J Ind Med. 2016;59(3):178–85.
6. Bach PB, Kattan MW, Thornquist MD, Kris MG, Tate RC, Barnett MJ, Hsieh LJ, Begg CB. Variations in lung cancer risk among smokers. J Natl Cancer Inst. 2003;95(6):470–8.
7. Spitz MR, Hong WK, Amos CI, Wu X, Schabath MB, Dong Q, Shete S, Etzel CJ. A risk model for prediction of lung cancer. J Natl Cancer Inst. 2007;99(9):715–26.
8. Gevenois PA, de Maertelaer V, Madani A, Winant C, Sergent G, De Vuyst P. Asbestosis, pleural plaques and diffuse pleural thickening: three distinct benign responses to asbestos exposure. Eur Respir J. 1998;11(5):1021–7.

9. Tiitola M, Kivisaari L, Zitting A, Huuskonen MS, Kaleva S, Tossavainen A, Vehmas T. Computed tomography of asbestos-related pleural abnormalities. Int Arch Occup Environ Health. 2002;75(4):224–8.
10. Mastrangelo G, Marangi G, Ballarin MN, Fadda E, Scoizzato L, Fedeli U, Marchiori L, Valentini F. Lung cancer risk in past asbestos workers a few decades after exposure cessation and prospects for screening. Arch Environ Occup Health. 2016;71(4):237–44.
11. Sverzellati N, Silva M, Calareso G, Galeone C, Marchiano A, Sestini S, et al. Low-dose computed tomography for lung cancer screening: comparison of performance between annual and biennial screen. Eur Radiol. 2016;26(11): 3821–9.
12. Fagerstrom KO. Measuring degree of physical dependence to tobacco smoking with reference to individualization of treatment. Addict Behav. 1978;3(3–4):235–41.
13. Pastorino U, Boffi R, Marchiano A, Sestini S, Munarini E, Calareso G, Boeri M, Pelosi G, Sozzi G, Silva M, et al. Stopping smoking reduces mortality in low-dose computed tomography screening participants. J Thoracic Oncol. 2016;11(5):693–9.
14. Remy-Jardin M, Sobaszek A, Duhamel A, Mastora I, Zanetti C, Remy J. Asbestos-related pleuropulmonary diseases: evaluation with low-dose four-detector row spiral CT. Radiology. 2004;233(1):182–90.
15. Meirelles GS, Kavakama JI, Jasinowodolinski D, Nery LE, Terra-Filho M, Rodrigues RT, Neder JA, Napolis LM, Bagatin E, D'Ippolito G, et al. Pleural plaques in asbestos-exposed workers: reproducibility of a new high-resolution CT visual semiquantitative measurement method. J Thorac Imaging. 2006;21(1):8–13.
16. Paris C, Thierry S, Brochard P, Letourneux M, Schorle E, Stoufflet A, Ameille J, Conso F, Pairon JC, National AM. Pleural plaques and asbestosis: dose- and time-response relationships based on HRCT data. Eur Respir J. 2009;34(1):72–9.
17. Hansell DM: Imaging of diseases of the chest, 5th ed. / David M. Hansell ... [et al.]. edn. [Edinburgh?]: Mosby; 2010.
18. Goldstraw P, Crowley J, Chansky K, Giroux DJ, Groome PA, Rami-Porta R, Postmus PE, Rusch V, Sobin L, International Association for the Study of Lung Cancer International Staging C, et al. The IASLC lung cancer staging project: proposals for the revision of the TNM stage groupings in the forthcoming (seventh) edition of the TNM classification of malignant tumours. J thoracic Oncol. 2007;2(8):706–14.
19. Brims FJ, Murray CP, de Klerk N, Alfonso H, Reid A, Manners D, Wong PM, Teh J, Olsen N, Mina R, et al. Ultra-low-dose chest computer tomography screening of an asbestos-exposed population in Western Australia. Am J Respir Crit Care Med. 2015;191(1):113–6.
20. Murray CP, Wong PM, Teh J, de Klerk N, Rosenow T, Alfonso H, et al. Ultra low dose CT screen-detected non-malignant incidental findings in the Western Australian Asbestos Review Programme. Respirology. 2016;21(8): 1419–24.
21. Markowitz SB, Levin SM, Miller A, Morabia A. Asbestos, asbestosis, smoking, and lung cancer. New findings from the north American insulator cohort. Am J Respir Crit Care Med. 2013;188(1):90–6.
22. Mastrangelo G, Ballarin MN, Bellini E, Bicciato F, Zannol F, Gioffre F, Zedde A, Tessadri G, Fedeli U, Valentini F, et al. Asbestos exposure and benign asbestos diseases in 772 formerly exposed workers: dose-response relationships. Am J Ind Med. 2009;52(8):596–602.
23. Baumann F, Buck BJ, Metcalf RV, McLaurin BT, Merkler DJ, Carbone M. The presence of asbestos in the natural environment is likely related to Mesothelioma in young individuals and women from southern Nevada. J thoracic Oncol. 2015;10(5):731–7.
24. Ferrante D, Mirabelli D, Tunesi S, Terracini B, Magnani C. Pleural mesothelioma and occupational and non-occupational asbestos exposure: a case-control study with quantitative risk assessment. Occup Environ Med. 2016;73(3):147–53.
25. Wheeler DC, Burstyn I, Vermeulen R, Yu K, Shortreed SM, Pronk A, Stewart PA, Colt JS, Baris D, Karagas MR, et al. Inside the black box: starting to uncover the underlying decision rules used in a one-by-one expert assessment of occupational exposure in case-control studies. Occup Environ Med. 2013;70(3):203–10.
26. Cox CW, Rose CS, Lynch DA. State of the art: imaging of occupational lung disease. Radiology. 2014;270(3):681–96.
27. Tockman MS. Clinical detection of lung cancer progression markers. J Cell Biochem Suppl. 1996;25:177–84.
28. Melamed MR. Lung cancer screening results in the National Cancer Institute new York study. Cancer. 2000;89(11 Suppl):2356–62.
29. Niklinski J, Niklinska W, Chyczewska E, Laudanski J, Naumnik W, Chyczewski L, Pluygers E. The epidemiology of asbestos-related diseases. Lung Cancer. 2004;45(Suppl 1):S7–S15.
30. Ledda C, Pomara C, Bracci M, Mangano D, Ricceri V, Musumeci A, Ferrante M, Musumeci G, Loreto C, Fenga C, et al. Natural carcinogenic fiber and pleural plaques assessment in a general population: a cross-sectional study. Environ Res. 2016;150:23–9.
31. Bach PB, Elkin EB, Pastorino U, Kattan MW, Mushlin AI, Begg CB, Parkin DM. Benchmarking lung cancer mortality rates in current and former smokers. Chest. 2004;126(6):1742–9.
32. Wille MM, Thomsen LH, Petersen J, de Bruijne M, Dirksen A, Pedersen JH, Shaker SB. Visual assessment of early emphysema and interstitial abnormalities on CT is useful in lung cancer risk analysis. Eur Radiol. 2016; 26(2):487–94.
33. Sverzellati N, Randi G, Spagnolo P, Marchiano A, Silva M, Kuhnigk JM, La Vecchia C, Zompatori M, Pastorino U. Increased mean lung density: another independent predictor of lung cancer? Eur J Radiol. 2013;82(8):1325–31.
34. Mascalchi M, Picozzi G, Falchini M, Vella A, Diciotti S, Carrozzi L, et al. Initial LDCT appearance of incident lung cancers in the ITALUNG trial. Eur J Radiol. 2014;83(11):2080–6.

Napsin A levels in epithelial lining fluid as a diagnostic biomarker of primary lung adenocarcinoma

Akifumi Uchida[1], Takuya Samukawa[1], Tomohiro Kumamoto[1], Masahiro Ohshige[1], Kazuhito Hatanaka[2], Yoshihiro Nakamura[3], Keiko Mizuno[1], Ikkou Higashimoto[1], Masami Sato[3] and Hiromasa Inoue[1*]

Abstract

Background: It is crucial to develop novel diagnostic approaches for determining if peripheral lung nodules are malignant, as such nodules are frequently detected due to the increased use of chest computed tomography scans. To this end, we evaluated levels of napsin A in epithelial lining fluid (ELF), since napsin A has been reported to be an immunohistochemical biomarker for histological diagnosis of primary lung adenocarcinoma.

Methods: In consecutive patients with indeterminate peripheral lung nodules, ELF samples were obtained using a bronchoscopic microsampling (BMS) technique. The levels of napsin A and carcinoembryonic antigen (CEA) in ELF at the nodule site were compared with those at the contralateral site. A final diagnosis of primary lung adenocarcinoma was established by surgical resection.

Results: We performed BMS in 43 consecutive patients. Among patients with primary lung adenocarcinoma, the napsin A levels in ELF at the nodule site were markedly higher than those at the contralateral site, while there were no significant differences in CEA levels. Furthermore, in 18 patients who were undiagnosed by bronchoscopy and finally diagnosed by surgery, the napsin A levels in ELF at the nodule site were identically significantly higher than those at the contralateral site. In patients with non-adenocarcinoma, there were no differences in napsin A levels in ELF. The area under the receiver operator characteristic curve for identifying primary lung adenocarcinoma was 0.840 for napsin A and 0.542 for CEA.

Conclusion: Evaluation of napsin A levels in ELF may be useful for distinguishing primary lung adenocarcinoma.

Keywords: Lung cancer diagnosis, Primary lung adenocarcinoma, Epithelial lining fluid, Biomarkers, Bronchoscopy

Background

Lung cancer is one of the most common malignant tumours and carries a high mortality rate [1]. The recent increased use of chest computed tomography (CT) has resulted in more frequent incidental detection of peripheral lung nodules, and the most common malignant finding is primary lung adenocarcinoma [2, 3]. Some novel tumour markers and imaging tests are useful for lung cancer [4], but these markers have inadequate diagnostic accuracy. Various circulating tumour markers for primary lung adenocarcinoma have been identified. Carcinoembryonic antigen (CEA) and sialyl Lewis Xi antigen (SLX) are clinically established and useful for the management of primary lung adenocarcinoma. However, their values in serum are not suitable for screening or diagnosis of early-stage primary lung adenocarcinoma due to low sensitivity and specificity [5–7].

The pathological diagnosis of primary lung adenocarcinoma is usually based on tissue or cytological samples obtained by bronchoscopy. However, collection of such samples is sometimes difficult due to the location and size of the nodule or the condition of the patient [2, 8]. CT-guided needle biopsy and thoracoscopic lung biopsy are useful alternative methods, although the invasiveness of both procedures is a disadvantage [9, 10]. Therefore, it is crucial to develop novel diagnostic tools, including other

* Correspondence: inoue-pulm@umin.net
[1]Department of Pulmonary Medicine, Graduate School of Medical and Dental Sciences, Kagoshima University, 8-35-1 Sakuragaoka, Kagoshima 890-8520, Japan
Full list of author information is available at the end of the article

biomarkers and techniques for sample collection, for the accurate diagnosis of primary lung adenocarcinoma.

Bronchoscopic microsampling (BMS) has attracted attention as a new diagnostic tool for lung cancer (Fig. 1) [11]. With the BMS technique it is possible to obtain epithelial lining fluid (ELF), the liquid which covers the bronchial wall and alveolus, without the need for saline injection [12]. ELF is transported toward the trachea by ciliary movement, and for diagnostic purposes it is not necessary for ELF to contact the tumour directly. Biochemical substances, including biochemical markers, tumour makers, tumour-derived nucleic acids and drug concentrations, can be measured by analysing ELF without the invasiveness or sample dilution required when testing bronchoalveolar lavage fluid [11, 13–19]. Of note, a previous study reported that measurement of CEA and cytokeratin fragment 19 in ELF was a beneficial diagnostic adjunct in patients with a small peripheral lung nodule [11].

Napsin A, an aspartic protease, is mainly expressed in alveolar type II cells. Previous studies have shown that napsin A is present and active in the alveolar space [20–22]. Immunohistochemical reactivity for napsin A is positive in most cases of primary lung adenocarcinoma, but negative in most cases of squamous cell carcinoma as well as adenocarcinoma of other organs. Its local expression was reported to be useful for identifying the lung origin of metastatic adenocarcinoma [23, 24]. In comparison with napsin A, CEA showed less sensitivity and specificity for histologically diagnosing lung adenocarcinoma using immunohistochemical biomarkers [25].

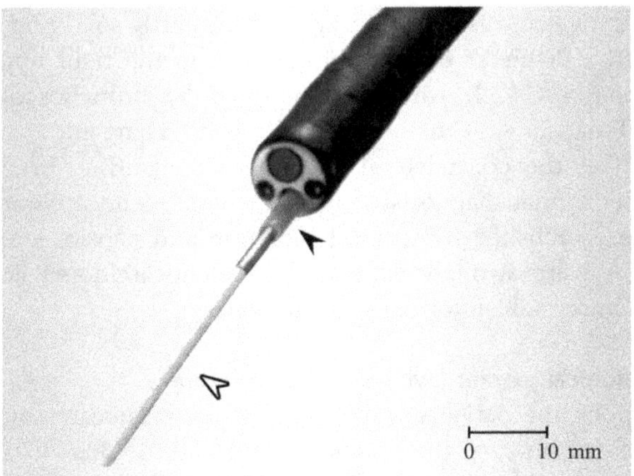

Fig. 1 Bronchoscopic microsampling (BMS) procedure. The BMS probe consists of a polyethylene outer sheath (black arrowhead) and an inner cotton fiber rod probe attached to a 30-mm-long stainless steel guide wire (white arrowhead). The probe is guided to the affected lesion in the subsegmental bronchus thorough the bronchoscope channel and the inner fiber rod probe (white arrowhead) is placed on the bronchial membrane as near as possible to the lung nodule. BMS: bronchoscopic maicrosampling

Based on these findings, we hypothesised that napsin A levels in ELF at the primary lung adenocarcinoma site would be increased. To test this hypothesis, we compared napsin A levels in ELF at the malignant nodule site with those at the unaffected contralateral site. Furthermore, we measured CEA levels in ELF and compared the diagnostic usefulness of ELF-derived napsin A and CEA.

Methods

Study design

Patients with an indeterminate peripheral lung nodule who had bronchoscopy at Kagoshima University Medical and Dental Hospital from December 2012 to September 2016 were enroled in this study. We planned to analyse subjects who required surgical resection of the primary lung cancer. The selection criterion for the present study was the presence of a peripheral lung nodule with a diameter of less than 30 mm that was anticipated to be resectable with indications for surgery via bronchoscopy. Written informed consent for this study was obtained before bronchoscopy. This study was approved by the institutional review board of Kagoshima University Medical and Dental Hospital and the committee's reference number was 24-71. A final definitive histological diagnosis of primary lung adenocarcinoma was made by surgical resection in all patients. For serum marker analysis, healthy volunteers with normal chest radiographs and who had provided written informed consent were matched for gender and age and enrolled in the study as a control group.

Microsampling probe and procedure

The BMS probe used was the BC-401C (Fig. 1, Olympus Co., Tokyo, Japan). ELF samples were obtained both from a subsegmental bronchus as near as possible to the nodule, using fluoroscopy, and from the contralateral subsegmental bronchus using first the BMS technique followed by endobronchial ultrasound sonography and fluoroscopy with subsequent transbronchial lung biopsy. The BMS method was performed as previously described [12]. After inserting a bronchoscope, the BMS probe in the outer sheath was inserted through the bronchoscope and the inner probe was advanced from the outer sheath toward the affected lesion at the subsegmental bronchus, and then the inner probe was placed on the bronchial membrane for 10 s to absorb the ELF. The inner probe was then immediately withdrawn into the outer sheath. This procedure was repeated three times. We also obtained ELF from the corresponding subsegmental bronchus of the contralateral lung as an internal control. After the BMS procedures, the inner probe tips were frozen at −80 °C. They were weighed and then ELF was extracted by stirring for 1 min following the addition of 3 mL of saline. The tips were then dried and weighed again to measure the ELF volume and calculate the dilution factor.

Measurement

The napsin A levels in both ELF (ELF-napsin A) and serum (serum-napsin A) were measured by enzyme-linked immunosorbent assay with the Human Napsin A Assay Kit (Immuno-Biological Laboratories Co., Gunma, Japan). The CEA levels in ELF (ELF-CEA) were determined by chemiluminescent enzyme immune assay with Lumipulse Presto CEA (Fujirebio Inc., Saitama, Japan), and those in serum (serum-CEA) were quantified by electro-chemiluminescence immune assay with Cobas 800 (Roche Diagnostics K.K., Tokyo, Japan). Both ELF-napsin A and ELF-CEA were expressed per unit volume after correction for the dilution factor.

Statistical analysis

The patients who were diagnosed as other than primary lung adenocarcinoma were treated as non-adenocarcinoma. Data were analysed using SPSS version 23 software (IBM SPSS, Chicago, USA). Differences in serum-napsin A and serum-CEA between patients with primary lung adenocarcinoma and those in the control group were analysed by the Mann-Whitney U test. Differences in the variables related to ELF-napsin A and ELF-CEA between the nodule site and contralateral site in the patients who underwent bronchoscopy were compared by the nonparametric Wilcoxon signed-rank test, since the data were not normally distributed. Differences in ELF-napsin A at the nodule site between the patients with primary lung adenocarcinoma and those with non-adenocarcinoma were analysed by the Mann-Whitney U test. The data for each histological subtype of primary lung adenocarcinoma were compared using the nonparametric Kruskal-Wallis analysis of variance test. Correlations were examined using Spearman's correlation test. Statistical significance was defined as $P < 0.05$. Receiver operating characteristic (ROC) curve analysis was used to assess the ability of ELF-napsin A and ELF-CEA, respectively, to predict the diagnosis of primary lung adenocarcinoma. In ROC analyses, the ELF values at the contralateral site in patients with primary lung adenocarcinoma and at the bilateral sites in patients with non-adenocarcinoma were treated as negative controls. The difference between the areas under the ROC curves (AUCs) for ELF-napsin A and ELF-CEA were performed with EZR version 1.36 (Saitama Medical Center, Jichi Medical University, Saitama, Japan), which is a graphical user interface for R (The R Foundation for Statistical Computing, Vienna, Austria). Any samples with values below the lower limit of quantification were assigned a value of half of the lower quantification limit for analysis.

Result

Patients characteristics

We performed BMS in 43 consecutive patients according to our selection criteria. Of 43 patients, 3 patients could not have a surgery because of distant metastasis. Five patients refused surgery for definitive diagnosis. Finally, total 8 patients were excluded, the remaining 35 patients were included in the analysis.

All patients underwent BMS followed by surgical resection without complications, except for mycobacterium infection, allowing for the determination of histological features. Of 35 patients, 27 patients were diagnosed with primary lung adenocarcinoma, and two patients were diagnosed as primary lung adenosquamous carcinoma and combined large cell neuroendocrine carcinoma (LCNEC); LCNEC with adenocarcinoma, respectively. In patients with non-adenocarcinoma, two patients were diagnosed with primary lung squamous cell carcinoma, one patient was diagnosed as primary lung large cell carcinoma, and one patient was diagnosed with metastatic carcinoma from nasopharyngeal carcinoma. The other two patients were identified as mycobacterium tuberculosis and nontuberculous mycobacterial infection, respectively (Table 1).

Patients with primary adenocarcinoma were 48 to 80 years of age, with a median age of 67 years. In 11 patients, the diagnosis of primary lung adenocarcinoma was obtained by transbronchial lung biopsy or curettage, while the other 18 patients were diagnosed by surgical resection. The pathological stage was determined surgically to be stage IA in 25 patients, stage IB in three, and stage IIIA in one. The diameter of the primary nodule at surgery was 22 (9–36) mm, median (range). One representative case is shown in Fig. 2. This partly solid nodule with a diameter of 20 mm was seen in the right upper lobe on CT. It was not diagnosed by bronchoscopy. ELF-napsin A at the nodule site was 20911 ng·mL^{-1}, and that at the contralateral site was 370 ng·mL^{-1}. In this case, a final diagnosis of primary lung adenocarcinoma was established by surgical resection and napsin A and CEA were strongly expressed in adenocarcinoma cells on immunohistological examination.

Biological marker levels in ELF and serum

Among the patients with primary lung adenocarcinoma, ELF-napsin A at the nodule site was 11091 (326–55729) ng·mL^{-1} after correction for the dilution factor, while that at the contralateral site was 805 (180–5266) ng·mL^{-1}, indicating a significant difference ($P < 0.001$, Fig. 3a). Conversely, ELF-CEA at the nodule site was 135 (6–7799) ng·mL^{-1}, and that at the contralateral site was 158 (6–1806) ng·mL^{-1}, indicating no significant difference ($P = 0.634$, Fig. 3b). Furthermore, in 18 patients who were undiagnosed by bronchoscopy and finally diagnosed by surgery, ELF-napsin

Table 1 Clinical characteristics of patient cohort

Characteristics					
Primary lung adenocarcinoma	$n = 27$		Non-adenocarcinoma	$n = 6$	
LC with adenocarcinoma component	$n = 2$				
Age (median, IQR)	67,	12		75,	14
	number of patients	(%)		number of patients	(%)
Gender					
Male	15	51.7		4	66.7
Female	14	48.3		2	33.3
Smoking status					
never	13	44.8		2	33.3
ex-smoker	11	38.0		3	50.0
current	5	17.2		1	16.7
Pathological diagnosis by bronchoscopy					
yes	11	37.9		5	83.3
no	18	62.1		1	16.7
Pathological stage					
IA	25	86.2			
IB	3	10.3			
IIIA	1	3.5			
Histological subtype and diagnosis					
Primary lung adenocarcinoma			Primary lung squamous cell carcionoma	2	33.2
Adenocarcinoma in situ	1	3.5	Primary lung large cell carcionoma	1	16.7
Minimally invasive adenocaricinoma			Metastatic carcinoma from nasopharyngeal carcinoma	1	16.7
Non-mucinous	4	13.7			
Mucinous	1	3.5	Mycobacterium tuberculosis	1	16.7
Adenocarcinoma			Nontuberculous mycobacterial infection	1	16.7
Lepidic adenocarcinoma	2	6.8			
Acinar adenocarcinoma	3	10.3			
Papillary adenocarcinoma	14	48.2			
Solid adenocarcinoma	1	3.5			
Invasive mucinous adenocarcinoma	1	3.5			
Adenosquamous carcinoma	1	3.5			
Combined LCNEC	1	3.5			

LC Lung carcinoma, *IQR* Interquartile range, *LCNEC* Large cell neuroendocrine carcinoma
Data are presented as number or %, unless otherwise stated
Pathological stage is classified according to the TNM Classification of Malignancy Tumors, 7th Edition
Histological type is categorised according to the WHO Classification of Tumors of the Lung, Pleura, Thymus and Heart, Fourth Edition

A at the nodule site was 8438 (326–52337) ng·mL^{-1}, and that at the contralateral site was 704 (235–5266) ng·mL^{-1}. In this population there were identically significant differences between ELF-napsin A at the nodule site and those at the contralateral site ($P = 0.001$, Fig. 3c), as well as no difference between ELF-CEA at the nodule site, 135 (6–545) ng·mL^{-1}, and that at the contralateral site, 201 (6–1003) ng·mL^{-1} ($P = 0.571$, Fig. 3d).

In serum analysis, serum-napsin A in patients with primary lung adenocarcinoma was 16.1 (2.0–366.1) ng·mL^{-1}, and that in the control group was 23.3 (3.1–219.5) ng·mL^{-1}, indicating no significant difference ($P = 0.251$). Similarly, there was no difference between serum-CEA in patients with primary lung adenocarcinoma, 3.3 (0.4-15.7) ng·mL^{-1}, and that in the control group, 1.8 (0.6-9.1) ng·mL^{-1}, ($P = 0.056$).

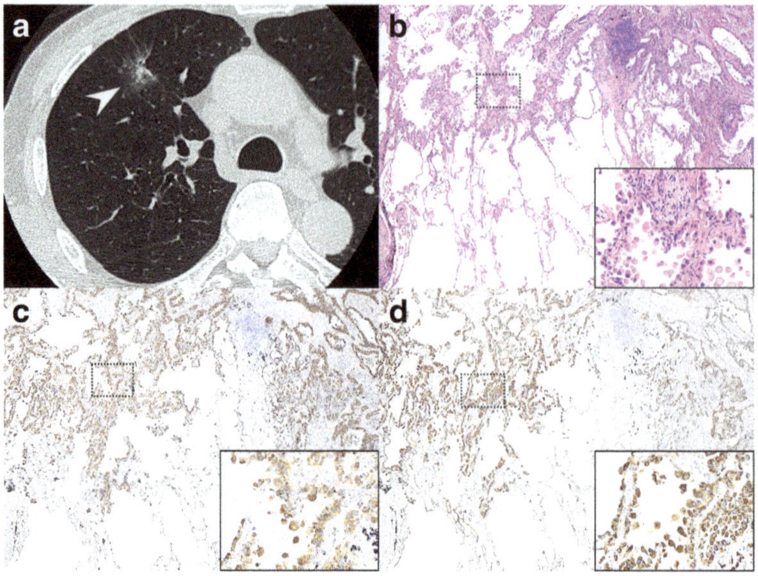

Fig. 2 Computed tomography (CT) and immunohistological findings in a representative case. **a** A lung CT image shows a 20-mm, partly solid, ground-glass opacity nodule (arrowhead) in the right upper lobe. **b** Minimally invasive adenocarcinoma. The cancer demonstrates predominant lepidic growth with <5-mm invasion. The cancer cells have polygonal cytoplasm and atypical nuclei (inset) (hematoxylin-eosin staining, original magnification ×40 and high magnification ×100). **c** Immunohistological staining for napsin A. Napsin A is strongly positive in adenocarcinoma cells (inset for greater detail) (original magnification ×40 and high magnification ×100). **d** Immunohistological staining for CEA. CEA is strongly positive in adenocarcinoma cells (inset for greater detail) (original magnification ×40 and high magnification ×100). CT: computed tomography; CEA: carcinoembryonic antigen

In patients with non-adenocarcinoma, ELF-napsin A at the nodule site was 2041 (398–5108) ng·mL^{-1}, and that at the contralateral site was 1719 (425–4186) ng·mL^{-1}, indicating no significant difference ($P = 0.463$, Fig. 4a). ELF-napsin A at the nodule site was significantly higher in primary lung adenocarcinoma than in non-adenocarcinoma ($P = 0.024$, Fig. 4b).

There was no significant difference in ELF-napsin A or ELF-CEA between histological subtypes of primary lung adenocarcinoma ($P = 0.919$ and $P = 0.590$, respectively). There was no significant difference in ELF-napsin A or ELF-CEA between smoking history and pathological stage (data not shown).

Relationship between ELF and other clinical parameters

There was no significant correlation between ELF-napsin A and serum-napsin A ($P = 0.916$, $r = 0.021$, Fig. 5a). There was no significant correlation between ELF napsin A and tumour sizes at surgery, however ELF-napsin A tended to rise as tumour sizes increased ($P = 0.053$, $r = 0.362$, Fig. 5b).

Diagnostic values of napsin A levels in ELF

We used ROC curve analysis to evaluate the sensitivity and specificity of ELF-napsin A and ELF-CEA as biomarkers for distinguishing primary lung adenocarcinoma (resected from 29 nodule sites) from normal tissue and non-adenocarcinoma (resected from 29 contralateral sites in primary lung adenocarcinoma and 12 bilateral sites in non-adenocarcinoma) (Fig. 6). The AUCs for nodule sites versus negative controls were 0.840 for ELF-napsin A and 0.542 for ELF-CEA (Table 2). The AUC of ELF-napsin A was significantly higher than that of ELF-CEA ($P < 0.001$). It was not possible to perform an ROC analysis for ELF-napsin A in combination with ELF-CEA using a binary logistic regression model, because the *p*-value of an ROC curve analysis for ELF-CEA was not significant. The optimal cut-off values for predicting the diagnosis of primary lung adenocarcinoma were 3280 ng·mL^{-1} for ELF-napsin A, with a sensitivity and specificity of 79.3% and 82.9%, respectively, and 82 ng·mL^{-1} for ELF-CEA, with sensitivity and specificity values of 75.9% and 34.1%, respectively (Table 2).

Discussion

In this study, we demonstrated that ELF-napsin A was a useful diagnostic marker for primary lung adenocarcinoma. ELF-napsin A at the nodule site was significantly higher in patients with primary lung adenocarcinoma. Moreover, except for three patients, ELF-napsin A at the nodule site was higher than that at the contralateral site. In the representative case shown in Fig. 2, many partly solid nodules could not be recognized on fluoroscopy or ultrasound sonography and were undiagnosed by bronchoscopy. Even in such patients, however, ELF-napsin A was significantly elevated. These findings suggested that in patients with elevated ELF-napsin A and no histological diagnosis of

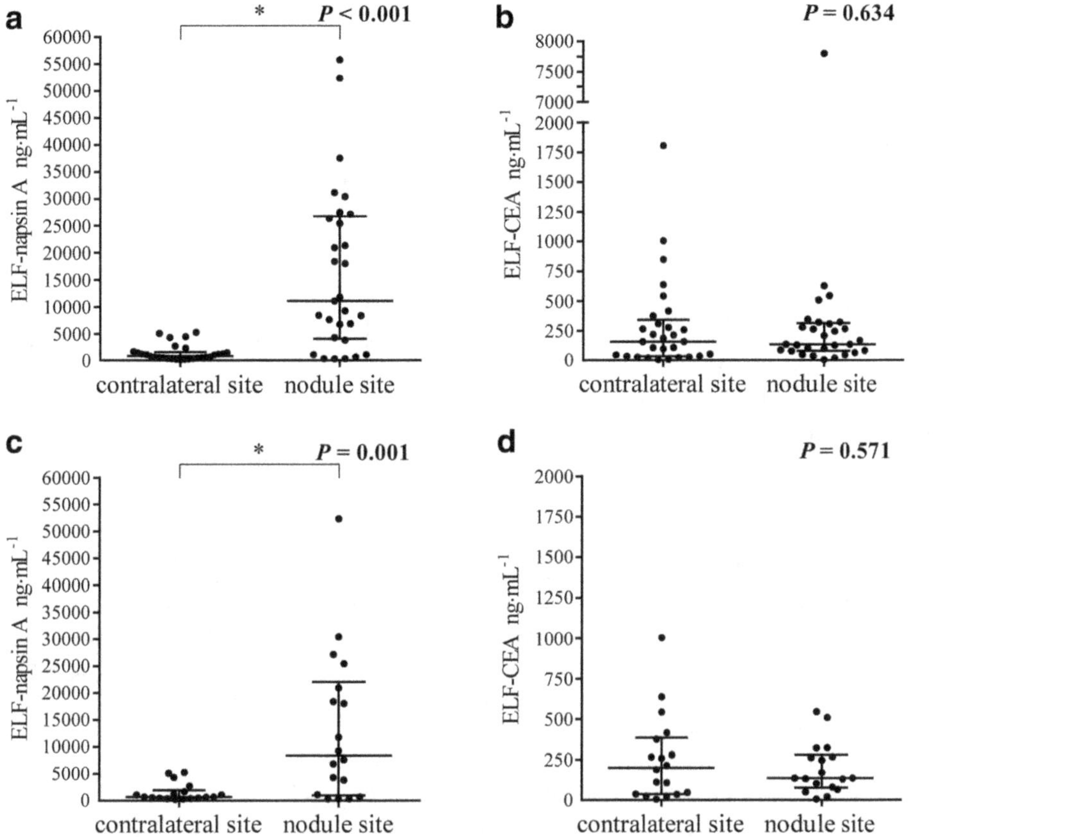

Fig. 3 Values of napsin A and CEA in ELF in the patients with primary lung adenocarcinoma. **a** Levels of napsin A in ELF (ELF-napsin A) in the patients with primary lung adenocarcinoma ($n = 29$, $P < 0.001$). **b** Values of CEA in ELF (ELF-CEA) in the patients with primary lung adenocarcinoma ($n = 29$, $P = 0.634$). **c** ELF-napsin A in the patients with primary lung adenocarcinoma who were undiagnosed by bronchoscopy and finally diagnosed by surgery ($n = 18$, $P = 0.001$). **d** ELF-CEA in the patients with primary lung adenocarcinoma who were undiagnosed by bronchoscopy and finally diagnosed by surgery ($n = 18$, $P = 0.571$). CEA: carcinoembryonic antigen; ELF: epithelial lining fluid

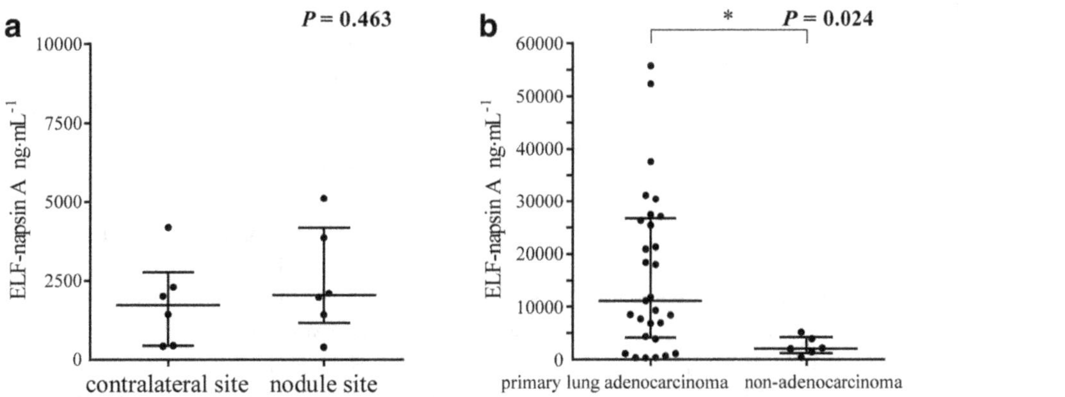

Fig. 4 Napsin A levels in ELF in patients with primary lung adenocarcinoma and those with non-adenocarcinoma. **a** Values of napsin A in ELF (ELF-napsin A) in the patients with non-adenocarcinoma ($n = 6$, $P = 0.463$). **b** ELF-napsin A at the nodule site in primary lung adenocarcinoma ($n = 29$) and in non-adenocarcinoma ($n = 6$) ($P = 0.024$). ELF: epithelial lining fluid

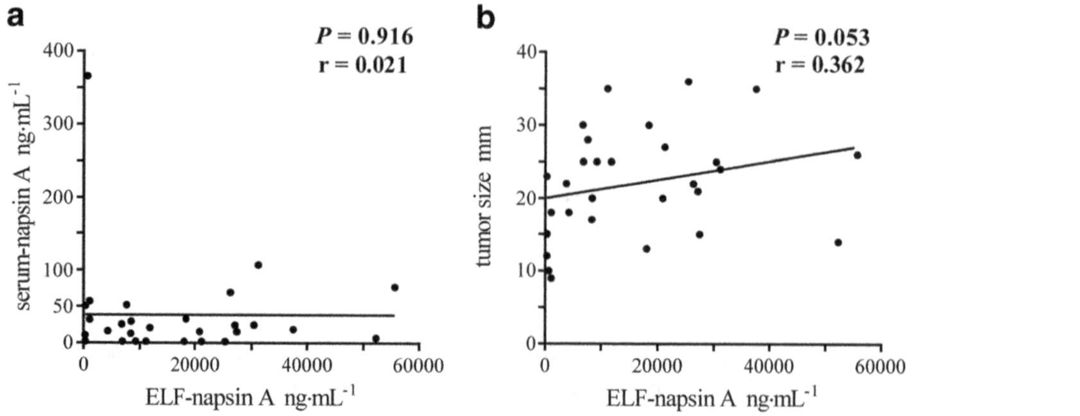

Fig. 5 Correlations of levels of napsin A in ELF. **a** Correlation between the levels of napsin A in ELF (ELF-napsin A) and the serum levels of napsin A (serum-napsin A) ($n = 28$, $P = 0.916$, $r = 0.021$). **b** Correlation between ELF-napsin A and the tumour size at surgery ($n = 29$, $P = 0.053$, $r = 0.362$). ELF: epithelial lining fluid

primary lung carcinoma by bronchoscopy, it is advisable to perform further evaluation with a high suspicion of primary lung adenocarcinoma. Furthermore, in ROC curve analysis, the AUC for ELF-napsin A was clearly higher than that for ELF-CEA, proving that ELF-napsin A is more valuable for diagnosing primary lung adenocarcinoma.

Because of the small diameters and complicated divergence patterns of bronchi, the detection rate of small lung nodules by bronchoscopy is not high. While the use of fluoroscopy, ultrasound sonography, and new bronchoscopy devices has gradually increased the rate of successful bronchoscopic diagnosis [8, 26–28], it is still not sufficient. If a definite diagnosis is not obtained by bronchoscopy, CT-guided needle biopsy or thoracoscopic lung biopsy are necessary, but both procedures are highly invasive and carry risks of grave complications [9, 10]. It is desirable to develop a diagnostic tool with fewer complications, more convenience, and higher sensitivity and specificity.

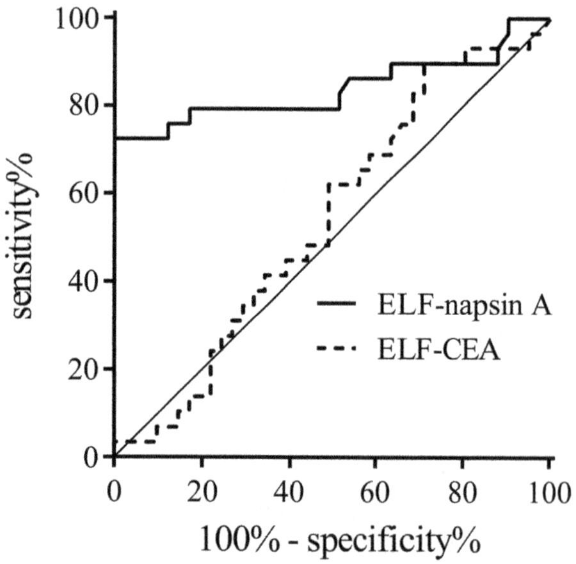

Fig. 6 Receiver operating characteristic (ROC) curve for napsin A and CEA in ELF. The ROC curves for napsin A in ELF (ELF-napsin A, solid line) and CEA in ELF (ELF-CEA, dashed line). The areas under the ROC curves are 0.840 for ELF-napsin A and 0.542 for ELF-CEA

The BMS technique, used to obtain ELF with bronchoscopy, is less invasive than bronchoalveolar lavage or transbronchial biopsy. Tumour-derived proteins and nucleic acids are contained in ELF close to a nodule, and the ELF is then transported toward the central bronchi by ciliary movement. As a result, the characteristics of a nodule can be evaluated by investigating ELF and direct access to the nodule is not necessary [11, 17–19]. A previous report found that the measurement of three biomarkers in ELF, namely CEA, cytokeratin fragment 19 and SLX, were useful for diagnosis of a small lung nodule [11]. But since these tumour markers are not specific for primary lung carcinoma, their utility for distinguishing primary lung carcinoma from metastatic cancer is uncertain. In contrast, napsin A is used as a diagnostic biomarker in immunohistochemical analyses for the purpose of discriminating between primary and metastatic lung carcinoma [23, 24].

In the present study, we demonstrated that ELF-napsin A at nodule sites was significantly higher than that at unaffected contralateral sites. The mechanism underlying this elevation in patients with primary lung adenocarcinoma is not known for certain, but it is probably due to overexpression of napsin A on primary lung adenocarcinoma tissue [29] in the alveolar space [20–22]. It may be that napsin A expressed by primary lung adenocarcinoma is released into the alveolar space and transported toward the central bronchi. The molecular weight of napsin A is approximately 38 kDa [30], while that of CEA is estimated to be 180 kDa [31]. This difference may account for the

Table 2 ROC analysis comparing ELF-napsin A and ELF-CEA

	AUC	95% CI, %	Cut off point	Sensitivity, %	Specificity, %	PPV, %	NPV, %	Positive LR	Negative LR
ELF-napsin A	0.840	72.8 to 95.3	3280 ng·mL^{-1}	79.3	82.9	76.7	85.0	4.64	0.25
ELF-CEA	0.542	40.7 to 67.8	82 ng·mL^{-1}	75.9	34.1	44.9	66.7	1.15	0.71

ELF Epithelial lining fluid, *CEA* Carcinoembryonic antigen, *AUC* Area under the ROC curve, *CI* Confidence interval, *PPV* Positive predictive value, *NPV* Negative predictive value, *LR* Likehood ratio

discrepancy in the detected levels of these markers in ELF. Furthermore, ELF-napsin A at nodule sites tended to rise according to increase in tumour size at surgery, suggesting that the expression of napsin A was greater with increased mass and secretory ability of primary lung adenocarcinoma, regardless of its histological subtype.

Serum-napsin A in patients with primary lung adenocarcinoma was not elevated compared with that in the control group. These results were consistent with our previous findings [32]. CEA is a commonly recommended biomarker in the management of lung cancer [33, 34]. But, because of its low sensitivity, it has not been generally recommended as a tool for the early screening of lung carcinoma, and it has been used as a potential prognostic biomarker and not a diagnostic biomarker. Moreover, CEA is not in itself a sufficiently strong indicator to guide treatment decisions for lung cancer [35]. A combination of biomarkers identifying primary lung adenocarcinoma may be helpful in distinguishing early-stage lung adenocarcinoma from benign lung disease, which presents as suspicious lung nodules.

The current study had several limitations. First, our sample size was small. Second, we could determine ELF-napsin A and ELF-CEA in cases of non-adenocarcinoma, including benign tumours and inflammation, in only a few patients. Last, the median diameter of primary lung adenocarcinoma at surgery was 22 mm. Therefore, our results should be confirmed in a larger cohort study, which includes various diseases and smaller-size lung nodules.

Conclusion

In summary, elevated napsin A levels in ELF were found in patients with primary lung adenocarcinoma, and the levels tended to rise as tumour size increased at surgery. Our findings suggest that napsin A levels in ELF may be clinically useful for distinguishing primary lung adenocarcinoma.

Abbreviations

AUC: Areas under the ROC curve; BMS: Bronchoscopic microsampling; CEA: Carcinoembryonic antigen; CT: Computed tomography; ELF: Epithelial lining fluid; ELF-CEA: CEA levels in ELF; ELF-napsin A: Napsin A levels in ELF; ROC: Receiver operating characteristic; serum-CEA: CEA levels in serum; serum-napsin A: Napsin A levels in serum; SLX: Sialyl Lewis Xi antigen

Acknowledgements

We thank Asami Harumatsu, Department of Pulmonary Medicine, Graduate School of Medical and Dental Sciences, Kagoshima University for their assistance in data collection.

Funding

This study was supported in part by Grants-in-Aid for Scientific Research from the Japan Society for the Promotion of Science (JSPS, KAKENHI grant 15 K09179).

Authors' contributions

AU, TS, MO and HI designed this study. AU, TK and MO contribute to the acquisition and analysis of data. AU, TS, KM, IH and HI contributed the data interpretation. KH, YN and MS revised this manuscript critically for important intellectual content. All authors read and approved the final manuscript.

Consent for publication

Witten informed consent for publication of all images in this manuscript was obtained from the patients.

Competing interests

Hiromasa Inoue reports grants from Astellas, AstraZeneca, Boehringer-Ingelheim, ChugaiPharm, GlaxoSmithKline, Pfizer, MerckSharp&Dohme, Teijin-Pharma, Torii, personal fees from Astellas, AstraZeneca, Boehringer-Ingelheim, Chugai-Pharm, GlaxoSmithKline, Kyorin, MerckSharp&Dohme, MeijiSeika-Pharma, Novartis, Otsuka, Pfizer, outside the submitted work.

Author details

[1]Department of Pulmonary Medicine, Graduate School of Medical and Dental Sciences, Kagoshima University, 8-35-1 Sakuragaoka, Kagoshima 890-8520, Japan. [2]Department of Pathology, Tokai University School of Medicine, 143 Shimokasuya, Isehara, Kanagawa, Japan. [3]Department of General Thoracic Surgery, Graduate School of Medical and Dental Sciences, Kagoshima University, 8-35-1 Sakuragaoka, Kagoshima, Japan.

References

1. World Health Organization. Cancer. Fact Sheet Number 297. www.who.int/mediacentre/factsheets/fs297/en/ Last updated February 2015. Accessed 10 Feb 2015.
2. Kennedy GT, Okusanya OT, Keating JJ, Heitjan DF, Deshpande C, Litzky LA, Albelda SM, Drebin JA, Nie S, Low PS, et al. The optical biopsy: a novel technique for rapid Intraoperative diagnosis of primary pulmonary Adenocarcinomas. Ann Surg. 2015;262(4):602–9.
3. Lim HJ, Ahn S, Lee KS, Han J, Shim YM, Woo S, Kim JH, Yie M, Lee HY, Yi CA. Persistent pure ground-glass opacity lung nodules >/= 10 mm in diameter at CT scan: histopathologic comparisons and prognostic implications. Chest. 2013;144(4):1291–9.

4. Slatore CG, Horeweg N, Jett JR, Midthun DE, Powell CA, Wiener RS, Wisnivesky JP, Gould MK. An official American Thoracic Society research statement: a research framework for pulmonary nodule evaluation and management. Am J Respir Crit Care Med. 2015;192(4):500–14.
5. Okada M, Nishio W, Sakamoto T, Uchino K, Yuki T, Nakagawa A, Tsubota N. Prognostic significance of perioperative serum carcinoembryonic antigen in non-small cell lung cancer: analysis of 1,000 consecutive resections for clinical stage I disease. Ann Thorac Surg. 2004;78(1):216–21.
6. Zenita K, Kirihata Y, Kitahara A, Shigeta K, Higuchi K, Hirashima K, Murachi T, Miyake M, Takeda T, Kannagi R. Fucosylated type-2 chain polylactosamine antigens in human lung cancer. Int J Cancer. 1988;41(3):344–9.
7. Satoh H, Ishikawa H, Kamma H, Yamashita YT, Takahashi H, Ohtsuka M, Hasegawa S. Serum sialyl lewis X-i antigen levels in non-small cell lung cancer: correlation with distant metastasis and survival. Clin Cancer Res. 1997;3(4):495–9.
8. Rivera MP, Mehta AC, Wahidi MM. Establishing the diagnosis of lung cancer: diagnosis and management of lung cancer, 3rd ed: American College of Chest Physicians evidence-based clinical practice guidelines. Chest. 2013; 143(5 Suppl):e142S–65S.
9. Wiener RS, Wiener DC, Gould MK. Risks of transthoracic needle biopsy: how high? Clin Pulm Med. 2013;20(1):29–35.
10. Wiener RS, Schwartz LM, Woloshin S, Welch HG. Population-based risk for complications after transthoracic needle lung biopsy of a pulmonary nodule: an analysis of discharge records. Ann Intern Med. 2011;155(3):137–44.
11. Watanabe M, Ishizaka A, Ikeda E, Ohashi A, Kobayashi K. Contributions of bronchoscopic microsampling in the supplemental diagnosis of small peripheral lung carcinoma. Ann Thorac Surg. 2003;76(5):1668–72. discussion 1673
12. Ishizaka A, Watanabe M, Yamashita T, Ogawa Y, Koh H, Hasegawa N, Nakamura H, Asano K, Yamaguchi K, Kotani M, et al. New bronchoscopic microsample probe to measure the biochemical constituents in epithelial lining fluid of patients with acute respiratory distress syndrome. Crit Care Med. 2001;29(4):896–8.
13. Ishizaka A, Matsuda T, Albertine KH, Koh H, Tasaka S, Hasegawa N, Kohno N, Kotani T, Morisaki H, Takeda J, et al. Elevation of KL-6, a lung epithelial cell marker, in plasma and epithelial lining fluid in acute respiratory distress syndrome. Am J Physiol Lung Cell Mol Physiol. 2004;286(6):L1088–94.
14. Koh H, Tasaka S, Hasegawa N, Asano K, Kotani T, Morisaki H, Takeda J, Fujishima S, Matsuda T, Hashimoto S, et al. Vascular endothelial growth factor in epithelial lining fluid of patients with acute respiratory distress syndrome. Respirology. 2008;13(2):281–4.
15. Kamiya K, Watanabe M, Kohno M, Izumi Y, Horinouchi H, Kawamura M, Shimada N, Nomori H. KL-6 and CEA levels in epithelial lining fluid microsamples predict response to gefitinib in patients with advanced non-small cell lung cancer. Respirology. 2011;16(6):976–82.
16. Kipnis E, Hansen K, Sawa T, Moriyama K, Zurawel A, Ishizaka A, Wiener-Kronish J. Proteomic analysis of undiluted lung epithelial lining fluid. Chest. 2008;134(2):338–45.
17. Kahn N, Kuner R, Eberhardt R, Meister M, Muley T, Winteroll S, Schnabel PA, Ishizaka A, Herth FJ, Poustka A, et al. Gene expression analysis of endobronchial epithelial lining fluid in the evaluation of indeterminate pulmonary nodules. J Thorac Cardiovasc Surg. 2009;138(2):474–9.
18. Yasuda H, Soejima K, Nakayama S, Kawada I, Nakachi I, Yoda S, Satomi R, Ikemura S, Terai H, Sato T, et al. Bronchoscopic microsampling is a useful complementary diagnostic tool for detecting lung cancer. Lung Cancer. 2011;72(1):32–8.
19. Kahn N, Meister M, Eberhardt R, Muley T, Schnabel PA, Bender C, Johannes M, Keitel D, Sultmann H, Herth FJ, et al. Early detection of lung cancer by molecular markers in endobronchial epithelial-lining fluid. J Thorac Oncol. 2012;7(6):1001–8.
20. Brasch F, Ochs M, Kahne T, Guttentag S, Schauer-Vukasinovic V, Derrick M, Johnen G, Kapp N, Muller KM, Richter J, et al. Involvement of napsin A in the C- and N-terminal processing of surfactant protein B in type-II pneumocytes of the human lung. J Biol Chem. 2003;278(49):49006–14.
21. Ueno T, Linder S, Na CL, Rice WR, Johansson J, Weaver TE. Processing of pulmonary surfactant protein B by napsin and cathepsin H. J Biol Chem. 2004;279(16):16178–84.
22. Woischnik M, Bauer A, Aboutaam R, Pamir A, Stanzel F, de Blic J, Griese M. Cathepsin H and napsin A are active in the alveoli and increased in alveolar proteinosis. Eur Respir J. 2008;31(6):1197–204.
23. Ueno T, Linder S, Elmberger G. Aspartic proteinase napsin is a useful marker for diagnosis of primary lung adenocarcinoma. Br J Cancer. 2003;88(8):1229–33.
24. Turner BM, Cagle PT, Sainz IM, Fukuoka J, Shen SS, Jagirdar J. Napsin A, a new marker for lung adenocarcinoma, is complementary and more sensitive and specific than thyroid transcription factor 1 in the differential diagnosis of primary pulmonary carcinoma: evaluation of 1674 cases by tissue microarray. Arch Pathol Lab Med. 2012;136(2):163–71.
25. Kim MJ, Shin HC, Shin KC, Ro JY. Best immunohistochemical panel in distinguishing adenocarcinoma from squamous cell carcinoma of lung: tissue microarray assay in resected lung cancer specimens. Ann Diagn Pathol. 2013;17(1):85–90.
26. Wang Memoli JS, Nietert PJ, Silvestri GA. Meta-analysis of guided bronchoscopy for the evaluation of the pulmonary nodule. Chest. 2012; 142(2):385–93.
27. Oki M, Saka H, Ando M, Asano F, Kurimoto N, Morita K, Kitagawa C, Kogure Y, Miyazawa T. Ultrathin Bronchoscopy with multimodal devices for peripheral pulmonary lesions. A randomized trial. Am J Respir Crit Care Med. 2015;192(4):468–76.
28. Mondoni M, Sotgiu G, Bonifazi M, Dore S, Parazzini EM, Carlucci P, Gasparini S, Centanni S. Transbronchial needle aspiration in peripheral pulmonary lesions: a systematic review and meta-analysis. Eur Respir J. 2016;48(1):196–204.
29. Sharma R, Wang Y, Chen L, Gurda GT, Geddes S, Gabrielson E, Askin F, Li QK. Utility of a novel triple marker (combination of TTF-1, Napsin-A and P40) in the subclassification of non-small cell lung carcinomas using fine needle aspiration cases. Hum Pathol. 2016;54:8–16.
30. Hirano T, Gong Y, Yoshida K, Kato Y, Yashima K, Maeda M, Nakagawa A, Fujioka K, Ohira T, Ikeda N, et al. Usefulness of TA02 (napsin A) to distinguish primary lung adenocarcinoma from metastatic lung adenocarcinoma. Lung Cancer. 2003;41(2):155–62.
31. Mitchell KF. A Carcinoembryonic antigen (CEA) specific monoclonal hybridma antibody that reacts only with high-molecular-weight CEA. Cancer Immunol Immunother. 1980;10:1–5.
32. Samukawa T, Hamada T, Uto H, Yanagi M, Tsukuya G, Nosaki T, Maeda M, Hirano T, Tsubouchi H, Inoue H. The elevation of serum napsin A in idiopathic pulmonary fibrosis, compared with KL-6, surfactant protein-a and surfactant protein-D. BMC Pulm Med. 2012;12:55.
33. Schneider J. Tumor markers in detection of lung cancer. Adv Clin Chem. 2006;42:1–41.
34. Lai RS, Hsu HK, Lu JY, Ger LP, Lai NS. CYFRA 21-1 enzyme-linked immunosorbent assay. Evaluation as a tumor marker in non-small cell lung cancer. Chest. 1996;109(4):995–1000.
35. Grunnet M, Sorensen JB. Carcinoembryonic antigen (CEA) as tumor marker in lung cancer. Lung Cancer. 2012;76(2):138–43.

21

Interventional bronchoscopy in malignant central airway obstruction by extra-pulmonary malignancy

Beomsu Shin[1], Boksoon Chang[2], Hojoong Kim[3] and Byeong-Ho Jeong[3*]

Abstract

Background: Interventional bronchoscopy is considered an effective treatment option for malignant central airway obstruction (MCAO). However, there are few reports of interventional bronchoscopy in patients with MCAOs due to extra-pulmonary malignancy. Therefore, the objective of this study was to investigate treatment outcomes and prognostic factors for bronchoscopic intervention in patients with MCAO due to extra-pulmonary malignancy.

Methods: We retrospectively analyzed consecutive 98 patients with MCAO due to extra-pulmonary malignancy who underwent interventional bronchoscopy between 2004 and 2014 at Samsung Medical Center (Seoul, Korea).

Results: The most common primary site of malignancy was esophageal cancer (37.9%), followed by thyroid cancer (16.3%) and head & neck cancer (10.2%). Bronchoscopic interventions were usually performed using a combination of mechanical debulking (84.7%), stent insertion (70.4%), and laser cauterization (37.8%). Of 98 patients, 76 (77.6%) patients had MCAO due to progression of malignancy, and 42 (42.9%) patients had exhausted all other anti-cancer treatment at the time of bronchoscopic intervention. Technical success was achieved in 89.9% of patients, and acute complications and procedure-related deaths occurred in 20.4% and 3.1% of patients, respectively. Reduced survival was associated with MCAO due to cancer other than thyroid cancer or lymphoma, mixed lesions, and not receiving adjuvant treatment after bronchoscopic intervention.

Conclusions: Bronchoscopic intervention could be a safe and effective procedure for MCAO due to end-stage extra-pulmonary malignancies. In addition, we identified possible prognostic factors for poor survival after intervention, which could guide clinicians select candidates that will benefit from bronchoscopic intervention.

Keywords: Interventional bronchoscopy, Malignant central airway obstruction, Extra-pulmonary malignancy

Background

Malignant central airway obstruction (MCAO) is clinically significant and is usually considered as a criterion for intervention; it is usually defined as ≥50% occlusion of the cross-sectional area of the trachea, mainstem bronchi, bronchus intermedius, or lobar bronchus [1]. MCAO can cause dyspnea, hemoptysis, atelectasis, and obstructive pneumonia, and is associated with decreased quality of life and increased mortality [2, 3]. However, treatments to resolve MCAOs have many limitations. Surgery is restrictively performed according to the location of the lesion, stage of the disease, and the general medical condition of each patient [4]. In addition, long periods of chemotherapy and radiation therapy may be needed to resolve airway obstruction [5]. On the other hand, bronchoscopic intervention can immediately alleviate symptoms related to airway obstruction and improve quality of life [1, 6, 7].

In total, 20–50% of patients with extra-pulmonary malignancy will have lung metastasis during their clinical course [8]. In addition, endobronchial metastases may occur in 1–4% of patients with extra-pulmonary malignancy [9, 10]. Finally, extra-pulmonary malignancy comprises 8–40% of all MCAO cases [1, 11, 12]. However, most studies have conducted analyses without classification based on primary malignancy sites, such as

* Correspondence: myacousticlung@gmail.com
[3]Division of Pulmonary and Critical Care Medicine, Department of Internal Medicine, Samsung Medical Center, Sungkyunkwan University School of Medicine, 81 Irwon-ro, Gangnam-gu, Seoul 06351, South Korea
Full list of author information is available at the end of the article

pulmonary and extra-pulmonary malignancies [1, 6, 11–15]. Based on these reports, there are limitations when managing patients with MCAO from an extra-pulmonary malignancy.

Herein, we conducted a retrospective study to evaluate the clinical outcomes and prognostic factors of bronchoscopic interventions in patients with MCAO due to extra-pulmonary malignancy.

Methods

Patients

We retrospectively reviewed all interventional bronchoscopy reports from January 2004 to December 2014 at Samsung Medical Center (a 1979-bed, tertiary care referral hospital in Seoul, South Korea) and identified 98 patients with MCAO due to extra-pulmonary malignancy. This study obtained approval from the institutional review board (IRB no. 2017-01-033) to review and publish information obtained from patient records. The need for informed consent was waived because patient information was anonymized and de-identified prior to analysis.

Airway intervention techniques

Airway anatomy was evaluated using chest computed tomography (CT) and, when possible, flexible bronchoscopy. MCAO was defined as ≥50% occlusion of the cross-sectional area of the trachea, main stem bronchi, bronchus intermedius, or lobar bronchus on the CT images or bronchoscopic findings [1].

Interventional bronchoscopy was performed according to standard techniques [16, 17]. After induction of general anesthesia, the patient was intubated with a rigid bronchoscope tube (Bryan Co., Woburn, MA, USA or Karl-Storz, Tuttlingen, Germany). Depending on the characteristics of airway obstruction (endobronchial lesion, extrinsic compression, and mixed lesion) and the medical condition of the patient, various combinations of airway intervention techniques were used, including mechanical debulking, laser, and insertion of silicone stents. Any endobronchial lesion was removed mechanically using rigid bronchoscope tubes and forceps. A neodymium-doped yttrium aluminum garnet laser (LaserSonics, Milpitas, CA, USA) or a diode laser (Biolitec, Ceralas®, Germany) were used to cauterize visible vessels before mechanical debulking or to ablate residual endobronchial tumor. Additionally, if needed, a silicone stent (Natural stent [M1S Co., Seoul, Korea] or Dumon stent [Novatech, La Ciotat, France]) was inserted to maintain airway patency against extrinsic compression or rapid progression [18].

Technical success was based on anatomic criteria, which were defined as the reopening of the airway lumen to > 50% of the normal cross sectional area and a connection to a viable area of distal lung by bronchoscopy [1]. If a physician successfully reopened a proximal airway, but then discovered distal lesions that occluded all segmental or subsegmental levels, this was classified as a technical failure [1].

Data collection

We retrospectively reviewed the medical records of all 98 patients. The following data were collected: demographic characteristics, primary site of malignancy, bronchoscopic findings (site of lesion, type of obstruction, and severity and length of stenosis), pre- and post-procedure treatment modalities, techniques applied during bronchoscopic interventions, procedure-related complications, and survival time.

Performance status was evaluated using the American Society of Anesthesiologists (ASA) physical status classification. Poor performance was defined as ≥ class 3 ASA physical status, which indicates severe systemic disease with functional limitation [19]. The severity of airway stenosis was determined using the Myer-Cotton stenosis grading system: Grade I, ≤50% luminal stenosis; Grade II, 51–70% luminal stenosis; Grade III, 71–99% luminal stenosis; and Grade IV, no lumen [20]. Respiratory distress was defined as worsening oxygenation or dyspnea after the procedure requiring additional oxygen supplies for at least 24 h. Excessive bleeding was defined as procedure-related bleeding which required transfusion or escalation in level of care.

Because all patients were in terminal stage with pulmonary metastasis from extra-pulmonary malignancy, the status of malignancy at the first bronchoscopic intervention was divided as follows. First, detection time of MCAO was divided as initial diagnosis of malignancy that had not yet been treated and disease progression of malignancy despite anti-cancer treatment. Second, we investigated the history of anti-cancer treatment after the first bronchoscopic intervention, and patients were divided into whether they received adjuvant treatment or not.

Statistical analysis

Data are presented as number (%) for categorical variables and median (interquartile range [IQR]) for continuous variables. The Kaplan–Meier method was used to estimate overall survival after the first bronchoscopic intervention. A multivariable Cox proportional hazard regression analysis was used to identify independent prognostic factors associated with overall survival. Because the total number of patients was not large enough to allow all variables to be analyzed, demographic data and variables that seemed to be directly related to the procedure and survival were selectively included in the analysis. The appropriateness of the proportional hazards assumption was evaluated using plots of the log minus log of Kaplan–Meier survival against the log of time. Statistical differences were considered significant at $P < 0.05$. All statistical analyses were performed using SPSS software (IBM SPSS Statistics ver. 22, Chicago, IL, USA).

Results

Baseline characteristics

Baseline characteristics of the study population are summarized in Table 1. Of the 98 patients, 60 (61.2%) were males. The median age was 63 (IQR, 54–72) years old and the median body mass index (BMI) was 21.1 kg/m^2 (IQR, 18.1–24.3 kg/m^2). Thirty-five patients (35.7%) had an ASA physical status ≥ class 3, and intubation before intervention was needed in 12 (12.2%) patients due to respiratory failure. The most common primary site of malignancy was esophageal cancer (37.9%), followed by thyroid cancer (16.3%), head & neck cancer (10.2%), renal cell carcinoma (7.1%), colorectal cancer (7.1%), and lymphoma (5.1%).

Characteristics of the MCAO site are summarized in Table 2. The most common site of MCAO was the trachea (63.3%), followed by the left main bronchus (21.4%)

Table 1 Baseline characteristics

Variables	*N* = 98
Age, years	63 (54–72)
Sex, male	60 (61.2)
Body mass index, kg/m^2	21.1 (18.1–24.3)
Comorbidity	
Diabetes mellitus	10 (10.2)
Chronic liver disease	8 (8.2)
Cerebrovascular disease	7 (7.1)
Congestive heart disease	6 (6.1)
Chronic pulmonary disease	3 (3.1)
Poor performance status[a]	35 (35.7)
Intubation due to respiratory failure before intervention	12 (12.2)
Primary site of malignancy	
Local extension	63 (64.4)
Esophageal cancer	37 (37.9)
Thyroid cancer	16 (16.3)
Head & neck cancer	10 (10.2)
Metastatic disease	35 (35.6)
Renal cell carcinoma	7 (7.1)
Colorectal cancer	7 (7.1)
Lymphoma	5 (5.1)
Others[b]	16 (16.3)

Data are presented as n (%) or the median (interquartile range)
[a]American Society of Anesthesiologists (ASA) physical status class ≥3 means severe systemic disease with functional limitation
[b]Sarcoma (*n* = 4), breast cancer (*n* = 3), hepatocellular carcinoma (*n* = 3), gastric cancer (*n* = 1), ovarian cancer (*n* = 1), neuroblastoma (*n* = 1), thymic cancer (*n* = 1), mesothelioma (*n* = 1), and peripheral nerve sheath tumor (*n* = 1)

Table 2 Bronchoscopic findings

Variables	*N* = 98
Site of lesion	
Single lesion	93 (94.9)
Trachea	62 (63.3)
Left main bronchus	21 (21.4)
Right main bronchus	6 (6.1)
Right bronchus intermedius	1 (1.0)
Lobar bronchus	3 (3.1)
Extended lesion	5 (5.1)
Trachea and each or both bronchi	3 (3.1)
Both main bronchi	2 (2.0)
Type of obstruction	
Endobronchial lesion	29 (29.6)
Extrinsic compression	15 (15.3)
Mixed lesion	54 (55.1)
Severity of stenosis (Myer and Cotton Grade)[a]	
II	25 (25.5)
III	55 (56.1)
IV	18 (18.4)
Length of MCAO[b], mm	30 (22–38)
Fistula between trachea and esophagus	8 (8.2)

Data are presented as n (%) or the median (interquartile range)
MCAO malignant central airway obstruction
[a]Categorization based on the percentage of reduction in cross-sectional area. Grade 1, ≤ 50% lumenal stenosis; Grade II, 51–70% lumenal stenosis; Grade III, 71–99% lumenal stenosis; Grade IV, no lumen
[b]Length of MCAO was defined as the sum of the length of the obstructive lesions more than Grade II

and the right main bronchus (6.1%). Mixed, endobronchial, and extrinsic obstructions were seen in 54 (55.1%), 29 (29.6%), and 15 (15.3%) patients, respectively. Most patients (74.5%) had ≥71% obstruction of cross sectional area (Grade III or IV). The median length of stenosis was 30 mm (IQR, 22–38 mm). Some patients (8.2%) had a fistula between the trachea and the esophagus.

Treatment modalities and complications

The median time from diagnosis of MCAO to bronchoscopic intervention was 0.4 months (IQR, 0.2-1.0 months) (Table 3). Bronchoscopic interventions were usually performed using a combination of treatment modalities, including mechanical debulking (84.7%), stent insertion (70.4%), and laser cauterization (37.8%). Thirty-five (35.7%) patients underwent bronchoscopic intervention more than twice during their clinical courses. Finally, only 10 patients (10.2%) had a technical failure. Of 22 patients who were diagnosed with MCAO as the initial diagnosis of malignancy, 7 (31.8%) patients did not receive adjuvant treatment after interventional bronchoscopy. Of 76 patients who were diagnosed with MCAO due to

Table 3 Treatment modalities and complications

Variables	N = 98
Time interval from diagnosis of MCAO to intervention, months	0.4 (0.2 – 1.0)
Treatment modalities	
Mechanical debulking	83 (84.7)
Silicone stent	69 (70.4)
Tube stent	65 (66.3)
Y stent	7 (7.1)
Laser	37 (37.8)
Tracheostomy	4 (4.1)
Number of interventional bronchoscopies	
1	63 (64.3)
≥ 2	35 (35.7)
Technical failure	10 (10.2)
MCAO as initial diagnosis of malignancy	22 (22.4)
No adjuvant treatment after interventional bronchoscopy	7 (7.1)
Adjuvant radiation therapy	10 (10.2)
Adjuvant chemotherapy	6 (6.1)
Adjuvant surgical resection	2 (2.0)
MCAO as disease progression of malignancy	76 (77.6)
No adjuvant treatment after interventional bronchoscopy	35 (35.7)
Adjuvant radiation therapy	28 (28.6)
Adjuvant chemotherapy	18 (18.4)
Adjuvant surgical resection	1 (1.0)
Acute complications	20 (20.4)
Respiratory distress	13 (13.3)
Excessive bleeding	10 (10.2)
Pneumothorax	3 (3.1)
Procedure-related death[a]	3 (3.1)
30-day mortality	13 (13.3)
Chronic complications	25 (25.5)
Mucostasis	19 (19.4)
Granulation tissue overgrowth	10 (10.2)
Stent migration	6 (6.1)

Data are presented as n (%) or the median (interquartile range)
MCAO malignant central airway obstruction
Patients could undergo more than one adjuvant treatment
Patients could have more than one complication
[a]Three patients died from tension pneumothorax, excessive bleeding, and pneumonia, respectively

progression of their malignancy, 35 (46.1%) did not receive adjuvant treatment after interventional bronchoscopy.

Acute complications included respiratory distress ($n = 13$), excessive bleeding ($n = 10$), and pneumothorax ($n = 3$) (Table 3). Procedure-related deaths occurred in three patients from tension pneumothorax, excessive bleeding, and pneumonia, respectively. Although chronic complications including mucostasis ($n = 19$), granulation tissue overgrowth ($n = 10$), and stent migration ($n = 6$) occurred not infrequently, most complications were manageable with additional procedures.

Survival and prognosis

Figure 1 shows the overall survival after bronchoscopic intervention according to primary site of malignancy, type of obstruction, and adjuvant treatment or not after interventional bronchoscopy. Median survival was 7 months and 30-day mortality was 13.3%. Survival rates at 1 year, 2 years, and 5 years were 34.7%, 22.4%, and 11.2%, respectively.

Table 4 shows independent prognostic factors related to mortality based on analysis with univariate and multivariate Cox proportional hazard regression. Because the plots of the log minus log of Kaplan–Meier survival against the log of time for all the variables seemed to be parallel, the hazards can be considered proportional. According to these analyses, overall survival was independently associated with primary site of malignancy, type of obstruction, and adjuvant treatment. Patients with thyroid cancer or lymphoma had better survival than those with other primary malignancies (adjusted hazard ratio [aHR], 0.245; 95% confidence interval [CI], 0.104–0.573; $P = 0.001$). Mixed lesions were significantly associated with worse survival compared to endobronchial lesions (aHR, 1.951; 95% CI, 1.084–3.510; $P = 0.026$). Patients with MCAO receiving adjuvant treatment had better survival than those with MCAO not receiving adjuvant treatment (aHR, 0.519; 95% CI, 0.301–0.895; $P = 0.018$).

Discussion

In patients with MCAO, bronchoscopic intervention can provide significant palliation [1, 21, 22]. In particular, bronchoscopic intervention may relieve life-threatening obstruction and provide better opportunities for other therapeutic modalities such as radiation and chemotherapy in patients with respiratory failure caused by MCAO [23]. This study revealed that bronchoscopic interventions such as mechanical debulking, laser, and stent insertion could be performed safely and successfully in most patients with MCAO due to extra-pulmonary malignancy. In addition, we found that poor survival was associated with primary malignancy site, mixed lesions, and not receiving adjuvant treatment after interventional bronchoscopy.

Recently, cancer survival has consistently increased because of advances in early detection and treatment and aging of the population [24]. In this respect, MCAO is importantly associated with a major reduction in quality of life and survival [3]. As the effectiveness of bronchoscopic intervention in patients with MCAO is well-

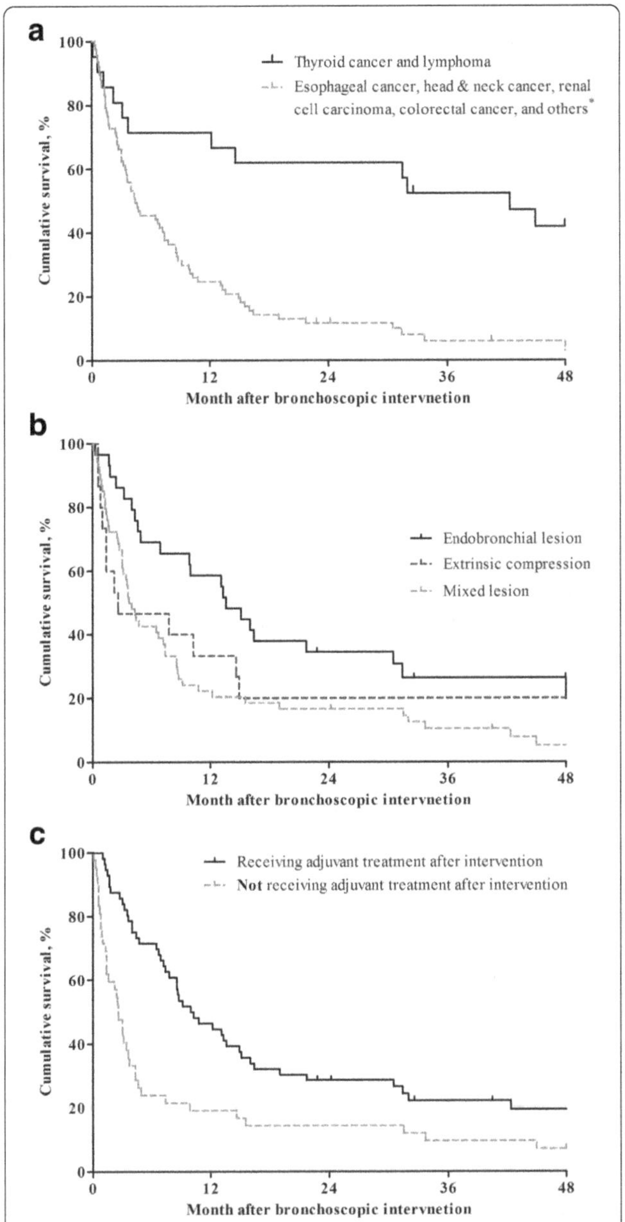

Fig. 1 Overall survival of patients after interventional bronchoscopy. Survival based on (**a**) primary site of malignancy, (**b**) type of obstruction, and (**c**) receiving adjuvant treatments or not after interventional bronchoscopy. MCAO, malignant central airway obstruction. *Sarcoma ($n = 4$), breast cancer ($n = 3$), hepatocellular carcinoma ($n = 3$), gastric cancer ($n = 1$), ovarian cancer ($n = 1$), neuroblastoma ($n = 1$), thymic cancer ($n = 1$), mesothelioma ($n = 1$), and peripheral nerve sheath tumor ($n = 1$)

known [1, 6, 11–14, 25, 26], bronchoscopic intervention is a preferred palliative therapy for relief of MCAO [21, 22]. However, most research is limited to patients with MCAO due to primary pulmonary malignancy [25, 26], or to a small proportion of patients with MCAO due to extra-pulmonary malignancy [1, 6, 11–15]. Furthermore, previous studies performed analysis without separating patients based on the primary site of malignancy. Although some reports targeted patients with MCAO due to extra-pulmonary malignancy, only a small number of patients were included [27–29]. For these reasons, previous reports were limited when analyzing treatment outcomes and prognostic factors in patients with MCAO due to extra-pulmonary malignancy.

In the present study, the technical success rate was 90.8%, and acute complication- and procedure-related mortality were 20.4% and 3.1%, respectively. Because there are few reports regarding bronchoscopic intervention in patients with MCAO due to extra-pulmonary malignancy, it is difficult to compare clinical outcomes with previous reports. Nonetheless, the technical success rate of the present study was as high as previous reports of interventional bronchoscopy in patients with MCAO due to mainly primary pulmonary malignancy, which was 88–100% [1, 6, 14, 25, 26]. However, acute complications and procedure-related mortality were slightly higher in the present study than in previous studies, which were 3–10% [6, 11, 25, 30] and 1% [6, 12, 14, 30], respectively. Considering that most of our patients had terminal-stage cancer and almost half of the patients had no further options for anti-cancer treatment in this study, we think that these technical success rates and complication rates are reasonable.

In this study, we also investigated prognostic factors associated with overall survival after the first bronchoscopic intervention. First, survival depends on the primary site of malignancy. We expected that patients with MCAO due to thyroid cancer (which is known to be slowly progressive) and lymphoma (known to have good response to chemoradiation therapy) would have better survival than those with MCAO due to other malignancies. Second, mixed lesions were a poor prognostic factor compared to endobronchial lesions. Mixed lesions frequently require a multimodal approach and can be associated with increased complications and mortality [15, 30]. Third, patients with MCAO not receiving adjuvant treatment after interventional bronchoscopy had a poor prognosis. As seen in previous studies, survival was poor among patients who had exhausted all options such as radiation, chemotherapy, and surgery before bronchoscopic intervention [6, 15, 25]. On the other hand, BMI, poor performance status, as evaluated by ASA score, intubation state before intervention, and detection time of MCAO were not significantly associated with increased mortality in our study. We hypothesize that this was because their poor general condition was rapidly resolved and did not influence long term survival after successful intervention. Thus, bronchoscopic intervention should not be limited to these populations.

This report has several limitations. First, selection bias may have influenced the significance of our results due

Table 4 Prognostic factors related to mortality

Variables	N	Univariable Cox regression		Multivariable Cox regression	
		Unadjusted HR (95% CI)	P	Adjusted HR (95% CI)	P
Age, years	–	0.996 (0.982–1.010)	0.596	1.005 (0.981 – 1.029)	0.679
Sex, male	60	1.224 (0.792–1.890)	0.363	0.721 (0.398 – 1.307)	0.282
Body mass index, kg/m^2	–	0.925 (0.869–0.984)	0.013	0.968 (0.901 – 1.041)	0.381
Poor performance status[a]	35	1.201 (0.776–1.859)	0.411	0.801 (0.470 – 1.363)	0.413
Intubation due to respiratory failure before intervention	12	1.308 (0.692–2.470)	0.409	1.110 (0.517 – 2.384)	0.788
Primary site of malignancy					
Esophageal, head & neck, renal, and colorectal cancer and others[b]	77	Reference		Reference	
Thyroid cancer and lymphoma	21	0.316 (0.174–0.575)	< 0.001	0.245 (0.104–0.573)	0.001
Site of lesion					
Single lesion	93	Reference		Reference	
Extended lesion	5	3.399 (1.333–8.663)	0.010	1.407 (0.433 – 4.571)	0.571
Type of obstruction					
Endobronchial lesion	29	Reference		Reference	
Extrinsic compression	15	1.261 (0.624–2.551)	0.518	0.879 (0.321–2.404)	0.802
Mixed lesion	54	1.914 (1.171–3.130)	0.010	1.951 (1.084–3.510)	0.026
Severity of stenosis (Myer and Cotton Grade)[c]					
II and III	80	Reference		Reference	
IV	18	1.057 (0.617–1.809)	0.841	0.556 (0.276 – 1.120)	0.100
Length of MCAO[d], mm	–	1.007 (0.989–1.024)	0.468	1.016 (0.988 – 1.044)	0.274
Number of interventional bronchoscopies					
1	63	Reference		Reference	
≥ 2	35	0.721 (0.461–1.129)	0.153	0.787 (0.461 – 1.342)	0.378
Detection time of MCAO					
Initial diagnosis of malignancy that have not yet been treated	22	Reference		Reference	
Disease progression of malignancy despite anti-cancer treatment	76	1.963 (1.146–3.362)	0.014	1.541 (0.710 – 3.347)	0.274
Adjuvant treatment after interventional bronchoscopy					
Not receiving adjuvant treatment	56	Reference		Reference	
Receiving adjuvant treatment	42	0.501 (0.327–0.768)	0.002	0.519 (0.301–0.895)	0.018

HR hazard ratio, *CI* confidential interval, *MCAO* malignant central airway obstruction

[a]American Society of Anesthesiologists (ASA) physical status class ≥3 means severe systemic disease with functional limitation

[b]Sarcoma ($n = 4$), breast cancer ($n = 3$), hepatocellular carcinoma ($n = 3$), gastric cancer ($n = 1$), ovarian cancer ($n = 1$), neuroblastoma ($n = 1$), thymic cancer ($n = 1$), mesothelioma ($n = 1$), and peripheral nerve sheath tumor ($n = 1$)

[c]Categorization based on the percentage of reduction in cross-sectional area. Grade 1, ≤ 50% lumenal stenosis; Grade II, 51–70% lumenal stenosis; Grade III, 71–99% lumenal stenosis; Grade IV, no lumen

[d]Length of MCAO was defined as the sum of the length of the obstructive lesions more than Grade II

to the retrospective design at a single center. Second, there have been advancements in treatment options for patients with terminal malignancy, such as chemoradiotherapy and supportive care throughout the study period. These advancements might have influenced recent patients, leading to slower disease progression and better survival than former patients. Third, there may be a lead-time bias in our results. Because all the patients were in terminal stage with pulmonary metastasis from extra-pulmonary malignancy at the time of diagnosis for MCAO, we divided all patients by detection time and receiving adjuvant treatment or not. Although we adjusted for these variables in the multivariable Cox proportional hazard regression analysis, lead-time bias may have influenced our results. Fourth, the number of patients was relatively small for multivariate analysis, including many prognostic variables. Therefore, interpretation of the main results will require caution. Finally, we could not evaluate spirometric data, quality of life, and symptom scores before and after treatment. This would be vital since the interventional procedures for MCAO are primarily palliative.

Conclusions

In conclusion, bronchoscopic intervention could be a safe and effective procedure for terminal stage cancer patients with extra-pulmonary malignancies with lung metastasis. Poor prognosis may be related with MCAO due to cancer other than thyroid cancer or lymphoma, mixed lesions, and no adjuvant treatment after bronchoscopic intervention. We hope that this study can help clinicians select candidates that will benefit from bronchoscopic intervention.

Funding
None.

Authors' contributions
BS has been involved in collection and assembly of data, data analysis and interpretation, and manuscript writing. BC has been involved in collection and assembly of data, data analysis and interpretation, and review. HK has been involved in conception and design and review. BHJ has been involved in conception and design, collection and assembly of data, data analysis and interpretation, manuscript writing, and review. All authors read and approved the final manuscript.

Consent for publication
Not applicable.

Competing interests
The authors declare that they have no competing interests.

Author details
[1]Department of Internal Medicine, Yonsei University Wonju College of Medicine, Wonju, South Korea. [2]Department of Pulmonary and Critical Care Medicine, Kyung Hee University Hospital at Gangdong, School of Medicine, Kyung Hee University, Seoul, South Korea. [3]Division of Pulmonary and Critical Care Medicine, Department of Internal Medicine, Samsung Medical Center, Sungkyunkwan University School of Medicine, 81 Irwon-ro, Gangnam-gu, Seoul 06351, South Korea.

References

1. Ost DE, Ernst A, Grosu HB, Lei X, Diaz-Mendoza J, Slade M, Gildea TR, Machuzak MS, Jimenez CA, Toth J, et al. Therapeutic bronchoscopy for malignant central airway obstruction: success rates and impact on dyspnea and quality of life. Chest. 2015;147(5):1282–98.
2. Macha HN, Becker KO, Kemmer HP. Pattern of failure and survival in endobronchial laser resection. A matched pair study. Chest. 1994;105(6):1668–72.
3. Walser EM, Robinson B, Raza SA, Ozkan OS, Ustuner E, Zwischenberger J. Clinical outcomes with airway stents for proximal versus distal malignant tracheobronchial obstructions. J Vasc Interv Radiol. 2004;15(5):471–7.
4. Wood DE. Management of malignant tracheobronchial obstruction. Surg Clin North Am. 2002;82(3):621–42.
5. Nihei K, Ishikura S, Kawashima M, Ogino T, Ito Y, Ikeda H. Short-course palliative radiotherapy for airway stenosis in non-small cell lung cancer. Int J Clin Oncol. 2002;7(5):284–8.
6. Jeon K, Kim H, Yu CM, Koh WJ, Suh GY, Chung MP, Kwon OJ. Rigid bronchoscopic intervention in patients with respiratory failure caused by malignant central airway obstruction. J Thorac Oncol. 2006;1(4):319–23.
7. Seijo LM, Sterman DH. Interventional pulmonology. N Engl J Med. 2001; 344(10):740–9.
8. Greelish JP, Friedberg JS. Secondary pulmonary malignancy. Surg Clin North Am. 2000;80(2):633–57.
9. Marchioni A, Lasagni A, Busca A, Cavazza A, Agostini L, Migaldi M, Corradini P, Rossi G. Endobronchial metastasis: an epidemiologic and clinicopathologic study of 174 consecutive cases. Lung Cancer (Amsterdam, Netherlands). 2014;84(3):222–8.
10. Kreisman H, Wolkove N, Finkelstein HS, Cohen C, Margolese R, Frank H. Breast cancer and thoracic metastases: review of 119 patients. Thorax. 1983;38(3):175–9.
11. Dalar L, Ozdemir C, Abul Y, Karasulu L, Sokucu SN, Akbas A, Altn S. Therapeutic bronchoscopic interventions for malignant airway obstruction: a retrospective study from experience on 547 patients. Medicine. 2016; 95(23):e3886.
12. Chen CH, Wu BR, Cheng WC, Chen CY, Chen WC, Hsia TC, Liao WC, Tu CY, Hsu WH. Interventional pulmonology for patients with central airway obstruction: an 8-year institutional experience. Medicine. 2017;96(2):e5612.
13. Amjadi K, Voduc N, Cruysberghs Y, Lemmens R, Fergusson DA, Doucette S, Noppen M. Impact of interventional bronchoscopy on quality of life in malignant airway obstruction. Respiration. 2008;76(4):421–8.
14. Razi SS, Lebovics RS, Schwartz G, Sancheti M, Belsley S, Connery CP, Bhora FY. Timely airway stenting improves survival in patients with malignant central airway obstruction. Ann Thorac Surg. 2010;90(4):1088–93.
15. Grosu HB, Eapen GA, Morice RC, Jimenez CA, Casal RF, Almeida FA, Sarkiss MG, Ost DE. Stents are associated with increased risk of respiratory infections in patients undergoing airway interventions for malignant airways disease. Chest. 2013;144(2):441–9.
16. Colt HG, Dumon JF. Airway stents. Present and future. Clin Chest Med. 1995; 16(3):465–78.
17. Kim H. Stenting therapy for stenosing airway disease. Respirology (Carlton, Vic). 1998;3(4):221–8.
18. Shin B, Kim K, Jeong BH, Eom JS, Song WJ, Kang HK, Kim H. Clinical significance of differentiating post-intubation and post-tracheostomy tracheal stenosis. Respirology (Carlton, Vic). 2017;22(3):513–20.
19. Owens WD, Felts JA, Spitznagel EL Jr. ASA physical status classifications: a study of consistency of ratings. Anesthesiology. 1978;49(4):239–43.
20. Myer CM 3rd, O'Connor DM, Cotton RT. Proposed grading system for subglottic stenosis based on endotracheal tube sizes. Ann Otol Rhinol Laryngol. 1994;103(4 Pt 1):319–23.
21. Mitchell PD, Kennedy MP. Bronchoscopic management of malignant airway obstruction. Adv Ther. 2014;31(5):512–38.
22. Guibert N, Mhanna L, Droneau S, Plat G, Didier A, Mazieres J, Hermant C. Techniques of endoscopic airway tumor treatment. J Thorac Dis. 2016;8(11): 3343–60.
23. Venuta F, Rendina EA, De Giacomo T, Mercadante E, Ciccone AM, Aratari MT, Moretti M, Coloni GF. Endoscopic treatment of lung cancer invading the airway before induction chemotherapy and surgical resection. Eur J Cardiothorac Surg. 2001;20(3):464–7.
24. Miller KD, Siegel RL, Lin CC, Mariotto AB, Kramer JL, Rowland JH, Stein KD, Alteri R, Jemal A. Cancer treatment and survivorship statistics, 2016. CA Cancer J Clin. 2016;66(4):271–89.
25. Guibert N, Mazieres J, Lepage B, Plat G, Didier A, Hermant C. Prognostic factors associated with interventional bronchoscopy in lung cancer. Ann Thorac Surg. 2014;97(1):253–9.
26. Stratakos G, Gerovasili V, Dimitropoulos C, Giozos I, Filippidis FT, Gennimata S, Zarogoulidis P, Zissimopoulos A, Pataka A, Koufos N, et al. Survival and quality of life benefit after endoscopic management of malignant central airway obstruction. J Cancer. 2016;7(7):794–802.
27. Fournel C, Bertoletti L, Nguyen B, Vergnon JM. Endobronchial metastases from colorectal cancers: natural history and role of interventional bronchoscopy. Respiration. 2009;77(1):63–9.
28. Chaussende A, Hermant C, Tazi-Mezalek R, Favrolt N, Hureaux J, Fournier C, Lorut C, Paganin F, Ngo MT, Vandemoortele T, et al. Endobronchial metastases from melanoma: a survival analysis. Clin Respir J. 2017;11(6): 1006–1011. (Epub 2016 Feb 25).
29. Dalar L, Ozdemir C, Sokucu SN, Karasulu L, Altin S. Bronchoscopic palliation to treat endobronchial metastasis of the tracheobronchial tree. Respir Investig. 2016;54(2):116–20.
30. Ost DE, Ernst A, Grosu HB, Lei X, Diaz-Mendoza J, Slade M, Gildea TR, Machuzak M, Jimenez CA, Toth J, et al. Complications following therapeutic bronchoscopy for malignant central airway obstruction: results of the AQuIRE registry. Chest. 2015;148(2):450–71.

Diaphragmatic parameters by ultrasonography for predicting weaning outcomes

Pongdhep Theerawit[1], Dararat Eksombatchai[2], Yuda Sutherasan[2*], Thitiporn Suwatanapongched[3], Charn Kiatboonsri[2] and Sumalee Kiatboonsri[2]

Abstract

Background: Diaphragmatic dysfunction remains the main cause of weaning difficulty or failure. Ultrasonographic measurement of diaphragmatic function can be used to predict the outcomes of weaning from mechanical ventilation. Our primary objective was to investigate the performance of various sonographic parameters of diaphragmatic function for predicting the success of weaning from mechanical ventilation.

Methods: We prospectively enrolled 68 adult patients requiring mechanical ventilation who were admitted to the intensive care unit from June 2013 to November 2013. The diaphragmatic inspiratory excursion, time to peak inspiratory amplitude of the diaphragm ($TPIA_{dia}$), diaphragmatic thickness (DT), DT difference (DTD), and diaphragm thickening fraction (TFdi) were determined by bedside ultrasonography performed at the end of a spontaneous breathing trial. A receiver operating characteristic curve was used for analysis.

Results: In total, 62 patients were analyzed. The mean $TPIA_{dia}$ was significantly higher in the weaning success group (right, 1.27 ± 0.38 s; left, 1.14 ± 0.37 s) than in the weaning failure group (right, 0.97 ± 0.43 s; left, 0.85 ± 0. 39 s) ($P < 0.05$). The sensitivity, specificity, positive predictive value, and negative predictive value of a $TPIA_{dia}$ of > 0.8 s in predicting weaning success were 92, 46, 89, and 56%, respectively. The diaphragmatic inspiratory excursion, DTD, and TFdi were associated with reintubation within 48 h. The P values were 0.047, 0.021, and 0. 028, and the areas under the receiver operating characteristic curve were 0.716, 0.805, and 0.784, respectively.

Conclusion: Among diaphragmatic parameters, $TPIA_{dia}$ exhibits good performance in predicting the success of weaning from mechanical ventilation. This study demonstrated a trend toward successful use of $TPIA_{dia}$ rather than diaphragmatic inspiratory excursion as a predictor of weaning from mechanical ventilation.

Keywords: Diaphragm ultrasound, Weaning, Spontaneous breathing trial, Diaphragmatic weakness, Diaphragmatic dysfunction

Background

Diaphragmatic dysfunction remains the main cause of weaning difficulty or failure. Its prevalence ranges from 33 to 95% [1–5]. Diaphragmatic dysfunction among patients hospitalized in the intensive care unit (ICU) is commonly attributed to critical illness polyneuropathy and myopathy [6]. Mechanical ventilation, even after a short period of time, can also induce diaphragmatic dysfunction by reducing the force that generates the capacity of the diaphragm, which may cause weaning difficulty. Diaphragmatic dysfunction can be worsened by disuse atrophy of both fast-twitch and slow-twitch myofibers of the diaphragm following the administration of a neuromuscular blocking agent [7–9].

Several parameters, including the rapid shallow breathing index (RSBI), vital capacity (VC), and maximum peak inspiratory pressure (PI_{MAX}), are routinely used to predict weaning failure from mechanical ventilation. However, the sensitivity, specificity, positive predictive value (PPV),

* Correspondence: sutherasan_yuda@yahoo.com
[2]Division of Pulmonary and Pulmonary Critical Care Medicine, Department of Medicine, Faculty of Medicine Ramathibodi Hospital, Mahidol University, Bangkok, 270 Rama 6 Road, Thung Phaya Thai, Ratchathewi, Bangkok 10400, Thailand
Full list of author information is available at the end of the article

negative predictive value (NPV), and cut-off values of these parameters are highly variable among studies. Moreover, these parameters do not directly reflect diaphragmatic function [10].

Although fluoroscopic examination of the diaphragm remains the gold standard for evaluation of diaphragmatic movement, it cannot be performed in patients in the ICU. Bedside ultrasound is being increasingly performed for real-time assessment of diaphragmatic movement. This technique allows qualitative and quantitative assessment of diaphragmatic function in terms of diaphragmatic thickness (DT) and diaphragmatic amplitude during contraction, which help to diagnose diaphragmatic weakness [11–14] and respiratory workload [12, 15] in patients in the ICU. Kim et al. [16] found that diaphragmatic excursion of < 10 mm or paradoxical movement is associated with weaning failure. DiNino et al. [17] suggested that diaphragm contractile function at the zone of apposition as measured by ultrasound may be useful for predicting extubation success or failure. Spadaro et al. [18] recently reported a new index, namely the diaphragmatic RSBI, which is calculated by substituting the tidal volume (TV) with the ultrasonographic evaluation of diaphragmatic displacement. This parameter is more accurate than the traditional RSBI for prediction of weaning failure [18].

To the best of our knowledge, quantitative assessment of both the right and left hemidiaphragms and comparison of these ultrasound parameters with conventional parameters have not been performed. We hypothesized that diaphragmatic parameters determined by bedside ultrasonography can predict the weaning outcome with better performance than conventional parameters. Therefore, we conducted this prospective study to investigate diaphragmatic function in patients in the ICU in terms of diaphragmatic motion and contractile function using bedside ultrasonography during the weaning period. We also evaluated the performance of these ultrasound parameters by comparison with conventional parameters routinely used to predict successful weaning from mechanical ventilation.

Methods

Study design and patient population

This prospective cross-sectional study was conducted at a tertiary-care, university-based hospital. The study was approved by the Ethical Clearance Committee on Human Rights Related to Research Involving Human Subjects, Faculty of Medicine Ramathibodi Hospital, Mahidol University (No. MURA2013/414/N_3SEP_{17}).

We consecutively enrolled adult patients aged > 18 years who were admitted to the medical or surgical ICU of Ramathibodi Hospital, Mahidol University from June 2013 to November 2013. All patients provided written informed consent prior to enrollment. When the patient was unable to provide consent because of consciousness disturbance, the next of kin provided written informed consent.

Inclusion and exclusion criteria

The inclusion criteria were as follows: 1) a requirement for intubation; 2) readiness for weaning from mechanical ventilation as defined by recovery from the cause of respiratory failure, a stable hemodynamic status, no requirement for a vasopressor, and no administration of sedative agents or neuromuscular blocking agents > 24 h before enrollment; and 3) readiness for respiration with a T-piece system.

The exclusion criteria were the presence of pneumothorax or ascites, a history of either neuromuscular disease or thoracic surgery, the presence of a tracheostomy tube, and poor image quality. The following baseline characteristics were recorded: age, sex, duration of mechanical ventilation, cause of respiratory failure, body mass index, and laboratory findings before extubation.

Measurements

In our units, there is no specific (written) criteria by which to determine the best time to start weaning and no formal guidelines for reducing support. In the present study, the patients' readiness to wean was assessed daily by clinical judgment of the attending intensivist and/or pulmonary physician. The primary physicians were blinded to the ultrasound results. The research team did not play a role in deciding whether a patient was to be extubated.

Exhaled TV, RSBI, VC, PI_{MAX}, and diaphragmatic parameters were measured in all participants at the end of a 2-h spontaneous breathing trial with a T-piece and zero pressure support (before extubation). We employed a hand-held Wright respirometer (Ferraris Medical Ltd., Hertford, Hertfordshire, England) to measure minute ventilation (MV). TV was calculated as MV divided by respiratory rate. The RSBI was the ratio between the respiratory rate (breaths/min) and TV (liters) [19]. Measurement of VC (slow VC) was performed in the upright position, after measurement of MV. During measurement of VC, each patient breathed until the end of inspiration, then exhaled to the approximate residual volume. This process was supervised by a pulmonary fellow. PI_{MAX} was measured with a negative inspiratory force meter, which is a calibrated device containing a unidirectional valve, attached to the end of an endotracheal tube (Instrumentation Industries, Inc., Bethel Park, PA, USA). PI_{MAX} was determined from the most negative pressure documented during 20 s of airway occlusion [19].

Transthoracic ultrasonography was performed at the bedside with a SonoSite M-Turbo (SonoSite Inc., Bothell, WA, USA) by a well-trained pulmonary physician. The examination was performed in both B- and anatomical M-modes. All examinations were carried out with patients in the supine position. We obtained diaphragmatic ultrasound values from three consecutive tidal breaths, and the average values were used for analysis.

The diaphragmatic inspiratory excursion and time to peak inspiratory amplitude of the diaphragm ($TPIA_{dia}$) of each hemidiaphragm (right $TPIA_{dia}$ and left $TPIA_{dia}$) were measured in M-mode using a 1- to 5-MHz ultrasound transducer during tidal breathing (Fig. 1) [20]. The measurement was performed via either a subcostal or intercostal approach in the mid-clavicular line, or in the right or left anterior axillary line. The liver or spleen was identified as a window for each hemidiaphragm. The ultrasound probe was placed in the direction in which the ultrasound beam reached the posterior third of the corresponding hemidiaphragm perpendicularly [15]. During inspiration, the normal diaphragm moved caudally toward the ultrasound transducer, which was recorded as an upward motion of the M-mode tracing. The amplitude of diaphragmatic inspiratory excursion was measured as the point of maximal height of inspiration in the M-mode tracing. The $TPIA_{dia}$ was defined as the time from the beginning of diaphragmatic contraction to the maximal amplitude of diaphragmatic inspiratory excursion as measured from the M-mode tracing.

DT was subsequently measured at the zone of apposition [15], which is the area of the diaphragm attached to the rib cage, at both end inspiration and end expiration using a 6–13 ultrasound transducer in M-mode (Fig. 2). The DT difference (DTD) was calculated by subtracting DT at end expiration from DT at end inspiration. The diaphragm thickening fraction (TFdi) was calculated as follows: (DTD)/(DT at end expiration) × 100 [21]. These data were not communicated to the patient care team during the study; they were stored on the hard disk of the ultrasound machine and later exported to files for further verification and analysis. All images were reviewed in terms of image quality by a pulmonary physician and a radiologist (P.T. and T.S.).

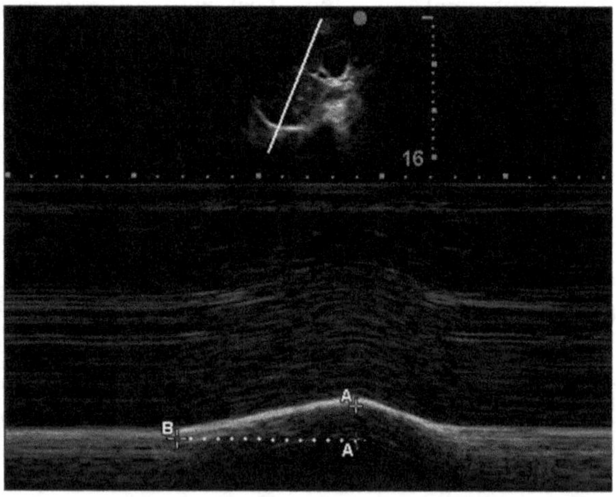

Fig. 1 Image showing measurement of the diaphragmatic inspiratory excursion and $TPIA_{dia}$ in M-mode ultrasound. The A-A is the height of diaphragmatic inspiratory excursion. The B-A is the $TPIA_{dia}$. $TPIA_{dia}$, time to peak inspiratory amplitude

Outcomes

The primary outcome was the diagnostic accuracy of diaphragmatic ultrasound parameters for predicting weaning success. Successful weaning from mechanical ventilation was defined as the ability to tolerate spontaneous breathing for at least 48 h without any level of assisted ventilation. Weaning failure was defined as the requirement for resumption of either invasive or noninvasive mechanical ventilation or reintubation within 48 h after extubation [16].

The secondary outcomes were the association between weaning parameters and diaphragmatic dysfunction [16], reintubation during admission, and reintubation within 48 h after extubation. Ultrasonographic diaphragmatic dysfunction was considered when each hemidiaphragm exhibited either vertical excursion of < 10 mm or the presence of paradoxical movement [16].

Statistical analysis

The patients were classified into two groups based on the primary outcome. All parameters were compared between the two groups. The unpaired Student's t-test was used to compare continuous variables, and the chi-square test was used to compare categorical variables. Data are presented as mean ± standard deviation for continuous variables with a normal distribution and as

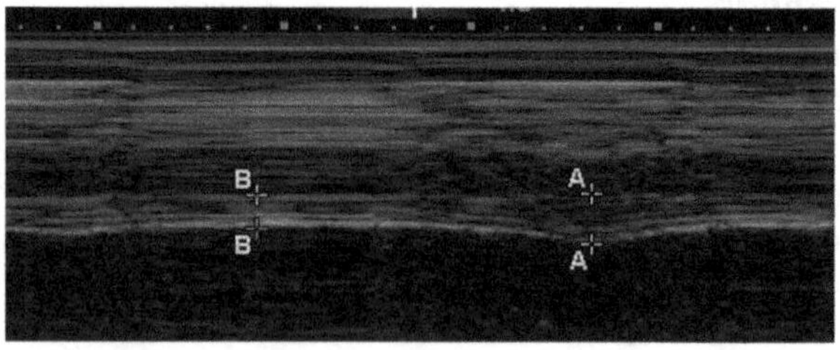

Fig. 2 Image illustrating the part of the diaphragm at the area of apposition for measurement of the diaphragmatic thickness (DT). The A-A is the DT at end inspiration, and the B-B is the DT at end expiration

median with interquartile range for variables without a normal distribution.

The variables associated with the primary and secondary outcomes were then analyzed with receiver operating characteristic (ROC) curves to determine their performance. Sensitivity and specificity were also analyzed to determine appropriate cut-off values of $TPIA_{dia}$ and RSBI.

To determine the correlation between diaphragmatic ultrasound values and weaning parameters, we used Pearson's correlation and presented the results as correlation coefficients. A P value of < 0.05 was considered statistically significant. Correlation coefficients of 0.00 to 0.19, 0.20 to 0.39, 0.40 to 0.59, 0.60 to 0.79, and 0.80 to 1.00 were considered to indicate very weak, weak, moderate, strong, and very strong correlations, respectively. We also performed subgroup analysis between patients with and without diaphragmatic dysfunction.

We analyzed inter-operator variability and intra-operator reproducibility of all diaphragmatic ultrasound parameters in 10 cases by two independent operators who were blinded. The former analysis was performed by Pearson's correlation, and the other was performed with intraclass correlations presented with the correlation coefficient, P value, and 95% confidence interval. All statistical analyses were performed using IBM SPSS Statistics for Windows, version 22.0 (IBM Corp., Armonk, NY, USA).

Results

In total, 68 patients were enrolled in our study. In six (9%) patients, however, the examination was not possible or was limited, resulting in poor image quality. These patients were finally excluded. The images of 62 patients were approved for analysis on the basis of quality. The numbers of patients with weaning success and reintubation are shown in Fig. 3. The patients' baseline characteristics are shown in Table 1. All diaphragmatic parameters obtained from the right and left hemidiaphragm were compared (Table 2), and no difference between the right and

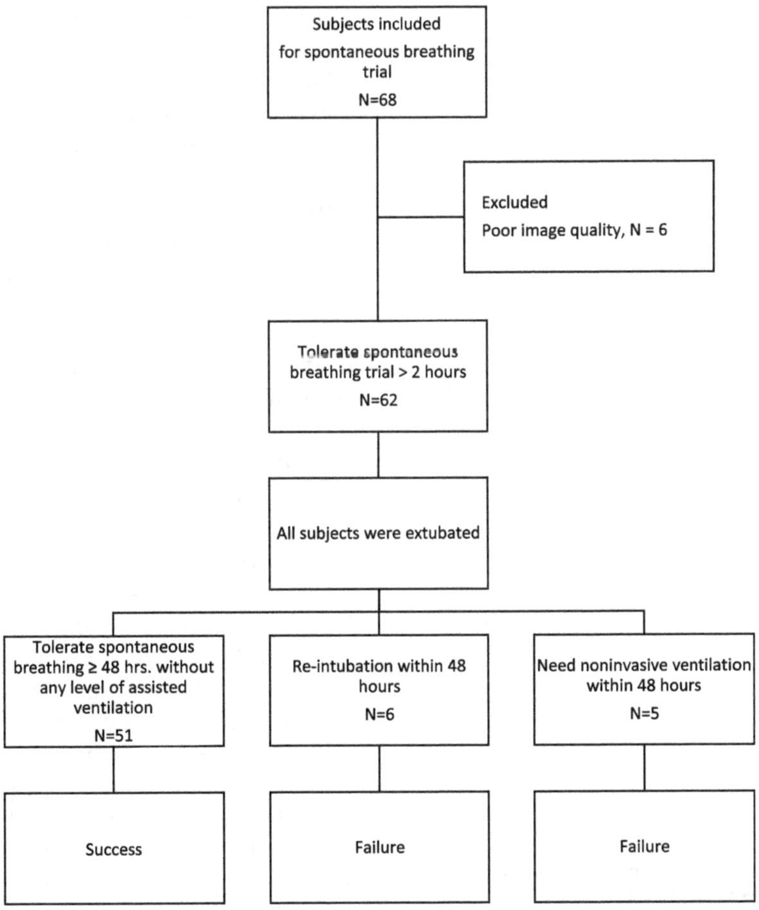

Fig. 3 Flow chart showing the number of patients with weaning success, weaning failure, and reintubation

Table 1 baseline characteristics

Demographic data	Value
Age (mean ± SD, years)	66.48 ± 16.7
Genders Male (n/%)	38/61
Body mass index (mean ± SD, kg/m^2)	22.5 ± 6.3
Medical patients (n/%)	42/68
Surgical patients (n/%)	20/32
APACHE II score (mean ± SD)	18.5 ± 7.2
Comorbidity (n/%)	
Hypertension	35/57
Diabetes	21/34
Chronic kidney disease	18/29
Ischemic heart disease	14/23
COPD	6/10
Hypothyroid	5/8
Adrenal insufficiency	3/5
Asthma	2/3
Reason for intubation (n/%)	
Neurological disease	10/16
Septic shock	10/16
Pneumonia	8/13
Heart disease	8/13
COPD exacerbation	4/7
Post-operative conditions	21/34
Laboratory findings (mean ± SD)	
Sodium (mmol/L)	135.9 ± 5.2
Potassium (mmol/L)	3.9 ± 0.59
Bicarbonate (mmol/L)	23.6 ± 4.5
Calcium (mmol/L)	7.9 ± 0.65
Magnesium (mmol/L)	1.97 ± 0.37
Phosphate (mmol/L)	4.6 ± 5.4
Albumin (g/dl)	24.8 ± 5.6
BUN (mg/dl)	29.3 ± 23.9
Creatinine (mg/dl)	1.9 ± 2.3
Hematocrit (%)	31.8 ± 5.5
Vital capacity (mean ± SD, L)	0.97 ± 0.4
Tidal volume (mean ± SD, L)	0.41 ± 0.2
PI_{MAX} (mean ± SD, mmHg)	40.7 ± 16.4
RSBI (mean ± SD, breath•min^{-1}/L)	60.2 ± 33.1
Duration of mechanical ventilation(days) [a]	2.8(1.1–5.7)
Length of stay (days)	
Intensive care stay[a]	4.8 (2.9–9.6)
Hospital stay[a]	13.3 (7.8–25.9)

APACHE II Acute Physiology and Chronic Health Evaluation II, *COPD* chronic obstructive airway disease, *BUN* blood urea nitrogen, *PI_{MAX}* Maximum peak inspiratory pressure, *RSBI* Rapid shallow breathing index
[a]present as median (inter quartile range)

Table 2 comparison between right and left diaphragmatic parameters

Ultrasonographic parameters	Right	Left	*P* value
Diaphragmatic inspiratory excursion (mm.)	13.5 ± 6.5	13.4 ± 6.2	0.87
$TPIA_{dia}$ (second)	1.2 ± 0.40	1.1 ± 0.39	0.08
Inspiratory DT (mm.)	3.8 ± 1.0	3.8 ± 1.0	0.33
Expiratory DT (mm.)	2.8 ± 0.7	2.8 ± 0. 6	0.52
DTD (mm.)	9.8 ± 4.9	10.1 ± 5.1	0.51
TFdi (%)	36 ± 17	35 ± 14	0.89

$TPIA_{dia}$ Time to peak inspiratory amplitude of diaphragm, *DT* diaphragmatic thickness, *DTD* Diaphragmatic thickness difference, *TFdi* diaphragm thickening fraction
All data are present as mean ± SD

left diaphragmatic parameters was seen. Consequently, we presented the ultrasound parameters according to the right hemidiaphragm.

With the exception of the potassium level, the demographic factors and laboratory findings did not differ significantly between the weaning success and failure groups (Table 3). The mean $TPIA_{dia}$ was significantly higher in the weaning success than failure group ($P < 0.05$). The RSBI during the spontaneous breathing trial was significantly lower in the weaning success than failure group ($P < 0.01$) (Table 3).

Table 4 shows the correlation coefficients between diaphragmatic and conventional parameters. The $TPIA_{dia}$ was significantly correlated with TV and inversely correlated with the RSBI (Fig. 4). There were moderate correlations between $TPIA_{dia}$ and VC, diaphragmatic inspiratory excursion and RSBI, and diaphragmatic inspiratory excursion and TV. The RSBI was inversely related to all diaphragmatic ultrasound parameters. For example, the lower the RSBI, the longer the $TPIA_{dia}$. There was no correlation between PI_{MAX} and any diaphragmatic ultrasound parameters.

Table 5 summarizes the sensitivity, specificity, PPV, and NPV of a $TPIA_{dia}$ of > 0.8 s and an RSBI of < 100 in predicting weaning success.

Regarding secondary outcomes, diaphragmatic inspiratory excursion, DTD, and TFdi were significantly lower in patients who underwent reintubation within 48 h. The *P* values were 0.047, 0.021, and 0.028, and the areas under the ROC curves were 0.716, 0.805, and 0.784, respectively. A diaphragmatic inspiratory excursion cut-off value of 12.85 mm provided a sensitivity of 83% and specificity of 55% for predicting reintubation within 48 h. The PPV and NPV of a diaphragmatic inspiratory excursion value of < 12.85 mm were 17 and 97%, respectively. A DTD of < 0.65 mm predicted reintubation within 48 h with a sensitivity and specificity of 83 and 77%, respectively. The PPV of a DTD of < 0.65 mm was 28%, and the NPV was 98%.

Table 3 comparison between success group and failure group

Parameters	Weaning success ($n = 51$)	Weaning Failure ($n = 11$)	*P* value	95% CI
Age (mean ± SD, years)	65.90 ± 17.05	69.18 ± 15.45	NS	−7.89 to 14.45
Gender (n/%)				
Female	33/65	5/45		
Male	18/35	6/55	NS	
BMI (mean ± SD, kg/m^2)	22.63 ± 6.18	21.91 ± 7.66	NS	−5.60 to 4.18
APACHE II score	18.29 ± 7.88	19.55 ± 2.34	NS	−3.58 to 6.08
Reason for intubation (n/%)				
Neurological disease	8/15.7	2/18.2	0.838	0.22 to 6.59
Septic shock	8/15.7	2/18.2	0.838	0.22 to 6.59
Pneumonia	6/11.8	2/18.2	0.623	0.29 to 9.62
Heart disease	6/11.8	2/18.2	0.623	0.29 to 9.62
COPD exacerbation	3/5.9	1/9.1	0.694	0.15 to 17.00
Post-operative conditions	19/37.3	2/18.2	0.305	0.07 to 1.92
TV (mean ± SD, ml.)	420.10 ± 207.48	370.91 ± 137.38	NS	− 82.17 to 180.55
VC (mean ± SD, L.)	1.01 ± 0.44	0.76 ± 0.34	NS	−0.05 to 0.54
RSBI	55.11 ± 25.02	83.84 ± 53.11	$P < 0.01$	−49.67 to −7.79
PI_{MAX} (mean ± SD, mmHg)	42.31 ± 17.17	32.50 ± 8.05	NS	−1.34 to 20.97
Electrolytes (mean ± SD)				
Sodium (mmol/L)	135.86 ± 5.03	136.00 ± 6.21	NS	−3.63 to 3.35
Potassium (mmol/L)	4.00 ± 0.57	3.46 ± 0.47	$P < 0.01$	0.17 to 0.92
Bicarbonate (mmol/L)	23.54 ± 4.63	23.81 ± 4.11	NS	−3.29 to 2.75
Magnesium (mmol/L)	1.97 ± 0.37	1.99 ± 0.43	NS	−0.32 to 0.28
Phosphate (mmol/L)	4.92 ± 5.82	3.01 ± 0.56	NS	−2.58 to 6.38
Calcium (mmol/L)	7.88 ± 0.63	8.06 ± 0.83	NS	−0.72 to 0.37
Albumin (g/dl)	25.29 ± 5.34	21.79 ± 6.26	NS	−0.72 to 7.72
Hematocrit (%)	32 ± 6	31 ± 4	NS	−4.79 to 2.58
Diaphragmatic inspiratory excursion (mean ± SD, mm.)				
Right	13.7 ± 5.6	12.4 ± 10.0	NS	−0.31 to 0.56
Left	13.5 ± 5.3	12.8 ± 09.6	NS	−0.35 to 0.48
$TPIA_{dia}$ (mean ± SD, second.)				
Right	1.27 ± 0.38	0.97 ± 0.43	$P < 0.05$	0.04 to 0.56
Left	1.14 ± 0.37	0.85 ± 0.39	$P < 0.05$	0.04 to 0.54
DTD (mean ± SD, mm.)				
Right	1.01 ± 0.46	0.84 ± 0.66	NS	−1.61 to 5.00
Left	1.05 ± 0.50	0.80 ± 0.48	NS	−0.84 to 5.82
TFdi (mean ± SD,%)				
Right	36 ± 15	33 ± 24	NS	−15.05 to 7.37
Left	37 ± 14	28 ± 13	NS	−18.16 to 0.65

COPD chronic obstructive airway disease, *APACHE II* acute physiology and chronic health evaluation II, *TV* Tidal volume, *VC* vital capacity, *RSBI* rapid shallow breathing index, PI_{MAX} Maximum peak inspiratory pressure, $TPIA_{dia}$ time to peak inspiratory amplitude, *DTD* diaphragmatic thickness difference, *TFdi* diaphragm thickening fraction

Nineteen of 62 (31%) patients had diaphragmatic dysfunction according to the criteria established by Kim et al. [16]. Patients who developed diaphragmatic dysfunction had a significantly higher RSBI and lower $TPIA_{dia}$, DTD, TFdi, TV, and PI_{MAX} (Table 6). The areas under the ROC curves of RSBI, $TPIA_{dia}$, DTD,

Table 4 Correlation coefficient among parameters

	TV	VC	RSBI	PI_{MAX}
Diaphragmatic inspiratory excursion	0.445*	0.217	−0.435*	0.077
$TPIA_{dia}$	0.639*	0.522*	− 0.703*	0.250
DTD	0.045	−0.017	−0.260ᵖ	0.166
TFdi	0.001	0.117	−0.218	0.237

TV Tidal volume, *VC* vital capacity, *RSBI* rapid shallow breathing index, PI_{MAX} Maximum peak inspiratory pressure, $TPIA_{dia}$ time to peak inspiratory amplitude, *DTD* diaphragmatic thickness difference, *TFdi* diaphragm thickening fraction
*P value < 0.01
ᵖP value < 0.05

TFdi, TV, VC, and PI_{MAX} for predicting diaphragmatic dysfunction were 0.720, 0.722, 0.697, 0.762, 0.700, 0.570, and 0.653, respectively.

The parameters that predicted reintubation during admission were PI_{MAX}, RSBI, VC, and $TPIA_{dia}$. The areas under the ROC curves were 0.725, 0.652, 0.735, and 0.710, respectively.

The intra-operator reproducibility analysis of TPIA in the two operators showed an intraclass correlation coefficient of 0.97 (95% confidence interval, 0.90–0.99; *P* < 0.001) and 0.92 (95% confidence interval, 0.70–0.98; P < 0.001), respectively. The inter-operator variability analysis between the two operators revealed a Pearson correlation coefficient ® of 0.95 (P < 0.001). The remaining parameters were analyzed as shown in Additional file 1: Table S1.

Discussion

Ultrasonography provides some advantages as a noninvasive diagnostic tool in critically ill patients, including availability at the bedside and avoidance of radiation hazards. The role of ultrasound in the assessment of diaphragm function has been studied [16] with the rationale that the diaphragm plays a crucial role in respiratory muscle endurance. However, data concerning its usefulness as a weaning predictor are limited [16, 17, 21–23]. We investigated the diagnostic performance of diaphragmatic function parameters assessed by ultrasonography to predict the success of weaning from mechanical ventilation.

The main findings of this study can be summarized as follows. 1) The prevalence of ultrasonographic diaphragmatic dysfunction was 31%. 2) The $TPIA_{dia}$ was a parameter that could be used to predict successful weaning from mechanical ventilation and had a strong correlation with the RSBI. 3) With respect to secondary outcomes, the diaphragmatic inspiratory excursion, DTD, and TFdi could predict reintubation within 48 h. 4) There was no difference between the right and left diaphragmatic parameters.

Diaphragmatic dysfunction is a common condition in the ICU and is associated with prolonged weaning from mechanical ventilation and weaning failure [16]. Jiang et al. [23] hypothesized that displacement of the liver/spleen as measured by ultrasonography can represent movement of the hemidiaphragms. They demonstrated that using a cutoff value of 1.1 cm can predict successful extubation [23]. Our study showed that the prevalence of diaphragmatic dysfunction in the medical and surgical ICU was 31%, which is in line with that reported by Kim et al. [16], who demonstrated that 29% of patients hospitalized in the medical ICU developed diaphragmatic dysfunction.

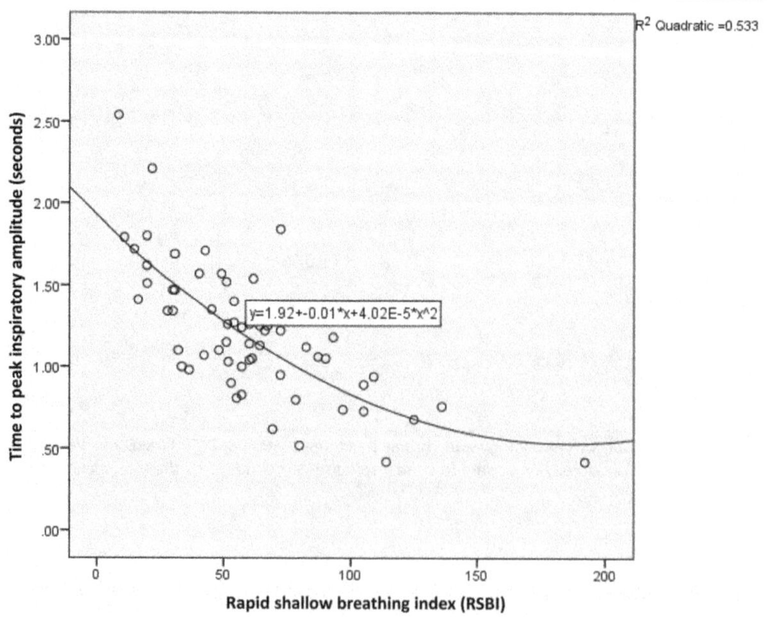

Fig. 4 Relationship between the RSBI and $TPIA_{dia}$. RSBI, rapid shallow breathing index; $TPIA_{dia}$, time to peak inspiratory amplitude

Table 5 Sensitivity, specificity, and negative and positive predictive values of ultrasonography and rapid shallow breathing index for predicting of weaning success

Parameters	Sensitivity	Specificity	Positive predictive value	Negative predictive value	Area under the curve
TPIA > 0.8 s	92.2	45.5	88.7	55.6	0.676
RSBI < 100	96.1	45.5	89.1	71.4	0.659

$TPIA_{dia}$ time to peak inspiratory amplitude, *RSBI* rapid shallow breathing index

Some previous investigators have performed only right hemidiaphragm ultrasound in the ICU because the acoustic window provided by the liver makes it easier to measure the parameters on this side [17, 21]. In the present study, we completed both right and left hemidiaphragm measurements without any difficulty. Nevertheless, we found that there was no significant difference between the right and left diaphragmatic parameters (Table 2). Therefore, measurement of the right hemidiaphragm may be more practical in clinical practice.

To the best of our knowledge, this is the first study to compare the performance of various diaphragmatic ultrasound-derived parameters with respect to weaning outcomes in critically ill patients. We also proposed a parameter, the $TPIA_{dia}$, to predict successful weaning from mechanical ventilation. We found that patients with a longer $TPIA_{dia}$ tended to have more successful weaning from mechanical ventilation, and we found a strong correlation between the $TPIA_{dia}$ and RSBI. This correlation suggests the presence of a relationship between $TPIA_{dia}$ and diaphragmatic strength. Physiologically, the strength and endurance of the diaphragm are not similar. Diaphragmatic strength refers to the capacity of the diaphragm to generate force, which is dependent on many factors such as diaphragm contractile activation, excitation–contraction coupling, central drive, nerve conductance, and neuromuscular transmission [24]. Endurance is defined as the ability of the diaphragm to sustain force over time. Our investigation suggests that the $TPIA_{dia}$ is associated with the strength of the diaphragm rather than its endurance.

In general, a more extended $TPIA_{dia}$ increases the diaphragmatic amplitude. Therefore, both parameters should display similar results. Although the diaphragmatic inspiratory excursion could predict reintubation, it could not predict weaning success. This result suggests that the diaphragmatic inspiratory excursion represents the endurance of the diaphragm rather than its strength. Why the inspiratory excursion showed a different result from the $TPIA_{dia}$ is not clear. However, we hypothesize that an individual patient may have his or her own inspiratory time and diaphragmatic amplitude for a required TV. This idea is supported by the relationship between the product of pressure created by respiratory muscle (Pmus) and the electrical activity of the diaphragm (EAdi) measured in neutrally adjusted ventilatory assist mode, as demonstrated in a study by Bellani et al. [25]. The authors showed a different Pmus/EAdi ratio in each patient and indicated that the patients had their own ratios. Consequently, we anticipate different $TPIA_{dia}$/diaphragmatic inspiratory excursion ratios among our patients, and they may have specific ratios of their own. Thus, we found a correlation coefficient of only 0.5 between the $TPIA_{dia}$ and diaphragmatic inspiratory excursion in an additional analysis. However, we need to further prove this hypothesis.

The $TPIA_{dia}$ showed an association with the success of breathing spontaneously without any assisted ventilation, whereas the DTD and TFdi were related to reintubation among the patients in our study. This can be explained by the fact that the DTD represents the endurance of the diaphragm, which is a major factor leading to reintubation. However, we could not explain why the diaphragmatic inspiratory excursion provides a similar result with respect to thickness difference parameters. The transdiaphragmatic pressure–time product needs further determination.

We found no correlation between PI_{MAX} and $TPIA_{dia}$ or other diaphragmatic ultrasound parameters. PI_{MAX} is

Table 6 a comparison between groups of diaphragmatic dysfunction and non- diaphragmatic dysfunction

Parameters	Diaphragmatic dysfunction ($n = 19$)	Non-diaphragmatic dysfunction ($n = 43$)	*P* value	95% CI
TV (mean ± SD, ml.)	318.68 ± 83.46	452.33 ± 218.34	< 0.05	29.87 to 237.41
VC (mean ± SD, L.)	838.89 ± 263.77	1019.30 ± 480.77	NS	−60.93 to 421.76
RSBI	79.53 ± 40.24	51.67 ± 25.63	< 0.01	−44.81to −10.92
PI_{MAX} (mean ± SD, mmHg)	33.72 ± 11.08	43.63 ± 17.45	< 0.05	0.98 to 18.83
$TPIA_{dia}$ (mean ± SD, second)	0.99 ± 0.33	1.31 ± 0.39	< 0.01	0.12 to 0.53
DTD (mean ± SD, mm.)	0.75 ± 0.50	1.08 ± 0.47	< 0.05	0.66 to 5.92
TFdi (mean ± SD,%)	25 ± 12	40 ± 16	< 0.01	6.79 to 23.69

TV Tidal volume, *VC* vital capacity, *RSBI* rapid shallow breathing index, *PI_{MAX}* Maximum peak inspiratory pressure, *$TPIA_{dia}$* time to peak inspiratory amplitude, *DTD* diaphragmatic thickness difference, *TFdi* diaphragm thickening fraction

a well-known index of respiratory muscle strength. However, some investigators have found that PI_{MAX} might be unreliable among patients in the medical ICU [26]. The most objective diagnostic test of respiratory muscle weakness is determination of the transdiaphragmatic pressure in response to phrenic nerve stimulation (PdiTw). Supinski et al. [27] investigated the correlation between PdiTw and PI_{MAX}. They found that when plotting PI_{MAX} against PdiTw, significant scatter was present between the two values, suggesting the unreliability of predicting PdiTw from the determination of PI_{MAX}. Nevertheless, each value is a predictor of both mortality and the duration of mechanical ventilation. This is in line with our study with respect to the fact that no correlation was found between PI_{MAX} and any diaphragmatic ultrasound parameters. The principles of measurement between these parameters are different. The PdiTw is affected by stimulation of the phrenic nerves, and diaphragmatic ultrasound evaluates mainly the diaphragm, whereas PI_{MAX} evaluates the inspiratory pressure by the contraction of all inspiratory muscles. Moreover, the diaphragmatic ultrasound examination and measurement of PdiTw were performed during submaximal breathing while measurement of PI_{MAX} was performed to assess the highest voluntary inspiratory muscle pressure generation.

Although the areas under the ROC curve of $TPIA_{dia}$ and the other ultrasound criteria were rather low in our study, they were at least equal to or better than the RSBI, the well-known criteria used in clinical practice. The area under the curve of the ultrasound criteria used to predict the weaning outcome varies from 0.68 to 0.79 among different studies [16, 22]. As evidenced by the quite low area under the curve of these ultrasound criteria indices, weaning failure depends on several clinical factors; for example, it can result not only from diaphragmatic dysfunction or critical illness myopathy but also excess mechanical load, impairment of respiratory mechanics, cardiovascular dysfunction, or an inability to clear secretions. Thus, a single diaphragmatic index might not be a perfect predictor, as shown in a study by Tenza-Lozano et al. [28]. They demonstrated that the area under the ROC curve of TFdi as a single predictor was 0.71. The performance of TFdi combined with lung ultrasound improved the prediction of weaning success with an AUC of 0.83, which supports our above-mentioned hypothesis [28]. Furthermore, we enrolled many patients of advanced age in the present study. The causes of weaning failure in older patients are multifactorial [29], and few specific parameters are available to predict weaning outcomes in this population [30]. Therefore, diaphragmatic parameters should be combined with other parameters for predicting weaning outcomes.

Since 1991, the RSBI has been used to predict weaning outcomes [19]. It exhibits the best performance compared with the CROP index, PI_{MAX}, and MV. However, the isolated RSBI may not be precise enough to predict weaning outcomes in patients undergoing prolonged mechanical ventilation [31]. The RSBI is a weaning predictor that measures the change in volume generated by all respiratory muscles while not specifically measuring the diaphragmatic contribution. A study by Kuo et al. [32] showed better performance of the RSBI at the 2-h time point of a spontaneous breathing trial than at the beginning. Consequently, the initial RSBI may not allow for proper assessment of patients with impaired diaphragmatic endurance but may be appropriate for assessment of impaired diaphragmatic strength. We did not find that the RSBI was associated with reintubation within 48 h after extubation in the present study.

Our study has some limitations. We enrolled both medical and postoperative patients in this study. Therefore, we cannot apply the results to specific diseases, such as chronic obstructive pulmonary disease. Further studies should be conducted to evaluate the role of $TPIA_{dia}$ in specific diseases. $TPIA_{dia}$ provided good sensitivity but low specificity for predicting successful weaning from mechanical ventilation, which means that there were some false-positives at low $TPIA_{dia}$ values. In other words, a given patient with a $TPIA_{dia}$ of ≤0.8 s could still have weaning success with an NPV of 56. However, a positive result that predicts weaning failure does not mean that the patient would have delayed weaning, but should be carefully evaluated during the weaning and extubation periods. Therefore, $TPIA_{dia}$ should be interpreted with caution and should be combined with other parameters. A validation cohort study should be conducted to confirm the results of our study. Furthermore, we analyzed the predictors of reintubation during hospital admission, and several uncontrolled variables could have interfered with the outcome (e.g., amount of secretion, consciousness level, or deterioration of the hemodynamic status).

Conclusions

Among diaphragmatic parameters, the $TPIA_{dia}$ exhibited good performance in predicting weaning outcomes and had a strong correlation with the RSBI. This study demonstrated a trend toward focusing on the $TPIA_{dia}$, rather than diaphragmatic inspiratory excursion, as a predictor of weaning from mechanical ventilation.

Additional file

Additional file 1: Table S1. Inter-operator variability and intra-operator reproducibility of diaphragmatic ultrasound parameters. *Analyzed by intraclass correlation and presented as intraclass correlation coefficient. **Analyzed by Pearson's correlation and presented as correlation coefficient *. All parameters exhibited a significant correlation ($P < 0.001$). $TPIA_{dia}$; Time to peak inspiratory amplitude of diaphragm, DT; diaphragmatic thickness.

Abbreviations

DT: Diaphragmatic thickness; DTD: Diaphragmatic thickness difference; ICU: Intensive care unit; MV: Minute ventilation; NPV: Negative predictive value; PdiTw: Transdiaphragmatic pressure in response to phrenic nerve stimulation; PI_{MAX}: Maximum peak inspiratory pressure; PPV: Positive predictive value; ROC: Receiver operating characteristic; RSBI: Rapid shallow breathing index; TFdi: Diaphragm thickening fraction; $TPIA_{dia}$: Time to peak inspiratory amplitude of diaphragm; TV: Tidal volume; VC: Vital capacity

Acknowledgments

We would like to express our gratitude to all involved internal medicine residents, pulmonary and critical care fellows, and pulmonary and critical care staff members and nurses for their contribution to this project. We also thank Angela Morben, DVM, ELS from Edanz Group (www.edanzediting.com/ac) for editing a draft of this manuscript.

Funding

Not applicable.

Authors' contributions

PT, DE, YS contributed to the study concept, design, planning, data acquisition, analyses, and manuscript preparation. PT, DE, YS and TS contributed to data acquisition and analysis, and interpretation of the data. PT, DE, YS, TS, CK, SK critically reviewed and revised the manuscript for important intellectual content. All authors reviewed the final version of the manuscript prior to submission and all accept responsibility for the integrity of the research process and findings. All authors read and approved the final manuscript.

Consent for publication

Not applicable.

Competing interests

The authors declare that they have no competing interests.

Author details

[1]Division of Critical Care Medicine, Department of Medicine, Faculty of Medicine Ramathibodi Hospital, Mahidol University, Bangkok, Thailand. [2]Division of Pulmonary and Pulmonary Critical Care Medicine, Department of Medicine, Faculty of Medicine Ramathibodi Hospital, Mahidol University, Bangkok, 270 Rama 6 Road, Thung Phaya Thai, Ratchathewi, Bangkok 10400, Thailand. [3]Department of Diagnostic and Therapeutic Radiology, Faculty of Medicine Ramathibodi Hospital, Mahidol University, Bangkok, Thailand.

References

1. de Letter MA, Schmitz PI, Visser LH, Verheul FA, Schellens RL, Op de Coul DA, et al. Risk factors for the development of polyneuropathy and myopathy in critically ill patients. Crit Care Med. 2001;29:2281–6.
2. Coakley JH, Nagendran K, Yarwood GD, Honavar M, Hinds CJ. Patterns of neurophysiological abnormality in prolonged critical illness. Intensive Care Med. 1998;24:801–7.
3. Coakley JH, Nagendran K, Honavar M, Hinds CJ. Preliminary observations on the neuromuscular abnormalities in patients with organ failure and sepsis. Intensive Care Med. 1993;19:323–8.
4. Berek K, Margreiter J, Willeit J, Berek A, Schmutzhard E, Mutz NJ. Polyneuropathies in critically ill patients: a prospective evaluation. Intensive Care Med. 1996;22:849–55.
5. Leijten FS, De Weerd AW, Poortvliet DC, De Ridder VA, Ulrich C, Harink-De Weerd JE. Critical illness polyneuropathy in multiple organ dysfunction syndrome and weaning from the ventilator. Intensive Care Med. 1996;22:856–61.
6. Chawla J, Gruener G. Management of critical illness polyneuropathy and myopathy. Neurol Clin. 2010;28:961–77.
7. Jaber S, Petrof BJ, Jung B, Chanques G, Berthet JP, Rabuel C, et al. Rapidly progressive diaphragmatic weakness and injury during mechanical ventilation in humans. Am J Respir Crit Care Med. 2011;183:364–71.
8. Levine S, Nguyen T, Taylor N, Friscia ME, Budak MT, Rothenberg P, et al. Rapid disuse atrophy of diaphragm fibers in mechanically ventilated humans. N Engl J Med. 2008;358:1327–35.
9. Hooijman PE, Beishuizen A, Witt CC, de Waard MC, Girbes AR, Spoelstra-de Man AM, et al. Diaphragm muscle fiber weakness and ubiquitin-proteasome activation in critically ill patients. Am J Respir Crit Care Med. 2015;191:1126–38.
10. Nemer SN, Barbas CS, Caldeira JB, Carias TC, Santos RG, Almeida LC, et al. A new integrative weaning index of discontinuation from mechanical ventilation. Crit Care. 2009;13:R152.
11. Kocis KC, Radell PJ, Sternberger WI, Benson JE, Traystman RJ, Nichols DG. Ultrasound evaluation of piglet diaphragm function before and after fatigue. J Appl Physiol (1985). 1997;83:1654–9.
12. Vivier E, Mekontso Dessap A, Dimassi S, Vargas F, Lyazidi A, Thille AW, et al. Diaphragm ultrasonography to estimate the work of breathing during non-invasive ventilation. Intensive Care Med. 2012;38:796–803.
13. Gottesman E, McCool FD. Ultrasound evaluation of the paralyzed diaphragm. Am J Respir Crit Care Med. 1997;155:1570–4.
14. Lloyd T, Tang YM, Benson MD, King S. Diaphragmatic paralysis: the use of M mode ultrasound for diagnosis in adults. Spinal Cord. 2006;44:505–8.
15. Matamis D, Soilemezi E, Tsagourias M, Akoumianaki E, Dimassi S, Boroli F, et al. Sonographic evaluation of the diaphragm in critically ill patients. Technique and clinical applications. Intensive Care Med. 2013;39:801–10.
16. Kim WY, Suh HJ, Hong SB, Koh Y, Lim CM. Diaphragm dysfunction assessed by ultrasonography: influence on weaning from mechanical ventilation. Crit Care Med. 2011;39:2627–30.
17. DiNino E, Gartman EJ, Sethi JM, McCool FD. Diaphragm ultrasound as a predictor of successful extubation from mechanical ventilation. Thorax. 2014;69:423–7.
18. Spadaro S, Grasso S, Mauri T, Dalla Corte F, Alvisi V, Ragazzi R, et al. Can diaphragmatic ultrasonography performed during the T-tube trial predict weaning failure? The role of diaphragmatic rapid shallow breathing index. Crit Care. 2016;20:305.
19. Yang KL, Tobin MJ. A prospective study of indexes predicting the outcome of trials of weaning from mechanical ventilation. N Engl J Med. 1991;324:1445–50.
20. Pasero D, Koeltz A, Placido R, Fontes Lima M, Haun O, Rienzo M, et al. Improving ultrasonic measurement of diaphragmatic excursion after cardiac surgery using the anatomical M-mode: a randomized crossover study. Intensive Care Med. 2015;41:650–6.
21. Ferrari G, De Filippi G, Elia F, Panero F, Volpicelli G, Apra F. Diaphragm ultrasound as a new index of discontinuation from mechanical ventilation. Crit Ultrasound J. 2014;6:8.
22. Zambon M, Greco M, Bocchino S, Cabrini L, Beccaria PF, Zangrillo A. Assessment of diaphragmatic dysfunction in the critically ill patient with ultrasound: a systematic review. Intensive Care Med. 2017;43:29–38.
23. Jiang JR, Tsai TH, Jerng JS, Yu CJ, Wu HD, Yang PC. Ultrasonographic evaluation of liver/spleen movements and extubation outcome. Chest. 2004;126:179–85.
24. Ottenheijm CA, Heunks LM, Dekhuijzen RP. Diaphragm adaptations in patients with COPD. Respir Res. 2008;9:12.
25. Bellani G, Mauri T, Coppadoro A, Grasselli G, Patroniti N, Spadaro S, et al. Estimation of patient's inspiratory effort from the electrical activity of the diaphragm. Crit Care Med. 2013;41:1483–91.
26. Multz AS, Aldrich TK, Prezant DJ, Karpel JP, Hendler JM. Maximal inspiratory pressure is not a reliable test of inspiratory muscle strength in mechanically ventilated patients. Am Rev Respir Dis. 1990;142:529–32.

27. Supinski GS, Westgate P, Callahan LA. Correlation of maximal inspiratory pressure to transdiaphragmatic twitch pressure in intensive care unit patients. Crit Care. 2016;20:77.
28. Tenza-Lozano E, Llamas-Alvarez A, Jaimez-Navarro E, Fernandez-Sanchez J. Lung and diaphragm ultrasound as predictors of success in weaning from mechanical ventilation. Crit Ultrasound J. 2018;10:12.
29. Fujii M, Iwakami S, Takagi H, Itoigawa Y, Ichikawa M, Iwakami N, et al. Factors influencing weaning from mechanical ventilation in elderly patients with severe pneumonia. Geriatr Gerontol Int. 2012;12:277–83.
30. Azeredo LM, Nemer SN, Barbas CS, Caldeira JB, Noe R, Guimaraes BL, et al. The integrative weaning index in elderly ICU subjects. Respir Care. 2017;62: 333–9.
31. Verceles AC, Diaz-Abad M, Geiger-Brown J, Scharf SM. Testing the prognostic value of the rapid shallow breathing index in predicting successful weaning in patients requiring prolonged mechanical ventilation. Heart Lung. 2012;41:546–52.
32. Kuo PH, Wu HD, Lu BY, Chen MT, Kuo SH, Yang PC. Predictive value of rapid shallow breathing index measured at initiation and termination of a 2-hour spontaneous breathing trial for weaning outcome in ICU patients. J Formos Med Assoc. 2006;105:390–8.

Automated computed tomographic scoring of lung disease in adults with primary ciliary dyskinesia

Trieu-Nghi Hoang-Thi[1,6], Marie-Pierre Revel[1], Pierre-Régis Burgel[2], Laurence Bassinet[3], Isabelle Honoré[2], Thong Hua-Huy[4], Charlotte Martin[1], Bernard Maitre[3] and Guillaume Chassagnon[1,5*]

Abstract

Background: The present study aimed to develop an automated computed tomography (CT) score based on the CT quantification of high-attenuating lung structures, in order to provide a quantitative assessment of lung structural abnormalities in patients with Primary Ciliary Dyskinesia (PCD).

Methods: Adult (≥18 years) PCD patients who underwent both chest CT and spirometry within a 6-month period were retrospectively included. Commercially available lung segmentation software was used to isolate the lungs from the mediastinum and chest wall and obtain histograms of lung density. CT-density scores were calculated using fixed and adapted thresholds based on various combinations of histogram characteristics, such as mean lung density (MLD), skewness, and standard deviation (SD). Additionally, visual scoring using the Bhalla score was performed by 2 independent radiologists. Correlations between CT scores, forced expiratory volume in 1 s (FEV_1) and forced vital capacity (FVC) were evaluated.

Results: Sixty-two adult patients with PCD were included. Of all histogram characteristics, those showing good positive or negative correlations to both FEV_1 and FVC were SD ($R = -0.63$ and -0.67; $p < 0.001$) and Skewness ($R = 0.67$ and 0.67; $p < 0.001$). Among all evaluated thresholds, the CT-density score based on MLD + 1SD provided the best negative correlation with both FEV_1 ($R = -0.68$; $p < 0.001$) and FVC ($R = -0.71$; $p < 0.001$), close to the correlations of the visual score ($R = -0.60$; $p < 0.001$ for FEV_1 and $R = -0.62$; $p < 0.001$, for FVC).

Conclusions: Automated CT scoring of lung structural abnormalities lung in primary ciliary dyskinesia is feasible and may prove useful for evaluation of disease severity in the clinic and in clinical trials.

Keywords: Computed tomography, Primary ciliary dyskinesia, Kartagener syndrome, Bronchiectasis

Background

Primary ciliary dyskinesia (PCD) is a rare genetic disorder characterized by defective ciliary structure and/or function, leading to inadequate mucociliary clearance and chronic oto-sino-pulmonary disease [1–3]. Organ laterality is also affected in almost half the patients [2]. Defective mucociliary airway clearance leads to recurrent and chronic bacterial infections of the lower respiratory tract, and to bronchiectasis [2].

Computed tomography (CT) is the gold standard method for the diagnosis of bronchiectasis, but its utility for monitoring PCD is not yet established [4, 5]. Correlations between CT structural changes and disease severity (lung function) have rarely been studied in PCD, especially in adults [5–13]. However, a large retrospective study recently suggested that a larger disease burden on CT may predict lung function decline in adults with PCD, indicating that CT assessment of lung structural abnormalities might be of value [5].

Most authors who have attempted to quantify bronchial disease in patients with PCD have used visual scoring methods initially designed to assess lung structural changes in patients with cystic fibrosis (CF), but the

* Correspondence: gchassagnon@gmail.com
[1]Radiology Department, Groupe Hospitalier Cochin-Hôtel Dieu, AP-HP, Université Paris Descartes - Sorbonne Paris Cité, Paris, France
[5]Center for Visual Computing, CentraleSupelec, Gif-sur-Yvette, France
Full list of author information is available at the end of the article

correlation between these visual scores and forced expiratory volume in 1 s (FEV_1) remains controversial in patients with PCD [7–14]. For example, Boon et al. reported a good negative correlation between a visual CT score and FEV_1 ($R = -0.63$, $P < 0.001$), whereas Cohen-Cymberknoh et al.found no correlation at all ($R = -0.36$, $P = 0.61$) [11, 12].

Although bronchiectasis, bronchial wall thickening, mucus plugging and mosaic perfusion are present in both PCD and CF, their relative predominance differs between the two diseases. Mosaic perfusion and small-airway mucus plugging predominate in PCD, meaning that their respective weight in the overall CT score should not be the same as in CF [5, 11]. This may be why some authors failed to find a correlation between visual scores and spirometry in PCD patients. Furthermore, visual scores suffer from several limitations, including the need for dedicated training and subjectivity in the assessment of CT changes [15].

Most lung structural changes in PCD, especially bronchial wall thickening, mucus plugging, consolidations and atelectasis are likely to increase lung attenuation and to modify the density histogram characteristics, which can be extracted from the CT images. On the density histogram, the mode corresponds to the most highly represented attenuation value; and skewness describes the asymmetry of the density curve, which is shifted to the right when there is an increase of lung density or to the left in case of decrease. Additionally, high-attenuating structures can be quantified by using a thresholding approach similar to that used to measure emphysema on CT, except that the latter is based on the quantification of low-attenuating lung areas, with attenuation values below minus 950 Hounsfield units (HU) [16]. The quantification of high-attenuating structural changes in the lungs, also using a thresholding approach has been reported to show good correlation with FEV_1 in patients with CF [17].

We postulated that disease severity in PCD might also be assessed by quantifying high-attenuating lung structures and by analysing changes in the lung density distribution. We therefore developed an automated CT scoring method based on histogram characteristic analysis and threshold-based quantification of high-attenuating lung structures in patients with PCD.

Methods

Patients

This retrospective study, performed in two accredited PCD reference centres, was approved by the Institutional Review Board of Société Pneumologie de Langue Française. The need for informed consent was waived, in accordance with French rules for retrospective observational studies.

All adult outpatients, with a diagnosis of PCD according to the ERS guidelines [18] were eligible if they had both chest CT exams of the whole thorax performed between November 2009 and July 2016 and spirometric measurements, both performed within a 6-month period. Exclusion criteria were the unavailability of CT images with a slice thickness ≤ 2 mm, reconstructed with a soft kernel, or the administration of iodinated contrast medium during the CT acquisition.

CT examinations

All CT examinations had been performed in the supine position at full inspiration, with usual acquisition parameters, allowing obtaining high resolution CT images of the whole thorax during a single breath hold. Five different 16-to-64 multislice CT devices from two different vendors (Somatom Sensation 16 and Somatom Definition DS, Siemens Healthcare, Erlangen, Germany; Lightspeed plus, Bright Speed 16 and Optima CT 660, GE Healthcare, Milwaukee, Wi) had been used, depending on the site and date of the CT examinations, all performed with equivalent acquisition parameters. The radiation dose resulting from each CT acquisition was evaluated by collecting the mean dose-length product (DLP) value from the dose reports.

Image analysis

Pulmonary situs type was identified as *solitus*, *inversus* or heterotaxy, based on the relationship between the upper-lobe bronchus and the ipsilateral pulmonary artery, and the morphology of the tracheobronchial tree [19]. CT images were also checked for prior lobectomy.

Lung structural changes were assessed by visual scoring and also by histogram analysis and thresholding of high attenuating lung structures.

Visual CT scoring was performed as follow

All the images were scored by one thoracic radiologist (CM) using the Bhalla score [20]. Twenty randomly selected examinations were also independently scored by a second radiologist (GC) to assess interobserver repeatability.

Automated CT scoring was performed as follows

First, the lungs were isolated from the mediastinum and chest wall using a commercially available, automated lung segmentation software (Myrian XP lung software version 1.19.1,Intrasense, Montpellier, France).

This allowed obtaining isolated whole lung volumes, for further density histogram analysis.

We also obtained separate volumes of the upper (right upper lobe and upper part of the left upper lung) and lower lungs (middle lobe, lingula, and lower lobes), after manual contouring of the fissures. This was only done for further comparison of the upper and lower lung CT-density scores. Otherwise, the process was fully automated.

The following histogram characteristics were analysed: mean lung density (MLD), mode (the most highly represented attenuation value), standard deviation (SD), kurtosis (sharpness of the density distribution), and skewness (asymmetry of the density distribution).

Lung structural changes having high attenuation values were quantified with a thresholding method, in order to obtain a CT-density score. Several threshold values were tested for their correlation with FEV_1 and forced vital capacity (FVC). Three fixed threshold values were tested (– 300, – 400 and – 500 HU), as well as eight adapted threshold values taking into account, for each CT examination, individual histogram features, known to be influenced by the inspiratory level [21, 22]. We hypothesized that adapted thresholds based on Mode or MLD or integrating SD might compensate for the changes of density distribution related to the level of inspiration.

The CT-density scores (one for each tested threshold value) were expressed as the proportion of lung showing attenuation values above the selected threshold. For instance, a CT-Density score value of 10 indicated that 10% of the lung had an attenuation value superior or equal to the threshold on CT.

More details about the whole procedure can be found on a previous work dedicated to automated scoring of CF lung structural changes [17].

Pulmonary function tests

Forced vital capacity (FVC) and forced expiratory volume in 1 s (FEV_1), expressed as the percentage of predicted values, were retrieved from the patients' files. Spirometry was performed as recommended by the American Thoracic Society/European Respiratory Society [23] and predicted values were calculated using the European Community for Steel and Coal reference values [24].

Statistical analysis

All analyses were done using the 'R' statistical software package (version 3.2.4, R Foundation, Vienna, Austria). Spearman's correlation coefficient was used to evaluate the correlations between visual scores, histogram characteristics, CT-density scores and spirometry measurements (FEV_1 and FVC). Spearman R values were interpreted as follows: < 0.4 = absent to weak correlation, 0.40–0.59 = moderate correlation, 0.60–0.79 = good correlation, > 0.8 = strong correlation. To evaluate the distribution of high attenuating lung structural changes, the CT-density scores of the upper lung portions (right upper lobe and upper component of the left upper lobe) were compared to those of the lower lung portions (middle lobe, lingula, and lower lobes), using Wilcoxon's paired test. Intraclass correlation coefficients (ICC) and Bland-Altman plots were used to assess interobserver repeatability of the visual scores. Excellent repeatability was assumed when the ICC was 0.8 or more.

Results

Patients

Between November 2009 and July 2016, 95 patients with a confirmed diagnosis of PCD were identified, of whom sixty-two patients were included in this study. Among the 33 excluded patients, 24 had no available CT examination, 6 patients had CT scans without soft kernel reconstruction or thin-slice images, and the interval between spirometry and CT exceeded 6 months in the remaining 3 cases (Fig. 1). For the 62 patients who were finally included, PCD diagnosis had been confirmed in 51 by electron microscopy of ciliary ultrastructure. The remaining 11 patients had Kartagener's syndrome with diffuse bronchiectasis and situs inversus on CT imaging, a combination of signs considered to validate PCD diagnosis [13].

Characteristics of the study population are presented in Table 1.

The mean ± SD age was 39 ± 15 years. Mean predicted FEV_1 was 67 ± 20% and mean predicted FVC was 80 ± 18%. Their correlation to patients' age was weak ($R = -0.32$, $p = 0.012$ for FEV_1) and ($R = -0.33$, $p = 0.008$ for FVC).

Regarding other characteristics, 37 patients (60%) had the usual arrangement of the pulmonary situs (*situs solitus*), while 24 (39%) had *situs inversus* and 1 (1%) had left isomerism.

Nineteen patients (31%) had previously undergone complete or partial lobectomy. The resections concerned the middle lobe in 15 patients (24%), the left lower lobe in 1 patient (2%), the middle lobe plus the left lower lobe

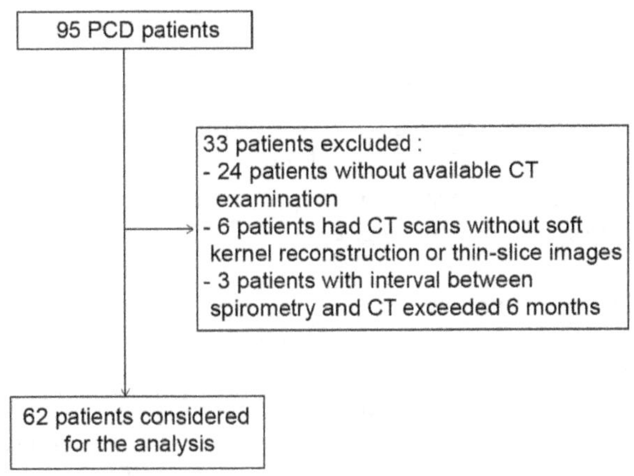

Fig. 1 Flow Chart

Table 1 Characteristics of the patients ($n = 62$)

Male/Female	32 / 30
Age, yr	39 (15)
Bronchial situs	
- solitus	37 (60)
- inversus	24 (39)
- left isomerism	1 (1)
Body mass index, kg/m^2	23.71 (4)
Percentage of predicted FEV$_1$	67 (20)
Percentage of predicted FVC	80 (18)
Median interval between spirometry and CT, months [interquartile range]	0 [0–16]

For quantitative variables, data are mean with standard deviation in parentheses
For qualitative variables, data are numbers of patients, and numbers in parentheses are percentages
Definition of abbreviations: CT computed tomography, *FEV$_1$* forced expiratory volume in 1 s, *FVC* forced vital capacity

in 2 patients (3%), and the middle lobe plus the lingula in the remaining patient (2%).

CT examinations

The median interval between CT and spirometry was 0 days [interquartile range: 0–29], 41 of the 62 CT scans being performed on the same day as spirometry. The mean DLP per CT scan was 200.3 ± 100.4 mGy.cm.

Visual CT score

The interobserver repeatability for the visual score was excellent (ICC = 0.84). Visual CT score, performed for all CT scans by one of the 2 radiologists, showed good correlation with FEV$_1$ ($R = -0.60$; $p < 0.001$) and FVC ($R = -0.62$; $p < 0.001$).

Histogram characteristics

Two histogram characteristics – kurtosis ($R = 0.56$; $p < 0.001$) and skewness ($R = 0.60$; $p < 0.001$)– showed a moderate to good correlation to FEV$_1$ (Table 2). The same two characteristics also correlated with FVC ($R = 0.65$; $p < 0.001$ and 0.67; $p < 0.001$, respectively). SD showed good negative correlation to both FEV1 ($R = -0.63$; $p < 0.001$) and FVC ($R = -0.67$; $p < 0.001$). Overall the correlations with FVC were slightly stronger than the correlations with FEV$_1$. Examples of variations in histogram shape according to pulmonary function are shown in Fig. 2.

CT-density scores

All CT-density scores showed moderate to good negative correlations with FEV$_1$ ($R = -0.54$ to -0.68; $p < 0.001$) and FVC ($R = -0.62$ to -0.71; $p < 0.001$) (Table 2). Overall, CT scores based on fixed thresholds showed weaker negative correlations with FEV$_1$ ($R = -0.51$ to -0.54; $p < 0.001$) and FVC ($R = -0.59$ to -0.62; $p < 0.001$)

Table 2 Correlations between spirometry, histogram characteristics and CT-density scores

	FEV$_1$		FVC	
	R	*P* value	R	*P* value
Histogram characteristics				
- MLD	−0.22	0.084	− 0.31	0.012
- Mode	0.14	0.285	0.11	0.397
- SD	−0.63	< 0.001	− 0.67	< 0.001
- Kurtosis	0.56	< 0.001	0.65	< 0.001
- Skewness	0.60	< 0.001	0.67	< 0.001
CT-density score with fixed thresholds				
- (−) 400 HU	−0.51	< 0.001	−0.59	< 0.001
- (−) 500 HU	−0.53	< 0.001	− 0.61	< 0.001
- (−) 600 HU	− 0.54	< 0.001	−0.61	< 0.001
CT-density score with adapted thresholds				
- MLD + 2 SD	−0.62	< 0.001	−0.67	< 0.001
- MLD + 1 SD	−0.68	< 0.001	− 0.71	< 0.001
- Mode + 500 HU	− 0.57	< 0.001	−0.64	< 0.001
- Mode + 400 HU	−0.60	< 0.001	− 0.65	< 0.001
- Mode + 300 HU	− 0.64	< 0.001	−0.70	< 0.001
- Mode + 3 SD	−0.54	< 0.001	− 0.62	< 0.001
- Mode + 2 SD	− 0.65	< 0.001	−0.70	< 0.001
- Mode + 1SD	−0.66	< 0.001	− 0.68	< 0.001

Definition of abbreviations: CT computed tomography, *FEV$_1$* forced expiratory volume in 1 s, *FVC* forced vital capacity, *HU* Hounsfield unit, *MLD* Mean Lung Density, *SD* Standard Deviation

than did CT-density scores based on adapted thresholds taking into account histogram characteristics. The strongest correlations were obtained using MLD + 1SD as threshold ($R = -0.68$; $p < 0.001$ for FEV$_1$ and $R = -0.71$ for FVC; $p < 0.001$) (Fig. 3). The correlations between CT score and PFTs were in the same range when considering each center separately: $R = -0.66$; $p < 0.001$ and -0.68; $p < 0.001$ for FEV1 and $R = -0.68$; $p < 0.001$ and -0.70; $p < 0.001$ for FVC. With this threshold value (MLD + 1SD), the automated score (CT-density score) correlated well with the visual score ($R = 0.70$, $p < 0.001$). Within the Bhalla visual score, the automated CT-density score correlated well with air wall thickening and mucus plugging- related items ($R = 0.64$ and 0.61, respectively; $p < 0.001$) and moderately with bronchiectasis-related items ($R = 0.58$; $p < 0.001$)".

The automated score values were significantly higher in the lower lungs (median: 8.83; interquartile range: 7.61–10.06) than in the upper lungs (median: 6.25; interquartile range: 5.57–6.81) ($p < 0.001$).

Results of automated CT scoring in patients with different FEV$_1$ and FVC values are illustrated in Figs. 4 and 5.

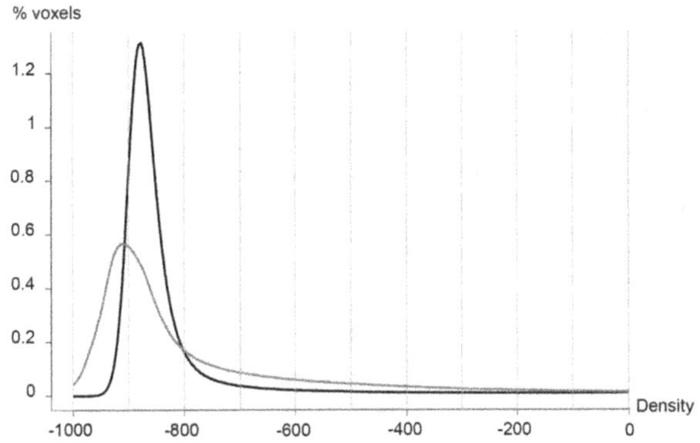

Fig. 2 Variation of histogram characteristics according to lung disease severity. Histogram of lung densities in a patient with mild disease (black line; FEV_1 = 81%; FVC = 101%;SD = 110.1; kurtosis =31.4). The histogram of lung densities in a patient with severe disease (grey line; FEV_1 = 25%; FVC = 54%) demonstrates higher scattering (SD = 213.9) and flattening (kurtosis = 6.7) of the curve

Discussion

To the best of our knowledge, the present manuscript describes the first automated CT scoring method designed to quantify lung changes associated with primary ciliary dyskinesia, based on the measurement of high-attenuating structures and considering histogram characteristics on CT. This approach is close to the quantification of emphysema, based on the measurement of low-attenuating lung areas. The method presented here has been previously validated in CF patients [17].

In the present cohort of 62 adults with PCD, the automated score correlated well with lung function (FEV_1 and FVC). Moreover, the value of the score was significantly different in the lower and upper portions of the lung, with higher score values in the lower part, consistent with the reported lower lung predominance of bronchial abnormalities in PCD patients [11].

Because the decline of lung function is slower in PCD than in CF, CT is less often performed. However, when performed, lung structural changes on follow-up CT need to be compared to previous images, which is complex in view of the high number of CT images with the modern multidetector technology. Rather than a subjective and time-consuming assessment, automated scoring provides an objective quantitative evaluation.

Regarding the thresholding method, we found that adapted thresholds based on histogram characteristics correlated better than fixed thresholds with the spirometric parameters. Lung attenuation is known to be influenced by parameters such as the level of inspiration, the kilovoltage, and the patient's position in the scan [21, 25, 26]. Expiration and, by extension, a lower level of inspiration, tend to flatten the CT density histogram, resulting in a higher SD and shifting of the curve towards higher density values, which increases Mode and MLD [26]. Instead of evaluating fixed thresholds alone, we postulated that inclusion of histogram characteristics in the threshold definition would compensate for variations not due to disease severity. Among the various thresholds tested here, MLD + 1SD gave the best results. This threshold is readily available, as most commercially available segmentation software programs provide both MLD and SD values.

One-third of our patients had previously undergone complete or partial lobectomy, even though bronchial abnormalities are not usually restricted to a single lobe in PCD and surgical resection is currently not considered an appropriate treatment for PCD [3]. This proportion is in line with the 41% prevalence reported by Kennedy et al. In this latter study, where visual CT scoring was performed, a maximal score was arbitrarily affected to the missing lung [14]. In our study, we only applied scoring to the existing lung and found good correlations of the visual score to FEV_1 and FVC, in the upper range of previously reported correlations (0.08 to − 0.63 for FEV_1 and − 0.38 to − 0.60 for FVC) [8, 10, 12]. The correlation of the CT-density score to FEV_1 and

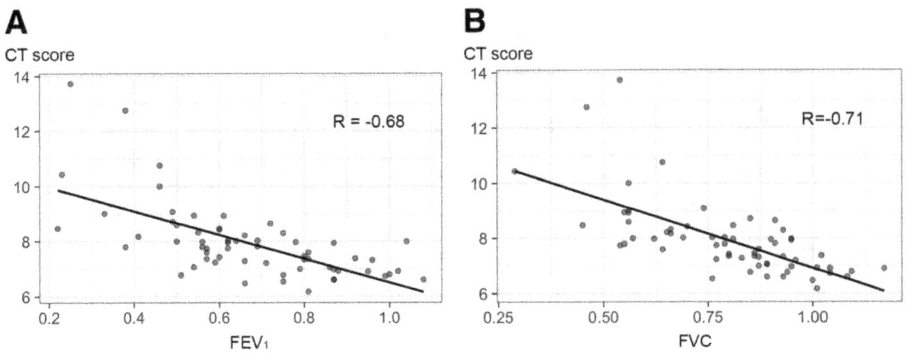

Fig. 3 Relationship between the CT-density score based on MLD + 1SD and lung functional parameters. **a** Relationship between CT-density score and FEV_1. **b** Relationship between CT-density score and FVC

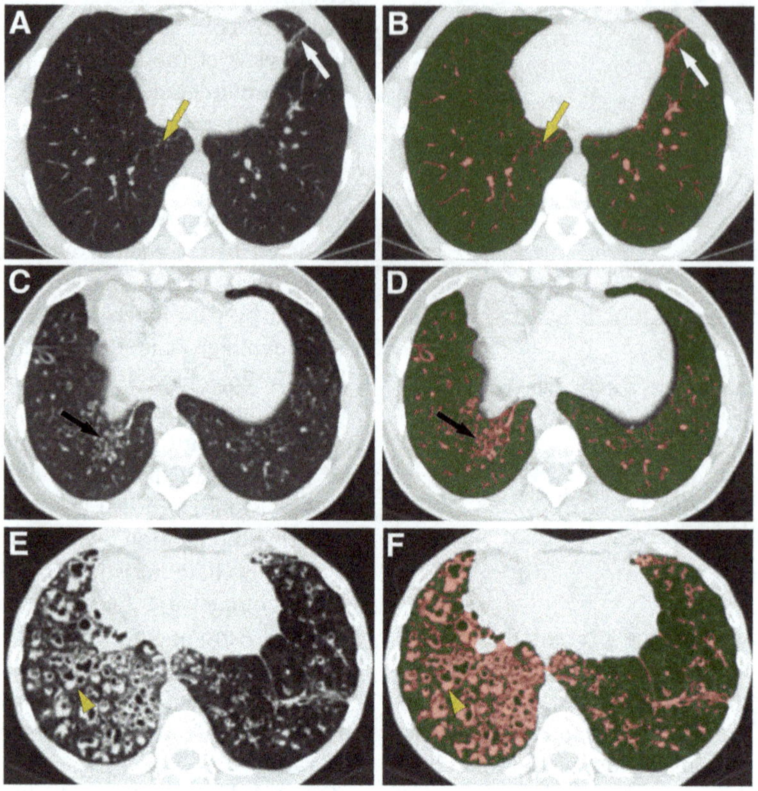

Fig. 4 CT-density scores in patients with increasing disease severity. Areas of high attenuation, using MLD + 1SD as threshold, are tagged in pink. **a**, **b** Patient with mild lung involvement (FEV_1 = 80%, CT score = 6.01): (**a**) Small areas of tree-in-bud (yellow arrow) and subsegmental atelectasis (white arrow) are seen on the native axial image. **b** Post-processed image, illustrating that these PCD-related abnormalities appear in pink, along with pulmonary vessels. **c**, **d** Patient with moderate lung involvement (FEV_1 = 60%, CT score = 8.37): areas of tree-in-bud (black arrow) seen on the native axial CT image (**c**) are more extensive and are pink-colored on the post-processed image (**d**) (**e**, **f**) Patient with severe lung involvement (FEV_1 = 25%, CT score = 13.72): (**e**) Visually, bronchial abnormalities (yellow arrowhead) predominantly affect the right lung on the native axial CT image. **f** Post-processed CT image. The CT-density score is 17.59 for the right lung and 10.87 for the left lung

FVC was in the same range, with the advantage of an automated method for the CT-density score.

Because most structural changes (e.g., bronchial wall thickening, mucus plugging) in PCD increase lung density, we based our automated scoring on the identification of high attenuating structures, leaving out empty bronchiectasis and mosaic perfusion. Thus, the automated score mainly quantifies potentially reversible, inflammatory changes such as mucoid impactions, bronchial wall thickening, bronchiolar nodules and consolidations,

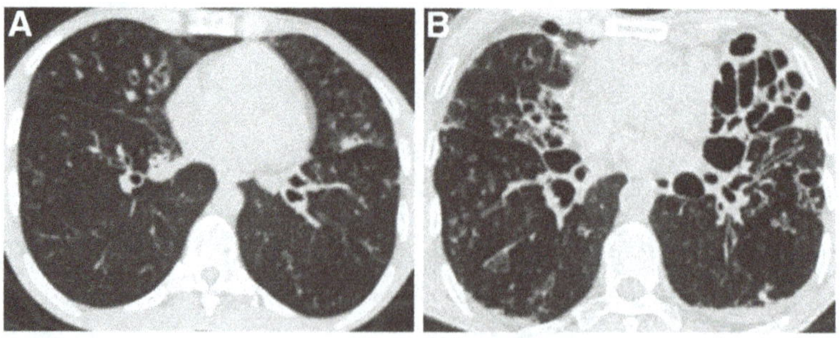

Fig. 5 Different imaging features in patients with similar FEV_1 values. **a** Patient with FEV_1 = 38% predicted and moderate bronchiectasis predominantly affecting the middle lobe. The CT-density score based on MLD + 1SD was 7.79. **b** Patient with FEV_1 = 38% predicted but much more severe bronchiectasis on visual assessment, especially in the lingula. The CT-density score based on MLD + 1SD was 12.75. These two examples show that CT imaging provides additional information to spirometry, especially regarding regional disease distribution (homogeneous versus heterogeneous), and the severity of bronchiectasis, which correspond to irreversible changes

whereas it does not consider irreversible changes (e.g., bronchiectasis). Based on these characteristics, we speculate variations in this score may prove useful in identifying worsening of bronchial disease (e.g., during pulmonary exacerbations) or improvement in bronchial patency (e.g., after recovery from a pulmonary exacerbation or due to the beneficial effect of therapy). Due to the unavailability of follow-up chest CT exams for most patients, we were not able to test this hypothesis and future longitudinal studies are needed.

Using our thresholding method, one drawback is that the pulmonary vessels are incorporated into the high-attenuating lung volume, which does not therefore correspond only to the diseased lung. However, differences in pulmonary vessel volume among patients had probably little influence on score variations compared to those due to the bronchial disease, given the good correlation between our score and spirometric parameters. Software capable of pulmonary vessel volume segmentation is being developed [27] and could be used to exclude the pulmonary vessels and improve the performance of the score.

Even though the automated score correlated well with the evaluated functional parameters, we also found that patients with similar FEV_1 values could have quite different CT phenotypes. We believe that quantitative assessment of structural changes is of interest in addition to PFT measurements for both cross-sectional evaluation and disease monitoring. For example, disease progression in CF has long relied on assessment of lung function decline whereas CT scan analysis clearly shows that structural abnormalities may appear without significant changes in FEV1 [28]. Thus, CT provides structural information which is complementary to spirometry in patients with CF and similar findings are likely occurring in patients with PCD. Calculating CT score does not imply additional procedures for the patients since it can be done from standard CT acquisitions performed as standard of care.

Our study has several limitations. Because this study was retrospective, the CT acquisition parameters were not standardized. This may have influenced the density thresholds. Standardized scanning protocols would probably improve the performance of the developed score. However, the fact that the scoring method can be applied to unstandardized CT examinations makes it suitable for daily clinical use. We did not perform longitudinal evaluation to determine whether changes in the automated CT score correlated with changes in pulmonary function, and whether, as previously suggested, CT-scored disease extent can predict the subsequent decline in pulmonary function. Indeed, our primary objective was to develop and validate an automated CT score by cross-sectional evaluation. Lastly, due to the relative rarity of PCD, it was not possible to split our population into a development and validation cohort. Thus, the developed method should further be validated in an independent cohort of PCD patients.

Conclusion

In conclusion, automated density–based CT scoring, together with histogram characteristic analysis, is feasible in PCD patients and correlates well with FEV_1 and FVC. MLD + 1SD offered the best correlations with both FEV_1 and FVC. Quantitative analysis of structural abnormalities on CT scans may prove useful for objectively evaluating lung disease changes in PCD, which may prove useful both in daily clinical use and as an outcome in clinical trials.

Abbreviations

CF: Cystic fibrosis; CT: Computed tomography; DLP: Dose-length product; FEV_1: Forced expiratory volume in 1 s; HU: Hounsfield units; ICC: Intraclass correlation coefficients; MLD: Mean lung density; PCD: Primary ciliary dyskinesia; SD: Standard deviation

Acknowledgments

not applicable

Funding

None

Authors' contributions

TTNH, MPR, PRB, BM and GC were involved in conception and design. TTNH, LB, IH, THH, CM and GC were involved in acquisition and analysis of the data. TTNH, MPR and GC were involved in drafting the manuscript. PRB, LB, IH, THH, CM and BM critically revised the work. All authors agreed to be accountable for all aspects of the work.

Consent for publication

not applicable

Competing interests

MPR and GC have made a patent application for the image analysis method presented in this article. The other authors declare that they have no competing interests.

Author details

[1]Radiology Department, Groupe Hospitalier Cochin-Hôtel Dieu, AP-HP, Université Paris Descartes - Sorbonne Paris Cité, Paris, France. [2]Pulmonary Department, Groupe Hospitalier Cochin-Hôtel Dieu, AP-HP, Université Paris Descartes - Sorbonne Paris Cité, Paris, France. [3]Service de Pneumologie et de Pathologie Professionnelle, DHU A-TVB, Centre Hospitalier Intercommunal de Créteil, Université Paris Est Créteil, Créteil, France. [4]Physiology Department, Groupe Hospitalier Cochin-Hôtel Dieu, AP-HP, Université Paris Descartes - Sorbonne Paris Cité, Paris, France. [5]Center for Visual Computing, CentraleSupelec, Gif-sur-Yvette, France. [6]Department Diagnostic Imaging, Vinmec International Hospital – Central Park, Ho Chi Minh City, Vietnam.

References

1. Afzelius BA. A human syndrome caused by immotile cilia. Science. 1976;193: 317–9.
2. Meeks M, Bush A. Primary ciliary dyskinesia (PCD). Pediatr Pulmonol. 2000; 29:307–16.
3. Honoré I, Burgel P-R. Primary ciliary dyskinesia in adults. Rev Mal Respir. 2016;33:165–89.
4. Barbato A, Frischer T, Kuehni CE, Snijders D, Azevedo I, Baktai G, et al. Primary ciliary dyskinesia: a consensus statement on diagnostic and treatment approaches in children. Eur Respir J. 2009;34:1264–76.
5. Shah A, Shoemark A, MacNeill SJ, Bhaludin B, Rogers A, Bilton D, et al. A longitudinal study characterising a large adult primary ciliary dyskinesia population. Eur Respir J. 2016;48:441–50.
6. Kennedy MP, Noone PG, Leigh MW, Zariwala MA, Minnix SL, Knowles MR, et al. High-resolution CT of patients with primary ciliary dyskinesia. AJR Am J Roentgenol. 2007;188:1232–8.
7. Santamaria F, Montella S, Tiddens HAWM, Guidi G, Casotti V, Maglione M, et al. Structural and functional lung disease in primary ciliary dyskinesia. Chest. 2008;134:351–7.
8. Maglione M, Bush A, Montella S, Mollica C, Manna A, Esposito A, et al. Progression of lung disease in primary ciliary dyskinesia: is spirometry less accurate than CT? Pediatr Pulmonol. 2012;47:498–504.
9. Magnin ML, Cros P, Beydon N, Mahloul M, Tamalet A, Escudier E, et al. Longitudinal lung function and structural changes in children with primary ciliary dyskinesia. Pediatr Pulmonol. 2012;47:816–25.
10. Pifferi M, Bush A, Pioggia G, Caramella D, Tartarisco G, Di Cicco M, et al. Evaluation of pulmonary disease using static lung volumes in primary ciliary dyskinesia. Thorax. 2012;67:993–9.
11. Cohen-Cymberknoh M, Simanovsky N, Hiller N, Gileles Hillel A, Shoseyov D, Kerem E. Differences in disease expression between primary ciliary dyskinesia and cystic fibrosis with and without pancreatic insufficiency. Chest. 2014;145: 738–44.
12. Boon M, Vermeulen FL, Gysemans W, Proesmans M, Jorissen M, De Boeck K. Lung structure-function correlation in patients with primary ciliary dyskinesia. Thorax. 2015;70:339–45.
13. Frija-Masson J, Bassinet L, Honoré I, Dufeu N, Housset B, Coste A, et al. Clinical characteristics, functional respiratory decline and follow-up in adult patients with primary ciliary dyskinesia. Thorax. 2017;72:154–60.
14. Kennedy MP, Omran H, Leigh MW, Dell S, Morgan L, Molina PL, et al. Congenital heart disease and other heterotaxic defects in a large cohort of patients with primary ciliary dyskinesia. Circulation. 2007;115: 2814–21.
15. Calder AD, Bush A, Brody AS, Owens CM. Scoring of chest CT in children with cystic fibrosis: state of the art. Pediatr Radiol. 2014;44:1496–506.
16. Gevenois PA, de Maertelaer V, De Vuyst P, Zanen J, Yernault JC. Comparison of computed density and macroscopic morphometry in pulmonary emphysema. Am J Respir Crit Care Med. 1995;152:653–7.
17. Chassagnon G, Martin C, Burgel P-R, Hubert D, Fajac I, Paragios N, et al. An automated computed tomography score for the cystic fibrosis lung. Eur Radiol. 2018.
18. Lucas JS, Barbato A, Collins SA, Goutaki M, Behan L, Caudri D, et al. European Respiratory Society guidelines for the diagnosis of primary ciliary dyskinesia. Eur Respir J. 2017;49:1601090.
19. Chassagnon G, Morel B, Carpentier E, Ducou Le Pointe H, Sirinelli D. Tracheobronchial branching abnormalities: lobe-based classification scheme. Radiographics. 2016;36:358-73.
20. Bhalla M, Turcios N, Aponte V, Jenkins M, Leitman BS, McCauley DI, et al. Cystic fibrosis: scoring system with thin-section CT. Radiology. 1991;179:783–8.
21. Goris ML, Zhu HJ, Blankenberg F, Chan F, Robinson TE. An automated approach to quantitative air trapping measurements in mild cystic fibrosis. Chest. 2003;123:1655–63.
22. Goris ML, Zhu HJ. Robinson TE. A critical discussion of computer analysis in medical imaging. Proc Am Thorac Soc. 2007;4:347–9.
23. Miller MR, Hankinson J, Brusasco V, Burgos F, Casaburi R, Coates A, et al. Standardisation of spirometry. Eur Respir J. 2005;26:319–38.
24. Quanjer PH, Tammeling GJ, Cotes JE, Pedersen OF, Peslin R, Yernault JC. Lung volumes and forced ventilatory flows. Report working party standardization of lung function tests, European Community for steel and coal. Official statement of the European Respiratory Society. Eur Respir J Suppl. 1993;16:5–40.
25. Robinson PJ, Kreel L. Pulmonary tissue attenuation with computed tomography: comparison of inspiration and expiration scans. J Comput Assist Tomogr. 1979;3:740–8.
26. Levi C, Gray JE, McCullough EC, Hattery RR. The unreliability of CT numbers as absolute values. AJR Am J Roentgenol. 1982;139:443–7.
27. Rudyanto RD, Kerkstra S, van Rikxoort EM, Fetita C, Brillet P-Y, Lefevre C, et al. Comparing algorithms for automated vessel segmentation in computed tomography scans of the lung: the VESSEL12 study. Med Image Anal. 2014;18: 1217–32.
28. Loeve M, Krestin GP, Rosenfeld M, de Bruijne M, Stick SM, Tiddens HA. Chest computed tomography: a validated surrogate endpoint of cystic fibrosis lung disease? Eur Respir J. 2013;42:844–57.

24

Malignant pleural mesothelioma: diagnostic value of medical thoracoscopy and long-term prognostic analysis

Li-Li Xu[†], Yuan Yang[†], Zhen Wang, Xiao-Juan Wang, Zhao-Hui Tong and Huan-Zhong Shi[*]

Abstract

Background: Malignant pleural mesothelioma (MPM) is marked by its difficult diagnosis and poor prognosis. Medical thoracoscopy (MT) is an effective and safe procedure for the diagnosis of exudative pleural effusions and many factors associated with poor prognosis of MPM. We conducted this study to investigate the value of MT for diagnosing of MPM and to identify prognostic factors for MPM patients.

Methods: From July 2005 through June 2014, a total of 833 patients with undiagnosed pleural effusions underwent MT and pleural biopsies were taken. Clinical data of all patients with MPM were retrospectively analyzed, and those with complete follow-up data were analyzed for prognostic factors.

Results: Eventually, MPM was the final diagnosis in 40 patients. Diagnostic efficiency of MT for MPM was 87.5%, since diagnosis of MPM failed to be established in 5 patients during the initial MT. Median survival was 17.1 mo (95% confidence interval: 13.6–20.7 mo). MT findings of pleural adhesion and plaques were adverse prognostic factors for MPM. In addition, old age, male gender, smoking history, histological type, poor staging, no treatment, low total protein level in pleural fluid, and computed tomographic findings such as pulmonary consolidation or infiltration, mediastinal lymphopathy, pulmonary mass or nodules, and pleural nodularity were also poor prognostic factors for MPM.

Conclusions: MT is safe with a high positive rate in the diagnosis of MPM, and pleural adhesion and plaques seen under MT may be the adverse prognostic factors for MPM. Multiple clinical characteristics can affect the survival of MPM patients.

Keywords: Malignant pleural mesothelioma, Medical thoracoscopy, Prognosis

Background

Malignant diffuse mesothelioma is a tumor arising from the mesothelial or submesothelial cells of the pleura, peritoneum, or pericardium. More than 80% of all mesothelioma originate in the pleura [1]. As malignant pleural mesothelioma (MPM) has been researched less than other primary neoplasms of the chest in the past few decades, it is of importance to study more about MPM, including its diagnosis and prognosis.

Clinical manifestations of mesothelioma are usually nonspecific. MPM is marked by its difficulty of diagnosis in the early stage. Because pleural effusion is usually the first clinical symptom of MPM, cytology of pleural effusion is often the first diagnostic examination to be performed. However, the accuracy of such an examination for the diagnosis of MPM is limited. The sensitivity of cytologic examination for a diagnosis of MPM was only 32% - 51.3% [2, 3]. Same problems are also observed in fine-needle biopsies or image-guided core needle biopsy. Medical thoracoscopy (MT) refers to the examination of the pleural space, and this procedure has been well documented to be highly sensitive of 87%–92.6% for diagnosing exudative pleural effusions with few complications which reported rates of 2% - 6% [4–6].

Once diagnosed as MPM, the median survival is short or only 4–16 mo [7–9]. Many factors associated with poor prognosis in patients with MPM, such as old age, poor

* Correspondence: shihuanzhong@sina.com
[†]Equal contributors
Department of Respiratory and Critical Care Medicine; Beijing Institute of Respiratory Medicine and Beijing Chaoyang Hospital, Capital Medical University, 8 Gongti Nanlu, Chaoyang District, Beijing 100020, China

performance status, advanced disease stage, thrombocytosis, chest pain, weight loss, asbestos exposure and long duration of symptoms [8, 10–13]. We conducted this study to investigate the usage of MT in the diagnosis of pleural effusion patients induced by MPM, and to identify general predictors of survival of MPM patients.

Methods

Patients

The study protocol was approved by the Institutional Review Boards for human studies of Beijing Chaoyang Hospital, China. Informed consents were not required as this was considered a review of clinical practice.

This study was a retrospective study. Between July 2005 and June 2014, a total of 833 patients with undiagnosed pleural effusions underwent MT and pleural biopsy was taken under direct visual control in the suspected areas such as pleural plaques and nodules, and systematically in several parts of the parietal pleura for mycobacterial, cytological, histological and immunohistochemical examination in our institution, and their detailed medical history, clinical presentation, laboratory examination results, and image data were recorded [6]. Only those data of pleural effusion patients with definite diagnosis of MPM were included in the current study, yielding 40 cases. Clinical stage was defined by the 7th TNM classification [14]. The initial MT followed by pathological and immunohistochemical analysis of pleural biopsy led to the definite diagnosis of MPM in 35 of 40 these patients. The remaining 5 MPE patients could not obtain the correct diagnose after the initial MT and the pleural biopsy only gave the result of non-specific pleurisy. After 8 mo follow-up, 2 of the 5 patients was diagnosed as MPE by the second MT, one was diagnosed by percutaneous needle lung biopsy, one was diagnosed by open-long biopsy and one was diagnosed by liver-biopsy [15]. Before MT, all patients underwent the initial diagnostic workup, which included a detailed medical evaluation, CT scans, pleural fluid analyses, and/or closed pleural biopsy examination.

Thoracoscopic procedures

MT was performed by chest physicians in our pulmonary procedural suite as described in our previous publications [6]. Pleural fluid and pleural biopsy samples obtained from each patient were analyzed. Cytological examination and biochemical parameters of pleural fluids and histopathological and immunohistochemical examination of pleural biopsies from all patients was performed. For pleural effusion, the effusion size of 300 ml - 500 ml was identified as small pleural effusion, the effusion size of 500 ml – 800 ml was identified as moderate pleural effusion, and the effusion size ≥800 ml was identified as large pleural effusion.

Follow-up

We followed up individual patients until their death. During the follow-up, the following information was required from the patients or relatives every month by telephone or personal interview: 1) the demographic characteristics of patients; 2) the therapeutic regimen (surgical excision, any chemotherapy, radiation therapy, or pleurodesis) after diagnosed with MPM; 3) the time of death.

Diagnostic criteria for MPM

Histopathology and immunohistochemistry review of all slides with at least one paraffin block representative pleural biopsy samples obtained through MT. The diagnosis of MPM was made by a panel of specialized pulmonary pathologists according to the current guideline [16]. MPM is divided into epithelioid, biphasic, and sarcomatoid subtypes on the basis of the predominant histomorphological growth pattern.

Statistical analysis

All analyses were performed with SPSS software (version 19. 0, SPSS Inc., Chicago, IL, USA). Data are presented as mean ± standard deviation (SD) or number with percentage. Descriptive statistical methods were used for data analysis.

We stratified patients by various factors including age, gender, smoking history, MT findings, histological type, staging, therapeutic regimen, TP of pleural fluid, LDH of pleural fluid and CT imagings. The rate of death was calculated for each level of the factor. MT findings, including pleural nodules, pleural hyperemia, pleural adhesion, pleural edema and pleural plaques, were examined to evaluate the relation with prognosis. The following other factors were also examined for the prognostic value: age, gender, smoking history, histological type, staging, treatment after diagnosed with MPM, laboratory levels of pleural fluid: total protein, lactate dehydrogenase and computed tomography (CT) imaging: pulmonary consolidation or infiltration, pulmonary atelectasis, mediastinal lymphopathy, pleural thickening, pulmonary mass or nodules, pleural nodularity.

Kaplan–Meier analyses were used and survival curves were plotted. Log rank test compared survival curves. Associations between possible prognostic variables and survival were estimated using Cox proportional hazards regression. All reported P values were two-sided and effects were considered significant if $P < 0.05$.

Results

Characteristics of patients with MPM

Between July 2005 and June 2014, 833 patients with undiagnosed pleural effusions successfully underwent MT, and pleural biopsy samples were obtained for diagnostic evaluation. Eventually, MPM was the final diagnosis in 40 patients. Patient characteristics are listed in Table 1. Thirty-five of 40

Table 1 Characteristics of study subjects with confirmed malignant pleural mesothelioma after medical thoracoscopy ($n = 40$)

Variables	Values
Age, yr., median (range)	62 (40–78)
Sex, male, n (%)	20 (50.0)
Symptom	
Dyspnea	26 (65.0)
Chest pain	19 (47.5)
Cough	11 (27.5)
Fatigue	6 (15.0)
Fever	3 (7.5)
CT imaging, n (%)	
Pulmonary consolidation or infiltration	20 (50.0)
Pulmonary atelectasis	19 (47.5)
Pleural thickening	17 (42.5)
Mediastinal lymphopathy	11 (27.5)
Pulmonary mass or nodules	11 (27.5)
Pleural nodularity	7 (17.5)
Effusion site, n (%)	
Right	19 (47.5)
Left	16 (40.0)
Bilateral	4 (10.0)
Effusion size, n (%)	
Large	20 (50.0)
Moderate	9 (22.5)
Small	11 (27.5)
Thoracoscopic findings, n (%)	
Pleural nodules	32 (80.0)
Pleural hyperemia	19 (47.5)
Pleural adhesion	15 (37.5)
Pleural edema	5 (12.5)
Pleural plaques	5 (12.5)
Histology type	
Epithelioid	14 (35.0)
Sarcomatoid	9 (22.5)
Biphasic	5 (12.5)
Undifferentiated	12 (30.0)

patients were diagnosed after pleural biopsy was taken by the initial MT. The remaining 5 patients could not get the correct diagnosis at the first time, we followed-up these patients and they were finally diagnosed as MPM [15].

As shown in Table 1, 20 patients were men and 20 were women, with their median age was 62 yrs., ranged from 40 yrs. to 78 yrs. The most common symptoms of MPM were dyspnea, chest pain, and cough. In 19 MPM patients, pleural fluid occurred on the right side, in 16 on the left, and in 4 both sides were affected. In either unilateral or bilateral effusion, the percentages of large, moderate, and small size of pleural effusions were 50%, 22.5%, and 27.5%, respectively. CT imaging revealed pulmonary consolidation or infiltration, pulmonary atelectasis, pleural thickening, mediastinal lymphopathy, pulmonary mass or nodules, and pleural nodularity.

MT findings and pathological study

Under MT, one or more abnormalities could be observed on the surface of parietal or/and visceral pleura in all patients studied. We observed pleural nodules in 32 patients, pleural hyperemia in 19, pleural adhesion in 15, pleural edema in 5 and pleural plaques in 5 (Table 1).

After MT, histological and immunohistochemical examinations, 14 of 40 patients were diagnosed with epithelioid, 9 sarcomatoid, 5 biphasic and 12 undifferentiated (Table 1).

Follow-up data of patients with MPM

Eventually, 33 of 40 patients were followed up until their death. The other 7 patients lost of follow-up. Median survival was 17.1 mo (95% confidence interval: 13.6–20. 7 mo), range from 1.0 mo to 69.9 mo; 9 patients survived less than 1 yr., 18 survived less than 2 yrs., and 6 survived more than 2 yrs.

Most patients were in the late stages of disease (stage III or IV of the TNM staging system), with 9 patients were in stage II and no one was in stage I when diagnosis of MPM was established. Chemotherapy was performed in 21 of 33 patients; chemotherapy and radiotherapy were performed in 3 patients. Other 9 patients were not given any antitumor therapy.

Assessment of prognostic factors for MPM

First of all, we focused on the prognostic value of MT findings, and noted that a statistically significant relation was detected on comparing overall survival and pleural adhesion and plaques with P-value of 0.016 and 0.023, respectively, with Hazard Ratio (95% Confidence Interval) of 0.277 (0.097–0.788) and 0.387 (0.170–0.879), respectively (Fig. 1).

Table 2 shows the univariate analyses of variables potentially impacting overall survival. Adverse prognostic factors included old age, male gender, smoking history, thoracoscopic findings such as pleural adhesion and plaques, histological type, poor staging and no treatment. Other adverse factors impacting prognosis like total protein level in pleural fluid and some CT findings were listed in Table 3.

Figure 2 shows Kaplan–Meier survival curves subclassified 6 variables of general condition. According to our analysis, a statistically significant relation was detected on comparing overall survival and age, gender and smoking history with P-value of 0.008, 0.020, and $<$ 0.

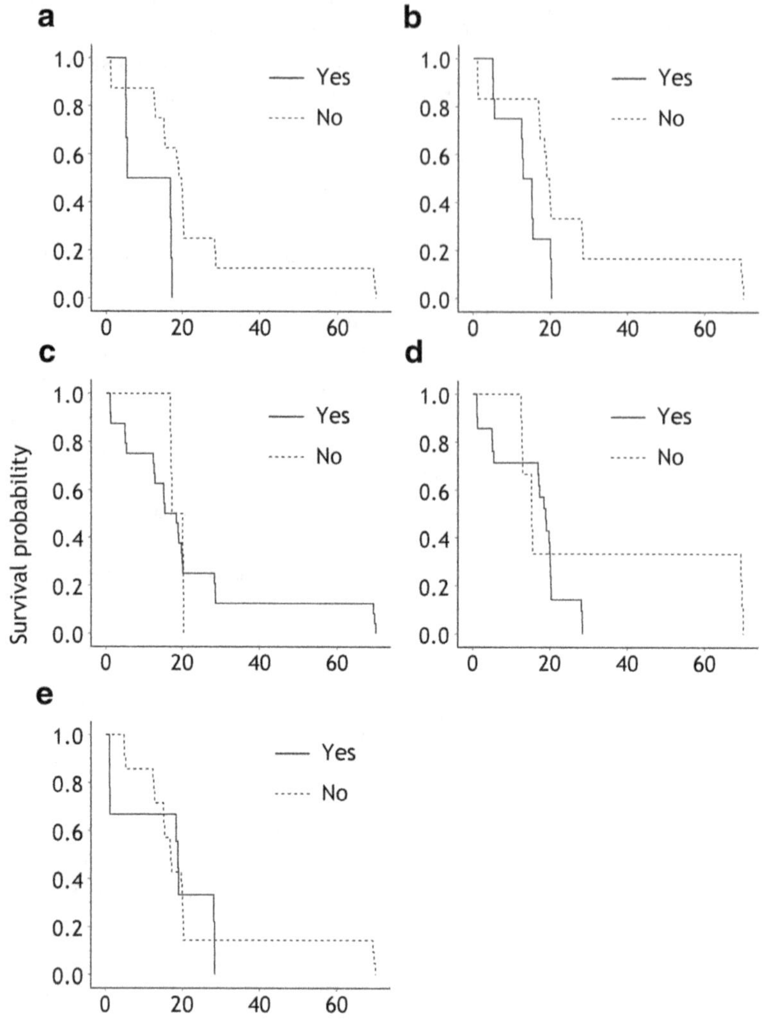

Fig. 1 Kaplan–Meier survival curves for prognostic factors of findings under medical thoracoscopy (log-rank test). (**a**) Pleural adhesion ($P = 0.010$), (**b**) pleural plaques ($P = 0.019$), (**c**) pleural nodules ($P = 0.985$), (**d**) pleural hyperemia ($P = 0.241$), and (**e**) pleural edema ($P = 0.814$)

001, respectively, and Hazard Ratio (95% Confidence Interval) of 1.81 (1.165–2.813), 0.346 (0.142–0.844) and 6.752 (2.418–18.855), respectively. A statistically relation was also detected on comparing overall survival and histological type, staging and treatment with *P*-value of < 0.001, < 0.001, and 0.001, respectively, and Hazard Ratio (95% Confidence Interval) of 0.095 (0.031–0.293), 21.042 (6.156–71.923) and 0.087 (0.021–0.359), respectively.

Figure 3 shows the Kaplan–Meier survival curves that some CT imaging may also be the adverse prognostic factors, such as pulmonary consolidation or infiltration, mediastinal lymphopathy, pulmonary mass or nodules and pleural nodularity, with *P*-value of 0.002, 0.006, 0. 003, and 0.043, respectively, and Hazard Ratio (95% Confidence Interval) of 0.191 (0.066–0.547), 0.230 (0. 080–0.661), 0.123(0.031–0.486) and 0.340 (0.120–0.964), respectively.

Discussion

The incidence of MPM has a growing tendency worldwide [17] and is likely to peak between the year 2015 and 2030 [18]. From July 2005 through June 2014, 833 patients with undiagnosed pleural effusions successfully underwent MT in our institute, 342 (41.1%) patients were confirmed to have malignant pleural effusion [6]. MPM (10.2%) is the second frequent cause of malignant pleural effusion. The most frequent cause is lung cancer (67.8%) [6].

Chest CT is commonly used in the preferred examination, which can display the surface of the whole pleura, the diaphragm and the lymph node [19]. The specificity of chest CT for identifying pleural tumors is about 88–95%, while the sensitivity is about 36–45% [20]. We noted in our study that MPM mainly appears as pulmonary consolidation or infiltration, as well pulmonary

Table 2 Association between clinic pathologic variables and survival

Prognostic factors	n	Median survival	Hazard Ratio	95% Confidence Interval	*P*
Age, yrs					
< 70	24	17.4			
≥ 70	9	5.1	1.81	1.165–2.813	0.008
Gender					
Male	12	13.0			
Female	21	20.0	0.346	0.142–0.844	0.020
Smoking history					
No smoking	21	20.0			
Smoking	12	5.4	6.752	2.418–18.855	< 0.001
Thoracoscopic findings					
Pleural nodules					
Yes	24	15.6			
No	6	17.4	1.009	0.399–2.554	0.985
Pleural hyperemia					
Yes	21	18.9			
No	9	15.3	0.573	0.223–1.468	0.246
Pleural adhesion					
Yes	6	5.4			
No	24	19.1	0.277	0.097–0.788	0.016
Pleural edema					
Yes	9	18.9			
No	21	17.1	0.908	0.404–2.038	0.814
Pleural plaques					
Yes	12	13.0			
No	18	19.1	0.387	0.170–0.879	0.023
Histological type					
Epithelioid	12	12.8			
Non-epithelioid	21	20.4	0.095	0.031–0.293	< 0.001
Staging					
I	0				
II	9	28.4			
III	15	17.1			
IV	9	3.0	21.042	6.156–71.923	< 0.001
Therapeutic regimen					
Chemotherapy	21	20.0			
Chemotherapy and radiotherapy	3	15.3			
No therapy	9	3.0	0.087	0.021–0.359	0.001

atelectasis on CT scan. Although it is still difficult in the tumor staging and distinguishing the diffuse pleural thickening from MPM [20], the images on CT scan can be used to guide subsequently biopsy and thus improve the diagnostic yield.

The diagnosis of MPM mainly relies on the pleural biopsy at present. Thoracoscopic pleural biopsy has become the most reliable method for the diagnosis of MPM for its comprehensive observation, accurately obtaining the tissue specimens, and the advantage of mini-invasive lesions [21]. In the present study, MPM was the final diagnosis in 40 patients with pleural effusion. Thirty-five of 40 patients were diagnosed by pleural biopsies which were taken during the initial MT, indicating that the diagnostic efficiency of MT

Table 3 Association between clinic variables and survival

Prognostic factors	n	Median survival	Hazard Ratio	95% Confidence Interval	*P*
TP of pleural fluid (g/L)					
< 40	12	3.2			
≥ 40	18	19.1	0.131	0.048–0.359	< 0.001
LDH of pleural fluid (IU/L)					
< 200	15	17.1			
≥ 200	15	15.3	1.276	0.591–2.753	0.535
CT imaging					
Pulmonary consolidation or infiltration					
Yes	9	3.0			
No	15	20.0	0.191	0.066–0.547	0.002
Pulmonary atelectasis					
Yes	18	13.0			
No	6	1.2	1.169	0.442–3.091	0.753
Mediastinal lymphopathy					
Yes	9	5.1			
No	15	20	0.230	0.080–0.661	0.006
Pleural thickening					
Yes	12	5.4			
No	12	13	0.693	0.288–1.666	0.412
Pulmonary mass or nodules					
Yes	9	5.1			
No	15	20.0	0.123	0.031–0.486	0.003
Pleural nodularity					
Yes	6	1.2			
No	18	13.0	0.340	0.120–0.964	0.043

TP total protein, *LDH* lactate dehydrogenase

for MPM is 87.5%. Our previous publication has reported that the overall diagnostic efficiency of MT for undiagnosed pleural effusions is 92.6% (771/833) [6]. The reason that MT has lower diagnostic efficiency for MPM may be multiple. Except the sampling error, this may, in part, be explained by the rapidly growing incidence of MPM, which can demonstrate various, misleading, histopathologic pitfalls, and the pleura is a common site for metastatic disease [22]. In addition, because neoplastic invasion of MPM occurs submesothelially, it may be difficult for a thoracoscopist to detect these areas on grossly normal appearing pleura [15]. To avoid this, biopsies should be taken as much as possible under the premise of no other side effects, especially in suspected areas such as pleural plaques and nodules. As a matter of fact, the diagnosis of MPM still requires a combination of clinical manifestations and other experimental results. MT as a real-time invasive procedure enables clinicians to improve tumor staging, particularly in the mediastinal region, by enabling the exact sampling point with adequate tissue for biopsy. Our current data support the consideration that MT is considered the best way for making diagnosis of MPM [23].

We analyzed survival in this retrospective cohort study of 40 patients diagnosed with MPM after MT in our hospital over a 10-yr period. Thirty-three patients with complete follow-up data were analyzed for variables potentially impacting overall survival. The median survival was 17.1 mo (95% confidence interval: 13.6–20.7 mo), range from 1.0 mo to 69.9 mo. Among the variables potentially affecting overall survival, first of all, pleural adhesion and plaques observed under MT are adverse prognostic factors for patients with MPM. These observations have not been mentioned in any one previous study. These results are reasonable since pleural biopsies were taken in the suspected areas under MT. This improves the authenticity of pleural biopsy and the diagnostic accuracy of histological types, which is related to the prognosis of MPM. We also noted that the other MT findings, such as pleural nodules, pleural hyperemia, and pleural edema, were not relative to prognosis of

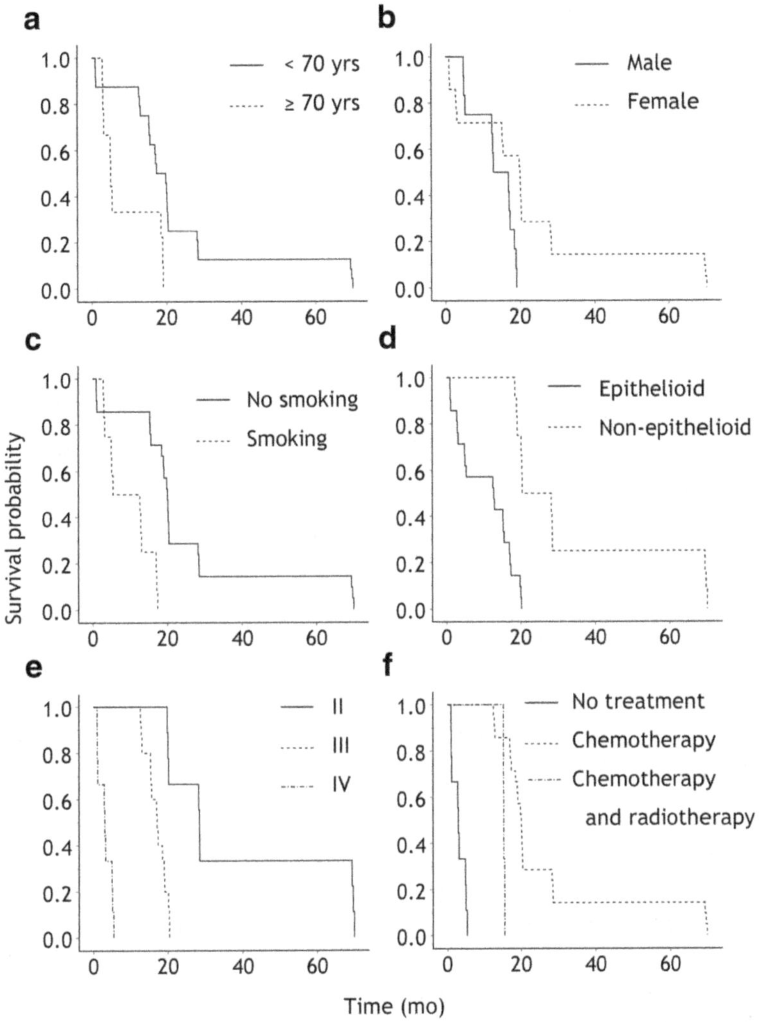

Fig. 2 Kaplan–Meier survival curves for prognostic factors of general conditions (log-rank test). (**a**) Two age groups ($P = 0.005$), (**b**) two groups for gender ($P = 0.015$), (**c**) two groups for smoking history ($P < 0.001$), (**d**) two groups for histological types ($P < 0.001$), (**e**) three groups for staging ($P < 0.001$), (**f**) three groups for treatment ($P < 0.001$)

MPM. This could be explained that these findings can also be commonly found in many other pleural diseases.

Old age and male gender have been recognized as negative prognostic factors [12, 13, 24, 25], such findings are also seen in the present study. As is well-known that smoking was an important cause of lung cancer incidence and global mortality [18, 26], this result should not be beyond expectations. However, no previous study investigated the relationship between survival and smoking history, as most doctors pay more attentions on relationship between survival and asbestos exposure. We found that MPM patients with a smoking history had worse survival. We also found that low total protein level in pleural fluid and some CT images, such as pulmonary consolidation or infiltration, mediastinal lymphopathy, pulmonary mass or nodules, and pleural nodularity were important poor prognostic factors of MPM. These findings may provide implications for poor prognosis and more aggressive treatment.

Our data revealed longer survival for MPM patients with the epithelioid type and this result is in line with many previous studies [11, 12, 14, 21, 24, 27]. The presence of an inflammatory stromal response demonstrated an association with improved survival [28]. The histological type influences the choice of therapeutic strategy and epithelioid type typically resulting in more aggressive medical procedures. Staging describes the anatomical extent of the neoplasm [14]. A statistically significant relation was detected on comparing overall survival and advanced stage in our study, as mediastinal nodal involvement has been recognized as a critical component of staging, with a detrimental effect on

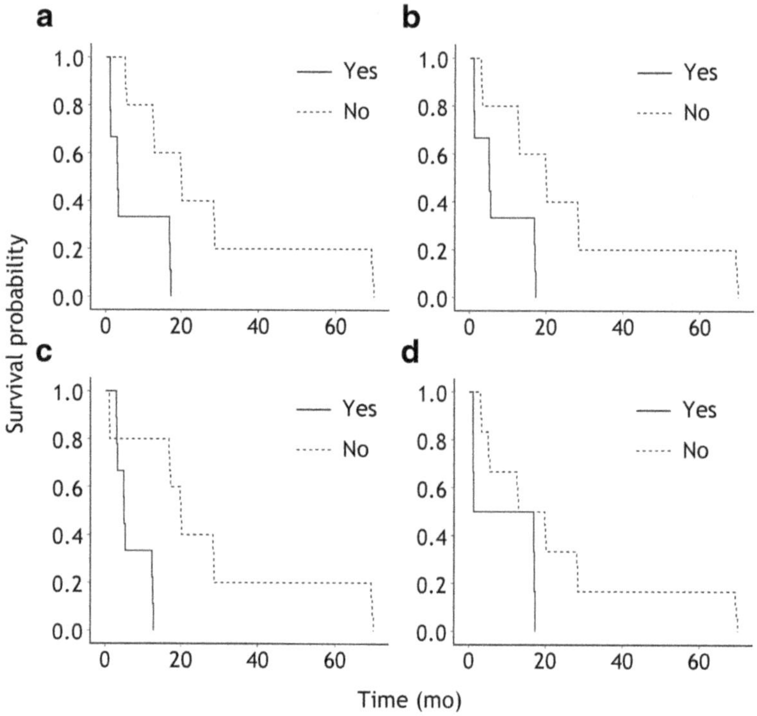

Fig. 3 Kaplan–Meier survival curves for prognostic factors of findings on computed tomography (log-rank test). (**a**) Pulmonary consolidation or infiltration ($P = 0.001$), (**b**) mediastinal lymphopathy ($P = 0.003$), (**c**) pulmonary mass or nodules ($P = 0.001$), (**d**) pleural nodularity ($P = 0.034$)

survival [29–32]. The fact that no patient was diagnosed in stage I and only 9 patients was diagnosed in stage II revealed the difficulty of the early diagnosis of MPM.

Our patients with no tumor treatment had worse survival than patients with chemotherapy or chemotherapy plus radiotherapy. The association between no treatment and a poor prognosis might merely because that no treatment was given only when patients were in advanced staging and poor overall condition that cannot support any treatment. None of the 33 patients were performed with surgical treatment, so the relationship between overall survival and surgical treatment cannot be analyzed.

Our study had some limitations. First, the study sample size was not large, with only 40 MPM patients diagnosed after MT were included in our study, and only 33 of 40 patients who provided follow-up data were analyzed for prognosis. Using a small sample increases the chance of assuming as true a false premise. Thus, chances are that the patients with proposed poor prognostic factors have no shorter lifetime compared to patients without these factors. Second, we could only analyzed the data from MPM patients who underwent MT procedure, and no data from the other control groups, such as the patients with cancers and benign pleural diseases, were available, it was therefore not possible to calculate the sensitivity and specificity of MT in diagnosing MPM. Third, none of 33 patients underwent surgery, thus the relationship between surgical intervention and overall survival cannot be analyzed. In addition, there is a potential selection bias to this retrospective study. Therefore, more prospective studies with a larger cohort of subjects are needed to support the present findings.

Conclusions

In summary, in view of difficulty of diagnosis and poor prognosis, the course of MPM remains aggressive and unfavorable. MT is safe with a high positive rate in the diagnosis of MPM, and pleural adhesion and plaques seen under MT may probably be the adverse prognostic factors of MPM. In addition, old age, male gender, smoking history, histological type, poor staging, no treatment, low total protein level in pleural fluid, and CT findings such as pulmonary consolidation or infiltration, mediastinal lymphopathy, pulmonary mass or nodules, and pleural nodularity may also be the poor prognostic factors for MPM. More prospective studies with a larger cohort of subjects are needed in the future to find the accurate prognostic factors for MPM.

Abbreviations

MPM: Malignant pleural mesothelioma; MT: Medical thoracoscopy; SD: standard deviation

Acknowledgements
Not applicable.

Take-home message
Medical thoracoscopy is useful for diagnosis and prognosis of malignant pleural mesothelioma.

Funding
This work was supported in part by grants from National Natural Science Foundation of China (No. 81730046 and No. 31470883), in part by the Beijing Municipal Administration of Hospitals' Mission Plan (No. SML20150301).

Authors' contributions
L.L.X., Y.Y., Z.W., X.J.W, Z.H.T. and H.Z.S. performed medical thoracoscopy. L.L.X. and Y.Y. worked in study abstraction, data analysis, and drafted manuscript. H.Z.S. designed the study, analyzed the result, and revised the manuscript. All authors read and approved the final manuscript.

Consent for publication
Not applicable.

Competing interests
The authors declare that they have no competing interests.

References
1. Delgermaa V, Takahashi K, Park EK, Le GV, Hara T, Sorahan T. Global mesothelioma deaths reported to the World Health Organization between 1994 and 2008. Bull World Health Organ. 2011;89(10):716–24. 724A-724C
2. Renshaw AA, Dean BR, Antman KH, Sugarbaker DJ, Cibas ES. The role of cytologic evaluation of pleural fluid in the diagnosis of malignant mesothelioma. Chest. 1997;111(1):106–9.
3. Rakha EA, Patil S, Abdulla K, Abdulkader M, Chaudry Z, Soomro IN. The sensitivity of cytologic evaluation of pleural fluid in the diagnosis of malignant mesothelioma. Diagn Cytopathol. 2010;38(12):874–9.
4. Casal RF, Eapen GA, Morice RC, Jimenez CA. Medical thoracoscopy. Curr Opin Pulm Med. 2009;15(4):313–20.
5. Medford AR, Bennett JA, Free CM, Agrawal S. Current status of medical pleuroscopy. Clin Chest Med. 2010;31(1):165–72. Table of Contents
6. Wang XJ, Yang Y, Wang Z, Xu LL, Wu YB, Zhang J, Tong ZH, Shi HZ. Efficacy and safety of diagnostic thoracoscopy in undiagnosed pleural effusions. Respiration. 2015;90(3):251–5.
7. Chahinian AP, Pajak TF, Holland JF, Norton L, Ambinder RM, Mandel EM. Diffuse malignant mesothelioma. Prospective evaluation of 69 patients. Ann Intern Med. 1982;96(6 Pt 1):746–55.
8. Alberts AS, Falkson G, Goedhals L, Vorobiof DA, Van der Merwe CA. Malignant pleural mesothelioma: a disease unaffected by current therapeutic maneuvers. J Clin Oncol. 1988;6(3):527–35.
9. Boutin C, Rey F, Gouvernet J, Viallat JR, Astoul P, Ledoray V. Thoracoscopy in pleural malignant mesothelioma: a prospective study of 188 consecutive patients. Part 2: prognosis and staging. Cancer. 1993;72(2):394–404.
10. Hasegawa S, Tanaka F. Malignant mesothelioma: current status and perspective in Japan and the world. Gen Thorac Cardiovasc Surg. 2008;56(7):317–23.
11. Baas P. Predictive and prognostic factors in malignant pleural mesothelioma. Curr Opin Oncol. 2003;15(2):127–30.
12. Curran D, Sahmoud T, Therasse P, van Meerbeeck J, Postmus PE, Giaccone G. Prognostic factors in patients with pleural mesothelioma: the European Organization for Research and Treatment of Cancer experience. J Clin Oncol. 1998;16(1):145–52.
13. Ruffie P, Feld R, Minkin S, Cormier Y, Boutan-Laroze A, Ginsberg R, Ayoub J, Shepherd FA, Evans WK, Figueredo A, Et A. Diffuse malignant mesothelioma of the pleura in Ontario and Quebec: a retrospective study of 332 patients. J Clin Oncol. 1989;7(8):1157–68.
14. Mineo TC, Ambrogi V. Malignant pleural mesothelioma: factors influencing the prognosis. Oncology (Williston Park). 2012;26(12):1164–75.
15. Yang Y, Wu YB, Wang Z, Wang XJ, Xu LL, Tong ZH, Shi HZ. Long-term outcome of patients with nonspecific pleurisy at medical thoracoscopy. Respir Med. 2017;124:1–5.
16. Scherpereel A, Astoul P, Baas P, Berghmans T, Clayson H, de Vuyst P, Dienemann H, Galateau-Salle F, Hennequin C, Hillerdal G, Le Pechoux C, Mutti L, Pairon JC, Stahel R, van Houtte P, van Meerbeeck J, Waller D, Weder W. Guidelines of the European Respiratory Society and the European Society of Thoracic Surgeons for the management of malignant pleural mesothelioma. Eur Respir J. 2010;35(3):479–95.
17. Cihan YB, Ozturk A, Arslan A, Deniz K, Baran M, Karaca H. ERCC1 as a biological marker guiding management in malignant pleural mesothelioma. Asian Pac J Cancer Prev. 2014;15(10):4117–23.
18. Neumann V, Loseke S, Nowak D, Herth FJ, Tannapfel A. Malignant pleural mesothelioma: incidence, etiology, diagnosis, treatment, and occupational health. Dtsch Arztebl Int. 2013;110(18):319–26.
19. Salahudeen HM, Hoey ET, Robertson RJ, Darby MJ. CT appearances of pleural tumours. Clin Radiol. 2009;64(9):918–30.
20. Tateishi U, Gladish GW, Kusumoto M, Hasegawa T, Yokoyama R, Tsuchiya R, Moriyama N. Cheste wall tumors: radiologic findings and pathologic correlation: part 2. Malignant tumors. Radiographics. 2003;23(6):1491–508.
21. Zhang W, Wu X, Wu L, Zhang W, Zhao X. Advances in the diagnosis, treatment and prognosis of malignant pleural mesothelioma. Ann Transl Med. 2015;3(13):182.
22. Greillier L, Cavailles A, Fraticelli A, Scherpereel A, Barlesi F, Tassi G, Thomas P, Astoul P. Accuracy of pleural biopsy using thoracoscopy for the diagnosis of histologic subtype in patients with malignant pleural mesothelioma. Cancer. 2007;110(10):2248–52.
23. Rodriguez PF. Diagnosis and treatment of malignant pleural mesothelioma. Arch Bronconeumol. 2015;51(4):177–84.
24. Herndon JE, Green MR, Chahinian AP, Corson JM, Suzuki Y, Vogelzang NJ. Factors predictive of survival among 337 patients with mesothelioma treated between 1984 and 1994 by the Cancer and leukemia group B. Chest. 1998;113(3):723–31.
25. Rusch VW. A proposed new international TNM staging system for malignant pleural mesothelioma from the international mesothelioma interest group. Lung Cancer. 1996;14(1):1–12.
26. Sugarbaker DJ, Flores RM, Jaklitsch MT, Richards WG, Strauss GM, Corson JM, DeCamp MM Jr, Swanson SJ, Bueno R, Lukanich JM, Baldini EH, Mentzer SJ. Resection margins, extrapleural nodal status, and cell type determine postoperative long-term survival in trimodality therapy of malignant pleural mesothelioma: results in 183 patients. J Thorac Cardiovasc Surg. 1999;117(1): 54–63. discussion 63-55
27. Nojiri S, Gemba K, Aoe K, Kato K, Yamaguchi T, Sato T, Kubota K, Kishimoto T. Survival and prognostic factors in malignant pleural mesothelioma: a retrospective study of 314 patients in the west part of Japan. Jpn J Clin Oncol. 2011;41(1):32–9.
28. Suzuki K, Kadota K, Sima CS, Sadelain M, Rusch VW, Travis WD, Adusumilli PS. Chronic inflammation in tumor stroma is an independent predictor of prolonged survival in epithelioid malignant pleural mesothelioma patients. Cancer Immunol Immunother. 2011;60(12):1721–8.
29. Richards WG, Godleski JJ, Yeap BY, Corson JM, Chirieac LR, Zellos L, Mujoomdar A, Jaklitsch MT, Bueno R, Sugarbaker DJ. Proposed adjustments to pathologic staging of epithelial malignant pleural mesothelioma based on analysis of 354 cases. Cancer. 2010;116(6):1510–7.
30. Flores RM, Routledge T, Seshan VE, Dycoco J, Zakowski M, Hirth Y, Rusch VW. The impact of lymph node station on survival in 348 patients with surgically resected malignant pleural mesothelioma: implications for revision of the American joint committee on Cancer staging system. J Thorac Cardiovasc Surg. 2008;136(3):605–10.
31. Ezzati M, Lopez AD. Estimates of global mortality attributable to smoking in 2000. Lancet. 2003;362(9387):847–52.
32. Hong S, Mok Y, Jeon C, Jee SH, Samet JM. Tuberculosis, smoking and risk for lung cancer incidence and mortality. Int J Cancer. 2016;139(11):2447–55.

25

Diagnostic and prognostic utility of mid-expiratory flow rate in older community-dwelling persons with respiratory symptoms, but without chronic obstructive pulmonary disease

Gülmisal Güder[1,2,3*], Susanne Brenner[2,3], Stefan Störk[2,3], Matthias Held[4], Berna DL Broekhuizen[1], Jan-Willem J Lammers[5], Arno W Hoes[1] and Frans H Rutten[1]

Abstract

Background: The maximal expiratory flow at 50 % of the forced vital capacity (MEF_{50}) is the flow where half of forced vital capacity (FVC) remains to be exhaled. A reduced MEF_{50} has been suggested as a surrogate marker of small airways disease. The diagnostic and prognostic utility of this easy to assess spirometric variable in persons with respiratory symptoms, but without COPD is unclear.

Methods: We used data from the UHFO-COPD cohort in which 405 community-dwelling persons aged 65 years or over, and a general practitioner's diagnosis of chronic obstructive pulmonary disease (COPD) underwent pulmonary function testing and echocardiography. In total 161 patients had no COPD according to the spirometric GOLD criteria. We considered MEF_{50} as reduced if < 60 % of predicted.

Results: Of the 161 patients without COPD (mean age 72 ± 5.7 years; 35 % male; follow-up 4.5 ± 1.1 years), 61 (37.9 %) had a reduced MEF_{50}. They were older, had more pack-years of smoking, more respiratory symptoms, and used more frequently inhaled medication than the remaining 100 subjects. A reduced MEF_{50} was nearly twice as often associated with newly detected heart failure (HF) at assessment (29.5 % vs. 15.6 %, $p = 0.045$). In age-and sex-adjusted Cox regression analysis, a reduced MEF_{50} was significantly associated with episodes of acute bronchitis (hazard ratio 2.54 95 % confidence interval (1.26; 5.13) $P = 0.009$), and in trend with pneumonia (2.14 (0.98; 4.69) $P = 0.06$) and hospitalizations for pulmonary reasons (2.28 (0.93; 5.62) $P = 0.07$).

Conclusions: In older community-dwelling persons with pulmonary symptoms but without COPD, a reduced MEF_{50} may help to uncover unrecognized HF, and identify those at a higher risk for episodes of acute bronchitis, pneumonia and hospitalizations for pulmonary reasons. Echocardiography and close follow-up should be considered in these patients.

* Correspondence: Gueder_G@ukw.de
[1]Julius Center for Health Sciences and Primary Care, University Medical Center Utrecht, Utrecht, The Netherlands
[2]Department of Internal Medicine I, Cardiology, University Hospital Würzburg, Oberdürrbacherstr. 6, D-97080 Würzburg, Germany
Full list of author information is available at the end of the article

Background

The maximal expiratory flow at 50 % of the forced vital capacity (MEF_{50}) is the flow where half of forced vital capacity (FVC) remains to be exhaled [1]. It corresponds to the forced expiratory flow at 50 % (FEF_{50}) and correlates highly with the maximum mid-expiratory flow (FEF25-75 %) [2]. As such, MEF_{50} indicates obstruction of small airways and may be used as a surrogate of early small airways disease defined by an abnormally low mid-expiratory flow in the presence of normal forced expiratory volume in 1 second (FEV_1), FVC, and FEV_1/FVC ratio [3].

The usefulness of forced expiratory flows to diagnose small airways disease is, however controversial, as intra-individual variability is high, even in healthy subjects [4, 5]. Especially in the presence of central obstructive ventilatory disorders such as COPD or asthma, forced expiratory flow parameters lack reproducibility and do not correlate well with other variables related to airway obstruction (as forced vital capacity, FVC and residual volume-total lung capacity index, (RV/TLC) [6, 7]. However, in absence of central obstructive disorders, e.g. in patients with symptoms suggestive of COPD but in whom COPD has been excluded spirometrically, a low maximal expiratory flow and small airways disease may strongly suggest an alternative diagnosis, e.g. primary bronchiolar disorders (bronchiolitis) or interstitial lung diseases with bronchiolar involvement [8]. Moreover, a low maximum expiratory flow might also direct differential diagnosis towards a non-pulmonary condition causing respiratory symptoms such as heart failure, either known or latent [9].

The aim of our analysis was to assess the prevalence and the potential prognostic value of a low post-dilatory $MEF_{50,}$ in older community-dwelling individuals with pulmonary symptoms of airways obstruction, but without COPD.

We assessed the relation of a low post-dilatory MEF_{50} with hitherto unknown heart failure, first episode of either acute bronchitis, pneumonia, hospitalizations for pulmonary reason, or all-cause mortality.

Methods

Study design and population

We made use of a data set derived from a prospective cohort study (UHFO-HF) investigating 405 patients aged ≥65 years with a clinical diagnosis of COPD in primary care. Population and study characteristics have been described in detail previously [10]. Patients clinically suspect of COPD but without spirometrically verified obstruction were recruited from 51 primary care practices and assessed in the outpatient clinic of the University Medical Center Utrecht, Netherlands. A standardized clinical examination, extensive pulmonary function testing (PFT), chest radiography, and echocardiography were performed in all participants [10]. Exclusion criteria comprised an already established diagnosis of heart failure, severe psychiatric disorder, immobility, and terminal illness with short life expectancy precluding study participation [10].

In 244 of 405 (60 %) patients from the original cohort COPD defined as a post-bronchodilator ratio of FEV1/FVC <0.7 according to the GOLD criteria could be spirometrically verified [11].

The present analysis refers to the remaining 161 patients with exclusion of a COPD diagnosis in spirometry. The study complied with the Declaration of Helsinki, and the Medical Ethics Committee of the University Medical Center Utrecht approved the study protocol. All participants gave their written informed consent.

Missing values

In four patients post-bronchodilator MEF_{50} values were missing. In these patients pre-bronchodilator measurements were used (two subjects with a $MEF_{50} < 60$ %, and two with a $MEF_{50} > 60$ % of predicted). Thus, the present study analyzes 161 patients without COPD.

Pulmonary function tests and definition of low MEF_{50}

Pre-and post-bronchodilator pulmonary function testing was performed with a fixed-volume bodyplethysmograph (Masterlab Jaeger, Würzburg, Germany). The post-bronchodilator test was assessed 30 minutes after inhalation of 40 µg of ipratropium bromide.

There are no published guidelines regarding normal values for MEF_{50}. We used 60 % of post-dilatory MEF_{50} predicted as cut-off in the presence of a post-dilatory FEV1/FVC ≥ 0.7 for defining low MEF_{50} [6]. Following the recommendations of the European Respiratory Society we used age, gender, and height for the calculation of the predicted values of all lung function parameters [12].

Blood test results

Laboratory results such as white blood cell count, haemoglobin, haematocrit, and serum aminoterminal pro-hormone B-type natriuretic peptide (NT-proBNP) were measured as part of the study assessment.

Echocardiography and definition of heart failure

Echocardiography was performed by two experienced cardiac sonographers using a Philips Sonos 5500 imaging system (Andover, MA, USA) and interpreted by a single cardiologist, who was blinded to clinical data [10]. Left ventricular ejection fraction (LVEF) was derived using Simpson's biplane or, when not possible, by single plane area–length method [13].

Left atrial volume was calculated by the biplane area–length method from apical four-and two-chamber views and indexed to the body surface area [14]. Mitral inflow and pulmonary venous inflow were measured with pulsed-wave Doppler echocardiography. Tissue Doppler was used to assess the sub-mitral movement of the septal wall, and a composite of abnormalities in diastolic function was employed to define diastolic dysfunction [15].

Presence or absence of heart failure was established by an expert panel consisting of two cardiologists, a pulmonologist, and a general practitioner using all available diagnostic information, including echocardiography and pulmonary function tests [10]. Heart failure was classified by the panel in line with the recommendations of the ESC guidelines on heart failure. The definition required presence of signs and symptoms suggestive of heart failure and additional criteria that led to the following subtypes: a) "heart failure with a reduced ejection fraction" when LVEF was reduced (arbitrarily defined as ≤45 %); b) "heart failure with preserved ejection fraction" when echocardiographically determined diastolic dysfunction was present and LVEF >45 %; of note, symptoms and/or signs should not, or insufficiently, be explained by co-incident pulmonary disease; and c) "right-sided heart failure" (cor pulmonale) when LVEF was >45 %, and the calculated pulmonary artery pressure >40 mmHg [10].

Follow-up and outcomes ascertainment

Patients included in the study were followed from April 2001 to June 2007 during a mean period of 4.3 (standard deviation 1.1) years. The follow-up data collection mode was described before [16]. In brief, the general practitioner's (GP) electronic medical files were scrutinized to obtain information on patient's drug prescription, pulmonary hospitalizations and survival status. Acute bronchitis was defined as an episode with bronchial wheezing and rhonchi for which the GP prescribed antibiotics and/or pulse prednisolon for 7 to 10 days.

Most episodes of pneumonia were diagnosed clinically by the GP and only occasionally confirmed by chest X-ray or sputum culture.

Data analysis

Continuous data were expressed as mean (standard deviation, SD) or median (quartiles). Group comparisons between patients with and without a $MEF_{50} < 60$ % of predicted were performed using Fisher's exact test or Mann–Whitney *U*-test, as appropriate (Tables 1 and 2). Correlations between MEF_{50} with other pulmonary function parameters were calculated with the Spearman rank order correlation coefficient (r). The strength of the correlation was graded using the following guide for the absolute value of r: 0.00-0.19 very weak; 0.20-0.39 weak; 0.40-0.59 moderate; 0.60-0.79 strong; 0.80-1.0 very strong.

Univariate, and age and sex adjusted multivariable Cox regression models were calculated for different outcomes (acute bronchitis, pulmonary hospitalizations, pneumonia, and all-cause mortality) and reported as hazard ratios (HR) with 95 % confidence intervals (CI). P values <0.05 were considered statistically significant. Data analysis was performed with SPSS 21 (IBM, Munich, Germany).

Results

Demographics of the patients with COPD according to the GOLD criteria

Patients excluded from our analysis (244 individuals with a GOLD diagnosis of COPD) were more often male (68 vs. 35 %, $P < 0.001$), and slightly older (73 [70; 77]) vs. 72 [67; 76] years $P = 0.016$) than the 161 patients included. All but one of the 243 patients with GOLD-COPD and available information on MEF had a post-dilatory $MEF_{50} < 60$ % of predicted confirming that a MEF_{50} below the chosen threshold is common in COPD.

Demographics of the patients without COPD according to the GOLD criteria

Table 1 lists the baseline characteristics of the 161 individuals under study, stratified by MEF_{50} </≥ 60 % of predicted. Patients with a low MEF_{50} (38 %) were older, had more pack-years of smoking, suffered more often from respiratory complaints, used more often inhaled medication (especially anticholinergics), and had higher leucocyte counts than subjects with a $MEF_{50} \geq 60$ %. Twenty-two of the 63 patients (35 %) with a low $MEF_{50} < 60$ % of predicted had a FEV1 and/or FVC % of predicted below 80 %. The remaining 41 participants (65 %) had normal values of FEV1 and FVC % of predicted.

Correlation between MEF_{50} and other pulmonary function test results

Patients with a low MEF_{50} had a normal total lung capacity (TLC), while the carbon monoxide (CO) diffusion capacity was lower than in those with a $MEF_{50} \geq 60$ % of predicted. Patients with a low MEF_{50} also had higher levels of total resistance, higher residual volume (RV) and larger RV/TLC ratio than subjects with a 'normal' MEF_{50} (Table 2). Reversibility of airway obstruction, defined as an increase of FEV1 levels > 200 ml and >12 % to baseline, did not differ between </≥ MEF_{50} 60 % of predicted.

Table 3 presents Spearman rank-order correlation coefficients for the association between MEF_{50} and other continuous pulmonary function test parameters. MEF_{50} correlated moderately to strongly with all pulmonary

Table 1 Characteristics of 161 patients with a GP's diagnosis of COPD, but with a post-dilatorory FEV1/FVC ratio > 0.7, divided in those with MEF_{50} < vs ≥ 60 % of predicted

	All, N = 161	MEF_{50} < 60 % of predicted, N = 63	MEF_{50} ≥ 60 % of predicted, N = 98	*p*-value
Demographics				
Male sex, %	34.8	30.2	37.6	0.40
Age, years	72 (67; 76)	73 (69; 79)	71 (66; 74)	0.002
Pack years smoking, years	2.3 (0; 28)	10 (0; 38)	0.6 (0; 20)	0.026
Body mass index, kg/m^2	27.0 (24.7; 30.0)	26.9 (24.7; 30.7)	27.1 (24.7; 29.7)	0.87
LVEF in %	60 (58; 60)	60 (56; 62)	60 (59; 60)	0.88
Systolic blood pressure, mmHg	154 (142; 164)	154 (144; 164)	153 (142; 165)	0.60
Comorbidities				
Hypertension; %	53.4	46.0	46.9	1.0
Atrial fibrillation, %	5.0	3.2	6.1	0.48
Diabetes, %	9.9	6.3	12.2	0.29
A history of asthma, %	12.4	14.3	11.2	0.63
Heart failure, %	20.5	28.6	15.3	0.048
Obesity	24.8	28.6	22.4	0.45
Symptoms				
Dyspnoea uphill, %	93.2	95.2	91.8	0.53
Dyspnoea while walking on level ground, %	43.5	58.7	33.7	0.002
Coughing >3 months, %	27.3	36.5	21.4	0.046
Wheezing, %	59	71.4	51.0	0.014
Phlegm production, %	42.9	49.2	38.8	0.20
Laboratory findings				
Hemoglobin, mmol/l	8.9 (8.3; 9.4)	8.9 (8.3; 9.2)	9.0 (8.4; 9.6)	0.24
Leucocytes /nl	7.3 (6.1; 8.7)	7.6 (6.8; 9.5)	7.0 (5.9; 8.2)	0.004
C-reactive protein, mg/l	3 (3; 6)	3.0 (3.0; 7.0)	3.0 (3.0; 5.8)	0.24
NT-proBNP, mg/dl	14.3 (8.1; 25.5)	16.8 (10.1; 29.3)	13.9 (7.0; 24.9)	0.078
Pharmacotherapy				
Diuretics	23.6	28.6	20.4	0.2
ACEi or ARB, %	23.6	25.4	22.4	0.71
Beta-blocker, %	13.7	11.1	15.3	0.49
Aspirin, %	23.0	27.0	20.4	0.34
Inhaled beta-2agonist, %	41.6	49.2	36.7	0.14
Inhaled anticholinergic, %	36	47.6	28.6	0.018
Inhaled corticosteroid, %	58.4	61.9	56.1	0.30
Chronic oral corticosteroid, %	1.9	4.8	0	0.058

Values are shown as median (quartiles) or percentages
Abbreviations: ACEi, angiotensin converting enzyme inhibitor; ARB, angiotensin II type 1 receptor blocker; obesity was defined as a body mass index ≥ 30 kg/m^2

function test results, except for TLC (no correlation) and RV (very weak correlation).

Association of low expiratory flow with newly detected heart failure

In total, N = 33 patients (20.5 %) were newly diagnosed with heart failure; N = 16 with heart failure with reduced ejection fraction, N = 17 with heart failure with preserved ejection fraction, and N = 0 isolated right-sided heart failure. A MEF_{50} < 60 % was associated with a new diagnosis of heart failure at the assessment: The incidence of newly diagnosed heart failure was 29.5 % in those with MEF_{50} < 60 % compared to 15.6 % in persons with a MEF_{50} ≥ 60 % of predicted (P = 0.045, Table 1).

Patients with a novel diagnosis of heart failure also had lower post-dilator $MEF_{75\,\%}$ of predicted (84 % [64; 103 %] vs. 97 % [86; 119 %], P = 0.03) than the 128 patients without heart failure, whereas peak expiratory flow and post-dilator

Table 2 Pulmonary function test results in patients with a MEF_{50} < vs ≥ 60 % of predicted

	All, N = 161	MEF_{50} < 60 % of predicted, N = 63	MEF_{50} ≥ 60 % of predicted, N = 98	*P* value
Post-dilator FEV1/FVC, %	76 (74; 81)	74 (71; 76)	80 (76; 85)	<0.001
FEV1, % of predicted	103 (89; 115)	85 (75; 102)	110 (101; 121)	<0.001
FVC, % of predicted	105 (91; 120)	93 (80; 112)	112 (100; 125)	<0.001
Post-dilator increase of FEV1 > 200 ml, %	13.7	17.5	11.2	0.35
Post-dilator increase of FEV1 > 200 ml and >12 %, %	11.8	14.3	10.2	0.46
Rtot, % of predicted	124 (86; 178)	165 (121; 213)	110 (76; 143)	<0.001
TLC, % of predicted	105 (97; 114)	103 (93; 112)	107 (97; 116)	0.18
TLC < 80 % of predicted, %	3.1	3.1	3.3	0.99
RV, % of predicted	108 (96; 126)	112 (100; 141)	107 (93; 120)	0.025
RV/TLC, %	102 (93; 115)	114 (101; 132)	98 (90; 106)	<0.001
DLCO, % of predicted	78 (67; 89)	70 (59; 80)	83 (75; 93)	<0.001
MEF_{25}, % of predicted	54 (38; 76)	38 (30; 46)	68 (54; 93)	<0.001
MEF_{50}, % of predicted	68 (49; 86)	47 (39; 55)	79 (70; 98)	<0.001
MEF_{75}, % of predicted	94 (74; 111)	75 (58; 91)	104 (91; 122)	<0.001
PEF, % of predicted	104 (88; 121)	98 (73; 108)	111 (96; 129)	<0.001

Data are shown as median (quartiles) or percentages. All pulmonary function test variables refer to post-dilatory values and are presented as percentage of predicted or as percentages

Abbreviations: FEV1, forced expiratory volume in 1 second; FVC, forced vital capacity; RV, residual volume; Rtot, total resistance; TLC, total lung capacity; DLCO, diffusion capacity of carbon monoxide; MEF maximum expiratory flow 25/50/75 % of the FVC remain to be exhaled; PEF peak expiratory flow

$MEF_{25\ \%}$ were not different between these two groups. Patients with heart failure had more often FEV1 values below 80 % of predicted than subjects without heart failure (27 % vs. 12 %, P = 0.05). The corresponding FVC values were also numerically but not statistically different (FVC below 80 % of predicted 21 vs. 11 %, P = 0.15).

Association of low MEF_{50} with prognosis

During follow-up, 34 patients experienced acute bronchitis and 27 patients a pneumonia, 21 patients were hospitalized for a pulmonary reason (pneumonia, bronchitis, acute exacerbation of newly diagnosed COPD), and 17 patients died (Table 4). In age-and sex-adjusted Cox regression analysis, a low MEF_{50} was significantly associated with acute bronchitis (2.54 (1.26; 5.13) P = 0.009) but not with pneumonia (2.14 (0.98; 4.69) P = 0.06), hospitalizations (2.28 (0.93; 5.62) P = 0.07, Table 5) or death (1.84 (0.68; 4.99) P = 0.23). If patients with heart failure (n = 33) were excluded from the analysis the associations became significant for all outcome measures except total mortality (Table 5).

Discussion

In this retrospective analysis of 161 older community-dwelling individuals with a clinical diagnosis of COPD but without spirometrically verified airways obstruction, we found that low maximum mid-expiratory flow (i.e., MEF_{50} < 60 % of predicted) was prevalent in 38 %. These patients had increased pulmonary resistance and residual volumes, and a higher RV/TLC index than subjects with a MEF_{50} ≥ 60 %. Further, a low MEF_{50} was associated with incident heart failure and predicted a higher risk for acute bronchitis during follow-up.

Small airways disease is frequently found in patients with airways obstruction as asthma or COPD [6]. In the present study we did not see differences in the prevalence of low MEF_{50} in patients with and without a history of asthma. However, since our patients were selected according to a GP's diagnosis of COPD, the prevalence of patients with a history of asthma was low (12 % in the total cohort). Reduced MEF is a characteristic feature of COPD [4]: in the original cohort of patients with verified COPD (244/405, data not shown) according to the GOLD

Table 3 Correlation between MEF_{50} and other pulmonary function parameters

	FEV1/ FVC	FEV1	FVC	Rtot	TLC	RV	RV/TLC	DLCO	MEF25 %	MEF75 %	PEF
r	0.62**	0.64**	0.46**	-0.63**	0.13	−0.18*	−0.58**	0.50**	0.84**	0.76**	0.59**

Spearman's correlation coefficients (r) between continuous values of MEF_{50} and other pulmonary function parameters (as % of predicted) with the Spearman's rank correlation test

* refers to p < 0.05 and **to p < 0.001

Table 4 Number of pulmonary events and all-cause deaths during a mean follow up of 4.5 years in patients with and without $MEF_{50} < 60$ % of predicted

	All (N = 161)	$MEF_{50} < 60$ % N = 63	$MEF_{50} \geq 60$ % N = 98	*P* value
Episodes of acute bronchitis, N (%)	34 (21.1 %)	20 (31.7 %)	14 (14.3 %)	0.01
Pneumonia, N (%)	27 (16.8 %)	15 (23.8 %)	12 (12.2 %)	0.08
Hospitalization for pulmonary reason, N (%)	21 (13.0 %)	12 (19.2 %)	9 (9.2 %)	0.09
All-cause death, N (%)	17 (10.6 %)	10 (15.9 %)	7 (7.1 %)	0.11

Absolute numbers of clinically relevant outcome measures during follow-up. *P* value refers to Fishers exact test

criteria, a $MEF_{50} < 60$ % of predicted was detected in 242 out of 243 persons (data not shown). In the remaining patient, MEF values were not available. The prognostic capacity of low MEF is thus not meaningful in patients with established airways obstruction.

Lower MEF values may also be found in the absence of airways obstruction, in primary bronchiolar disorders or interstitial lung disease, but also in systemic inflammatory diseases such as rheumatoid arthritis [8]. A low MEF is easily detectable with spirometry and relates to inflammation of the small non-cartilaginous bronchioles with an internal diameter of <2 mm and may well be an indicator of small airways disease or be considered as a precursor stage of COPD [6, 17, 18]. However, to determine the underlying pathophysiological substrate, histological investigation of lung biopsies or high resolution computer tomography scans would be needed, procedures that are not part of the routine assessment in clinical practice and thus were not available for this study [8, 19].

Expiratory flow volumes have previously been proposed as a tool for diagnosing extra-pulmonary restrictive disease [9]. Heart failure is such a condition as increased heart size and pulmonary congestion may simply reduce lung volumes [20]. In addition, pulmonary fluid overload in heart failure may cause or aggravate external bronchial obstruction with subsequent compromise of FEV1 [20, 21]. Thus, clinically and spirometrically, heart failure frequently mimics COPD. Indeed, in congestive heart failure, it has been repeatedly be shown that FEV1 values may be more reduced than corresponding FVC values, yielding FEV1/FVC ratios <0.70 in the absence of COPD [22, 23]. Importantly, this finding (i.e., pseudo-COPD) is not reproducible when the same individuals are re-assessed after recompensation under euvolemic conditions, calling for a more conscious use of spirometry in these cases [21, 24, 25]. Additionally, expiratory flow measurements may be more susceptible to heart failure than FEV1 or FEV1/FVC: in 29.5 % of the cases with a $MEF_{50} < 60$ % of predicted, previously unrecognized heart failure was detected. This is more than three times as high as might be expected in the general population aged > 65 years (estimated prevalence of heart failure in this age group 7-10 %) [26] and also higher than the percentage of newly detected cases of heart failure in the 244 patients with a GOLD-COPD diagnosis (prevalence 21 %) from the original cohort [10, 27]. Further 18 out of 33 patients (55 %) with previously unrecognized heart failure had a $MEF_{50} < 60$ % predicted, whereas only 9 (27 %) had a reduced FEV1 < 80 % predicted.

Although our study convincingly related a reduced MEF_{50} to clinically relevant outcomes, we acknowledge that the causality of these associations is not stringent. Some studies found that MEF_{50} was below average in subgroups of healthy never smokers [4, 5], or asymptomatic subjects [28]. Further, higher body mass index levels may attenuate MEF [29], but we observed no relation between body mass index levels and low MEF_{50} (Table 1).

Study limitations

The extensive pulmonary function testing with spirometry, bodyplethysmography, and CO diffusion measurements was performed only once at baseline, thus, time-dependent effects could not be addressed. Because histological investigations or chest CT scans

Table 5 Prognostic utility of $MEF_{50} < 60$ % of predicted in patients without COPD

	Acute bronchitis	Pneumonia	Hospitalization for pulmonary reasons	Death
Model 1	2.53 (1.28; 5.02) P = 0.008	2.11 (0.99; 4.51) P = 0.054	2.24 (0.94; 5.31) P = 0.07	2.17 (0.83; 5.71) P = 0.11
Model 2	2.54 (1.26; 5.13) P = 0.009	2.14 (0.98; 4.69) P = 0.06	2.28 (0.93; 5.62) P = 0.07	1.84 (0.68; 4.99) P = 0.23
Model 3	3.04 (1.36; 6.79) P = 0.007	2.66 (1.10; 6.40) P = 0.03	3.86 (1.25; 11.9) P = 0.019	1.97 (0.52; 7.36) P = 0.32

Hazard ratios with 95 % confidence intervals from Cox proportional hazard regression are presented. Median follow-up was 4.6 years. $MEF_{50} < 60$ % of predicted coded as "1"

Model 1: Unadjusted

Model 2: Adjusted for age and sex

Model 3: Adjusted for age and sex in the subgroup of 128 patients without heart failure

were not available in the GP setting of the current study, we were unable to assess small airways disease on a more pathophysiological basis. Further restrictive disorders might also account for MEF reduction. Patients with pulmonary restriction were not excluded in this study however, the prevalence in total cohort was low (3.1 %, N = 5) and there was no between group difference between patients with and without a MEF50 < 60 %.

Conclusions

In older community-dwelling patients with pulmonary symptoms but without central airway obstruction a low maximum MEF, easily obtained by spirometry, showed clinical utility to identify patients with previously undiagnosed heart failure and patients at risk for pulmonary events. Thus, MEF_{50} values should also be evaluated when obtaining spirometry in persons aged >65 years with shortness of breath.

Abbreviations

CI: Confidence intervals; COPD: Chronic Obstructive Pulmonary Disease; DLCO: Diffusion capacity of carbon monoxide; FEV1: Forced expiratory volume in 1 second; FVC: Forced vital capacity; GOLD: Global Initiative for Chronic Obstructive Lung Disease; GP: General practitioner; HF: Heart failure; HR: Hazard ratios; LVEF: Left ventricular ejection fraction; MEF_{50}: Maximal expiratory flow at 50 % of the forced vital capacity ; NT-proBNP: N-terminal pro-hormone B-type natriuretic peptide; PEF: Peak expiratory flow; PFT: Pulmonary function testing; RV: Residual volume; Rtot: Total resistance; SD: Standard deviation; TLC: Total lung capacity.

Competing interests

The authors declare that they have no competing interests.

Authors' contributions

GG analysed and interpreted the data and wrote the manuscript. SB, MH, BB and JL contributed significant intellectual content to the manuscript. AH helped to set up and design the study, and was instrumental in grant application, and contributed significant intellectual content to the manuscript. SS supervised data analysis and contributed significant intellectual content to the manuscript. FR designed the study, recruited patients, interpreted the data and wrote the manuscript. All authors read and approved the final manuscript.

Funding

We thank the participating patients, GP, and their assistants, including the general practices connected to the General Practice Network Utrecht (HNU). The original study was supported by a grant (number 904-61-144) from the Netherlands Organization for Scientific Research.
Analysis of this work was further supported by grants from the German Ministry of Education and Research (BMBF), Berlin, Germany [BMBF 01GL0304–Competence Network Heart Failure Germany; BMBF 01GI0205; BMBF 01EO1004–Comprehensive Heart Failure Center Würzburg]. GG was supported by a fellowship grant from the Medical Faculty of the University of Würzburg (Habilitationsstipendium). This publication was funded by the German Research Foundation (DFG) and the University of Würzburg in the funding programme Open Access Publishing.

Author details

[1]Julius Center for Health Sciences and Primary Care, University Medical Center Utrecht, Utrecht, The Netherlands. [2]Department of Internal Medicine I, Cardiology, University Hospital Würzburg, Oberdürrbacherstr. 6, D-97080 Würzburg, Germany. [3]Comprehensive Heart Failure Center, University of Würzburg, Würzburg, Germany. [4]Medical Mission Hospital, Department of Internal Medicine, Respiratory Medicine and Cardiology, Würzburg, Germany. [5]Department of Respiratory Medicine, University Medical Center Utrecht, Utrecht, The Netherlands.

References

1. Miller MR, Hankinson J, Brusasco V, Burgos F, Casaburi R, Coates A, et al. Standardisation of spirometry. Eur Respir J. 2005;26:319–38.
2. Bar-Yishay E, Amirav I, Goldberg S. Comparison of maximal midexpiratory flow rate and forced expiratory flow at 50 x% of vital capacity in children. Chest. 2003;123:731–5.
3. McFadden Jr ER, Linden DA. A reduction in maximum mid-expiratory flow rate. A spirographic manifestation of small airway disease. Am J Med. 1972;52:725–37.
4. Pellegrino R, Viegi G, Brusasco V, Crapo RO, Burgos F, Casaburi R, et al. Interpretative strategies for lung function tests. Eur Respir J. 2005;26:948–68.
5. Quanjer PH, Stanojevic S, Cole TJ, Baur X, Hall GL, Culver BH, et al. Multi-ethnic reference values for spirometry for the 3-95-yr age range: the global lung function 2012 equations. Eur Respir J. 2012;40:1324–43.
6. Burgel PR. The role of small airways in obstructive airway diseases. Eur Respir Rev. 2011;20:23–33.
7. Sorkness RL, Bleecker ER, Busse WW, Calhoun WJ, Castro M, Chung KF, et al. Lung function in adults with stable but severe asthma: air trapping and incomplete reversal of obstruction with bronchodilation. J Appl Physiol (1985). 2008;104:394–403.
8. Burgel PR, Bergeron A, De Blic J, Bonniaud P, Bourdin A, Chanez P, et al. Small airways diseases, excluding asthma and COPD: an overview. Eur Respir Rev. 2013;22:131–47.
9. Zanen P, Folgering H, Lammers JW. Flow-volumes indices as means to discriminate between intra-and extrapulmonary restrictive disease. Respir Med. 2005;99:825–9.
10. Rutten FH, Cramer MJ, Grobbee DE, Sachs AP, Kirkels JH, Lammers JW, et al. Unrecognized heart failure in elderly patients with stable chronic obstructive pulmonary disease. Eur Heart J. 2005;26:1887–94.
11. Vestbo J, Hurd SS, Agusti AG, Jones PW, Vogelmeier C, Anzueto A, et al. Global strategy for the diagnosis, management, and prevention of chronic obstructive pulmonary disease: GOLD executive summary. Am J Respir Crit Care Med. 2013;187:347–65.
12. Quanjer PH, Tammeling GJ, Cotes JE, Pedersen OF, Peslin R, Yernault JC. Lung volumes and forced ventilatory flows. Report Working Party Standardization of Lung Function Tests, European Community for Steel and Coal. Official Statement of the European Respiratory Society. Eur Respir J Suppl. 1993;16:5–40.
13. Schiller NB, Shah PM, Crawford M, DeMaria A, Devereux R, Feigenbaum H, et al. Recommendations for quantitation of the left ventricle by two-dimensional echocardiography. American Society of Echocardiography Committee on Standards, Subcommittee on Quantitation of Two-Dimensional Echocardiograms. J Am Soc Echocardiogr. 1989;2:358–67.
14. Tsang TS, Barnes ME, Gersh BJ, Bailey KR, Seward JB. Left atrial volume as a morphophysiologic expression of left ventricular diastolic dysfunction and relation to cardiovascular risk burden. Am J Cardiol. 2002;90:1284–9.
15. Garcia MJ, Thomas JD, Klein AL. New Doppler echocardiographic applications for the study of diastolic function. J Am Coll Cardiol. 1998;32:865–75.
16. Boudestein LC, Rutten FH, Cramer MJ, Lammers JW, Hoes AW. The impact of concurrent heart failure on prognosis in patients with chronic obstructive pulmonary disease. Eur J Heart Fail. 2009;11:1182–8.
17. Shaw RJ, Djukanovic R, Tashkin DP, Millar AB, Du Bois RM, Orr PA. The role of small airways in lung disease. Respir Med. 2002;96:67–80.
18. Mirsadraee M, Boskabady MH, Attaran D. Diagnosis of chronic obstructive pulmonary disease earlier than current Global Initiative for Obstructive Lung Disease guidelines using a feasible spirometry parameter (maximal-mid expiratory flow/forced vital capacity). Chron Respir Dis. 2013;10:191–6.

19. Hansell DM. Small airways diseases: detection and insights with computed tomography. Eur Respir J. 2001;17:1294–313.
20. Guder G, Brenner S, Stork S, Hoes A, Rutten FH. Chronic obstructive pulmonary disease in heart failure: accurate diagnosis and treatment. Eur J Heart Fail. 2014;16:1273–82.
21. Brenner S, Guder G, Berliner D, Deubner N, Frohlich K, Ertl G, et al. Airway obstruction in systolic heart failure–COPD or congestion? Int J Cardiol. 2013;168:1910–6.
22. Puri S, Dutka DP, Baker BL, Hughes JM, Cleland JG. Acute saline infusion reduces alveolar-capillary membrane conductance and increases airflow obstruction in patients with left ventricular dysfunction. Circulation. 1999;99:1190–6.
23. Guder G, Rutten FH. Comorbidity of heart failure and chronic obstructive pulmonary disease: more than coincidence. Curr Heart Fail Rep. 2014;11:337–46.
24. Guder G, Rutten FH, Brenner S, Angermann CE, Berliner D, Ertl G, et al. The impact of heart failure on the classification of COPD severity. J Card Fail. 2012;18:637–44.
25. Hawkins NM, Petrie MC, Jhund PS, Chalmers GW, Dunn FG, McMurray JJ. Heart failure and chronic obstructive pulmonary disease: diagnostic pitfalls and epidemiology. Eur J Heart Fail. 2009;11:130–9.
26. Tiller D, Russ M, Greiser KH, Nuding S, Ebelt H, Kluttig A, et al. Prevalence of Symptomatic Heart Failure with Reduced and with Normal Ejection Fraction in an Elderly General Population-The CARLA Study. PLoS One. 2013;8, e59225.
27. Hogg K, Swedberg K, McMurray J. Heart failure with preserved left ventricular systolic function; epidemiology, clinical characteristics, and prognosis. J Am Coll Cardiol. 2004;43:317–27.
28. Held M, Mittnacht M, Karl S, Kolb M, Jany B. Pulmonary and Cardiac Function in asymptomatic Obese Subjects and Changes following a Structured weight reduction Program: a Prospective Observational Study. PLoS One. 2014;9(9):e107480.
29. Lazarus R, Sparrow D, Weiss ST. Effects of obesity and fat distribution on ventilatory function: the normative aging study. Chest. 1997;111:891–8.

26

Tomographic findings of acute pulmonary toxoplasmosis in immunocompetent patients

Karina de Souza Giassi[1,2*], Andre Nathan Costa[3,4], Andre Apanavicius[3], Fernando Bin Teixeira[3], Caio Julio Cesar Fernandes[3,4], Alfredo Salim Helito[5] and Ronaldo Adib Kairalla[3,4]

Abstract

Background: Toxoplasmosis is one of the most common human zoonosis, and is generally benign in most of the individuals. Pulmonary involvement is common in immunocompromised subjects, but very rare in immunocompetents and there are scarce reports of tomographic findings in the literature. The aim of the study is to describe three immunocompetent patients diagnosed with acute pulmonary toxoplasmosis and their respective thoracic tomographic findings. Acute toxoplasmosis was diagnosed according to the results of serological tests suggestive of recent primary infection and the absence of an alternative etiology.

Case presentation: From 2009 to 2013, three patients were diagnosed with acute respiratory failure secondary to acute toxoplasmosis. The patients were two female and one male, and were 38, 56 and 36 years old. Similarly they presented a two-week febrile illness and progressive dyspnea before admission. Laboratory tests demonstrated lymphocytosis, slight changes in liver enzymes and high inflammatory markers. Tomographic findings were bilateral smooth septal and peribronchovascular thickening (100%), ground-glass opacities (100%), atelectasis (33%), random nodules (33%), lymph node enlargement (33%) and pleural effusion (66%). All the patients improved their symptoms after treatment, and complete resolution of tomographic findings were found in the followup.

Conclusion: These cases provide a unique description of the presentation and evolution of pulmonary tomographic manifestations of toxoplasmosis in immunocompetent patients. *Toxoplasma* pneumonia manifests with fever, dyspnea and a non-productive cough that may result in respiratory failure. In animal models, changes were described as interstitial pneumonitis with focal infiltrates of neutrophils that can finally evolve into a pattern of diffuse alveolar damage with focal necrosis. The tomographic findings are characterized as ground glass opacities, smooth septal and marked peribronchovascular thickening; and may mimic pulmonary congestion, lymphangitis, atypical pneumonia and pneumocystosis. This is the largest series of CT findings of acute toxoplasmosis in immunocompetent hosts, and the diagnosis should be considered as patients that present with acute respiratory failure in the context of a subacute febrile illness with bilateral and diffuse interstitial infiltrates with marked peribronchovascular thickening. If promptly treated, pulmonary toxoplasmosis can result in complete clinical and radiological recovery in immunocompetent hosts.

Keywords: Pulmonary toxoplasmosis, Chest, Toxoplasmosis

* Correspondence: ksgiassi@gmail.com
[1]Radiology Division, Hospital Sírio-Libanês, R. Dona Adma Jafet, 91, Bela Vista, SP 01308-050, Brazil
[2]Radiology Institute (InRad), University of São Paulo Medical School (FMUSP), Av. Dr. Enéas de Carvalho Aguiar, 44, Consolação, SP 05403-900, Brazil
Full list of author information is available at the end of the article

Background

Toxoplasma gondii is one of the most common human zoonosis, infecting approximately one-third of the world's population [1]. Although rare in Europe and in the USA, the seroprevalence for this obligate intracellular protozoan can reach 79% in males and 63% in females in Brazil [2]. Toxoplasmosis is generally benign and often goes unnoticed in healthy hosts; however, non-specific "flu-like" symptoms, hepatomegaly and diffuse lymphadenopathy may be associated with primary infection [2].

In adults, infection can result from the ingestion of undercooked or raw meat containing tissue cysts or from the consumption of water or food contaminated by oocysts that are excreted in the feces of infected cats [3,4]. Rarely, the parasite is also transmitted by blood transfusion or organ transplantation [5,6].

Pulmonary involvement in acute toxoplasmosis has been described in immunosuppressed patients [4-6], but is rare in immunocompetent subjects [7,8] Herein, we describe chest computed tomography (CT) findings in three immunocompetent patients with confirmed acute *T. gondii* infection and review the current literature.

Case presentation

From 2009 to 2013, three patients were diagnosed with acute respiratory failure secondary to acute toxoplasmosis with extensive lung involvement. Two of the patients were female, and one was male; the patients were 38, 56 and 36 years old, respectively. All three patients similarly presented to the emergency department with a two-week febrile illness and progressive dyspnea during the few days before admission without previous respiratory symptoms. The physical examinations revealed crackles in all patients and low oxygen saturation (SpO_2) values, ranging from 82% to 86%. One patient had splenomegaly. Regarding their medical history, two of the patients had Type 2 diabetes, one of whom had undergone bariatric surgery the year prior. The third patient was previously healthy. Laboratory test results were normal with the exception of lymphocytosis with atypical lymphocytes (in two patients), slight changes in liver enzymes and high inflammatory markers. The clinical and laboratory findings are summarized in Table 1. One patient was transferred from another hospital, where she was submitted to a lung biopsy and pleural drainage; unfortunately, we did not have access to these results.

The diagnosis of toxoplasmosis was made from serology (positive for IgM antibodies and low IgG avidity). In our institutions, real-time polymerase chain reaction-based assay to detect DNA of *T.gondii* is not available; therefore, serologic (IgM, IgG and IgG avidity) testing is our routine diagnosis method. All patients were investigated for immunodeficiency disorders (primary immunodeficiencies, hematological and non-hematological malignancies, and immunoglobulinopathies) and the use of immunosuppressive drugs. Regarding infectious differential diagnosis, all three patients had negative blood and urine cultures. Serology was performed for HIV, viral hepatitis (A, B and C), Epstein-Barr and cytomegalovirus in each one of the pacients and the results were negative. The lung biopsy culture, when performed, was negative for all microorganisms. Serology for *Mycoplasma pneumoniae* and *Chlamydia pneumonia* was performed in one of the patients; however, result was negative.

All patients underwent a chest CT scan, and the following CT abnormalities were found: bilateral smooth septal and peribronchovascular thickening (100%), ground-glass opacities (100%) (Figures 1 and 2), atelectasis (33%) and random nodules varying in size from 5 m to 2.5 cm (33%). Mediastinal findings were present in one patient and were characterized as paratracheal lymph node enlargement. Bilateral pleural effusions were noted in 2 patients (66%). The radiological findings are summarized in Table 2. Follow-up CT scans were obtained from one of the patients after complete resolution of the symptoms and demonstrated complete resolution of the findings (Figure 3A and B), and none of the patients presented respiratory or extra-pulmonary relapses.

Written informed consent was obtained from each of the patients regarding clinical and radiological data.

These three cases provide a remarkable description of the presentation and evolution of pulmonary tomographic manifestations of toxoplasmosis in immunocompetent patients.

Table 1 Clinical and laboratory findings of patients with acute pulmonary toxoplasmosis

Patient	Age	Year of diagnosis	Gender	Medical history	Symptoms	Leukocytes (cells/mm3)	Lymphocytes (cells/mm3)	CRP*	AST** UI/mL	ALT*** UI/mL
1	36	2013	Male	Type 2 diabetes and bariatric surgery	Fever, headache and dyspnea	13200	7500 (70 atypical)	35	217	314
2	56	2011	Female	Type 2 diabetes	Fever and progressive dyspnea	9.800	4.000	12	108	169
3	38	2009	Female	-	Fever, cough and dyspnea	11.350	6.700 (1.230 atypical)	26	190	229

*C-reactive protein. **Aspartate aminotransferase. ***Alanine aminotransferase.

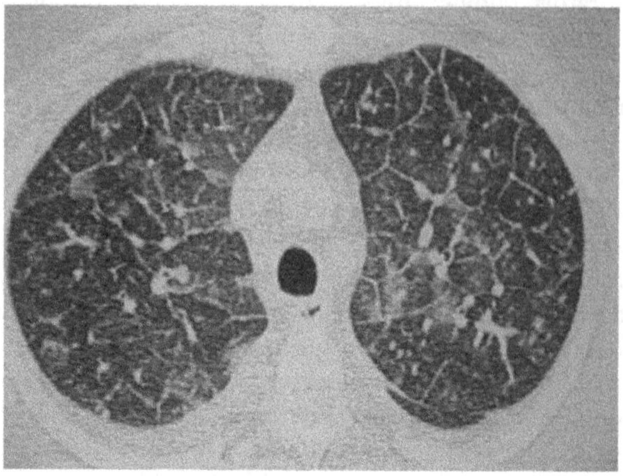

Figure 1 A 55 year-old female with pulmonary toxoplasmosis. Axial view of CT scan displays bilateral ground-glass opacities, interlobular and peribronchovascular smooth thickening and small bilateral pleural effusion.

Toxoplasma gondii is an obligate intracellular protozoan that belongs to the phylum Apicomplexa and subclass coccidia. This protozoan can assume three different forms: the oocyst, which releases sporozoites; the tissue cyst, which contains and may release bradyzoites; and the tachyzoite, which is a rapidly dividing, proliferative form of the parasite [1,2]. Felines are the definitive host, and human infection typically occurs via ingestion of undercooked meats containing tissue cysts or sporulated oocysts [1,2]. Tachyzoites can infect almost all nucleated cells in humans, residing and multiplying in host cells; the most commonly involved organs include the lymph nodes, brain, retinal cells, heart and lungs [8].

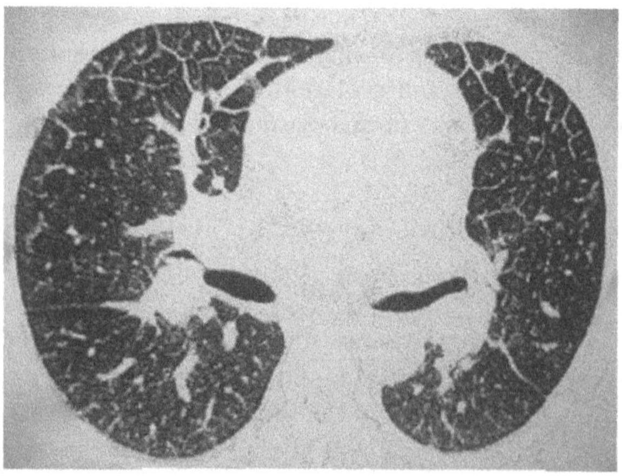

Figure 2 A 38-year-old male with pulmonary toxoplasmosis. Axial view of CT scan displays ground glass opacities and septal thickening.

The dissemination of rapidly dividing tachyzoites to various tissues represents either an acute infection (when these tachyzoites circulate via blood or lymphatic systems potentially infecting all cells and tissues) or the reactivation of a latent infection [1,2].

The activation of the systemic immune response and/ or antimicrobial therapy is usually sufficient to reduce the protozoan population, resulting in complete healing or occasionally a persistent chronic or latent infection state [2,7].

Acute toxoplasmosis with diffuse systemic and pulmonary involvement is most commonly related to immunocompromised patients. In this population, typical clinical findings include fever, lymph node enlargement, dyspnea and occasionally myalgia and gastrointestinal symptoms. The disease is very severe; cases of disseminated toxoplasmosis after stem cell transplantation (SCT) reach a mortality rate of 80% with a median survival time of 10 days post-diagnosis and 62.5 days post-allogeneic SCT [9].

In immunocompetent individuals, severe toxoplasmosis seems to be related to the pathogenicity of the microorganism strain. *T. gondii* strains from South America have atypical genotypes and higher diversity compared to the ones formerly described in North America and Europe. These atypical strains have been associated with a worse clinical involvement and outcome in mice and humans, due to its increased pathogenicity [9]. Indeed, most of the previous reported cases of severe toxoplasmosis and lung injury were reported in patients from these regions, or even patients infected by consumption of raw horsemeat imported from these regions [10].

In point of fact, lung involvement associated with *T. gondii* infection is rather rare in immunocompetent subjects, with only scarce descriptions in the medical literature. There are no recognized predisposing factors but, as discussed above, infections with more virulent strains, a high parasite burden, or even through inhalation of microorganisms are possible explanations [11,12].

Toxoplasma gondii pneumonia manifests with fever, dyspnea and a non-productive cough. In animal models, the earliest change following intravenous injection of infective tachyzoites is an interstitial pneumonitis with focal infiltrates of neutrophils, eosinophils and mononuclear cells. As the interstitial infiltrate spreads, the exudation of fibrin along with neutrophils and macrophages into alveolar spaces can occur. This can finally evolve into a pattern of diffuse alveolar damage with pneumocyte proliferation and focal necrosis [13,14].

Radiological abnormalities have been described in immunocompromised patients Chest radiographs demonstrates a reticulonodular infiltrate as a main finding, but nodular and coalescence opacities have also been described. In these patients, usual CT findings are bilateral and diffuse interstitial infiltrate with ground glass opacity

Table 2 CT findings of patients diagnosed with pulmonary toxoplasmosis

CT findings	Pulmonary	Mediastinal	Pleural
1	Diffuse GGO opacities, peribronchovascular and septal thickening, and nodules	-	Small bilateral effusion
2	Diffuse GGO opacities and peribronchovascular and septal thickening	Paratracheal lymph node enlargement	
3	Diffuse GGO opacities, peribronchovascular and septal thickening, and atelectasis		Small bilateral effusion

and slight and smooth thickening of the interlobular septa that might be indistinguishable from *Pneumocystis jirovecii* pneumonia in certain cases [15,16].

In immunocompetent subjects, former reports demonstrate diffuse interstitial infiltrate [17]. However, the CT patterns of pulmonary involvement have been poorly described in this population. Literature reports demonstrate diffuse ground-glass opacities with some degree of interlobular septal thickening and pulmonary nodules, associated or not to pleural effusion [12,13]. Our findings corroborate that the most prevalent findings are parenchymal abnormalities described as ground glass opacities, smooth septal and marked peribronchovascular thickening; as these findings were evident in all three patients. Atelectasis and nodules varying in size from 1.0 to 2.5 cm were also found, as was pleural effusion. Consequently, the main findings may mimic pulmonary congestion, lymphangitis, atypical pneumonia and pneumocystosis.

Conclusions

Because pulmonary toxoplasmosis is an uncommon infection, only a very limited number of cases are available to report in this study. Nevertheless, this is the largest series of CT findings of acute toxoplasmosis in immunocompetent hosts, and it raises concern that pulmonary toxoplasmosis should be considered as a differential diagnosis in immunocompetent patients that present with acute respiratory failure in the context of a subacute febrile illness.

Bilateral and diffuse interstitial infiltrates with marked peribronchovascular thickening with or without pleural effusion are the main tomographic patterns. Under these circumstances, a complete clinical history of raw or undercooked meat consumption or other potential exposures should be explored. If available, search for the specific strain of *T. gondii* should be attempted, as more virulent organisms seem to cause more severe organ compromise. Specific antimicrobial therapy with combination pyrimethamine, sulfadiazine and folinic acid should be instituted after a definitive diagnosis or in highly suspected cases [1,7] because the disease can have a potentially life-threatening course. If promptly treated, as demonstrated in the literature and our case series [5,17], pulmonary toxoplasmosis can result in complete lung recovery in immunocompetent hosts.

Consent

"Written informed consent was obtained from the patient for publication of this Case report and any accompanying images. A copy of the written consent is available for review by the Editor of this journal."

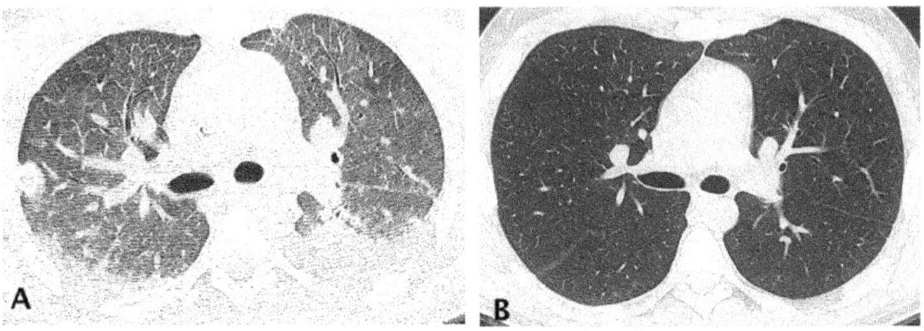

Figure 3 A 36-year-old male patient with pulmonary toxoplasmosis. Axial view of chest CT scan in **A** displays bilateral ground glass opacities and smooth septal and peribronchovascular thickening. In figure **B**, a complete resolution of the findings 3 months after treatment was evident.'

Competing interests
The authors declare that they have no competing interests.

Authors' contributions
KSG: wrote the draft of full-text, submitted the article. ANC:first revision of draft and data collection. AA: data collection. FBT: figure and table formatting, english revision. CJCF English revision. ASH: Draft revision. RAK: Final revision. All authors read and approved the final manuscript.

Author details
[1]Radiology Division, Hospital Sírio-Libanês, R. Dona Adma Jafet, 91, Bela Vista, SP 01308-050, Brazil. [2]Radiology Institute (InRad), University of São Paulo Medical School (FMUSP), Av. Dr. Enéas de Carvalho Aguiar, 44, Consolação, SP 05403-900, Brazil. [3]Pulmonary Division, Hospital Sírio-Libanês, R. Dona Adma Jafet, 91, Bela Vista, SP 01308-050, Brazil. [4]Pulmonary Division, Heart Institute (InCor), University of São Paulo Medical School (FMUSP), Av. Dr. Enéas de Carvalho Aguiar, 44, 2nd floor, block 1, Consolação, SP 05403-900, Brazil. [5]Hospital Sírio-Libanês, R. Dona Adma Jafet, 19, Bela Vista, SP 01308-050, Brazil.

References
1. Saadatnia G, Golkar M: **A review on human toxoplasmosis.** *Scand J Infect Dis* 2012, **44**(11):805–814.
2. Montoya JG, Liesenfeld O: **Toxoplasmosis.** *Lancet* 2004, **363**(9425):1965–1976.
3. Torgerson PR, Mastroiacovo P: **The global burden of congenital toxoplasmosis: a systematic review.** *Bull World Health Organ* 2013, **91**(7):501–508.
4. Ekman CC, Chiossi MF, Meireles LR, Andrade Junior HF, Figueiredo WM, Marciano MA, Luna EJ: **Case-control study of an outbreak of acute toxoplasmosis in an industrial plant in the state of São Paulo, Brazil.** *Rev Inst Med Trop Sao Paulo* 2012, **54**(5):239–244.
5. Carme B, Bissuel F, Ajzenberg D, Bouyne R, Aznar C, Demar M: **Severe acquired toxoplasmosis in immunocompetent adult patients in French Guiana.** *J Clin Microbiol* 2002, **40**(11):4037–4044.
6. Evans TG, Schwartzman JD: **Pulmonary toxoplasmosis.** *Semin Respir Infect* 1991, **6**:51–57.
7. Munir A, Zaman M, Eltorky M: **Toxoplasma gondii Pneumonia in a Pancreas Transplant Patient.** *South Med J* 2000, **93**(6):614–617.
8. Pomeroy C, Filice GA: **Pulmonary toxoplasmosis: a review.** *Clin Infect Dis* 1992, **14**(4):863–870.
9. Leal FE, Cavazzana CL, Andrade HF, Galisteo AJ, Mendonça JS, Kallas EG: **Toxoplasma gondii Pneumonia inmmunocompetent Subjects: Case Report and Review.** *Clin Infect Dis* 2007, **15**:44(6).
10. Sobanski V, Ajzenberg D, Delhaes L, Bautin N, Just N: **Severe toxoplasmosis in immunocompetent hosts: be aware of atypical strains.** *Am J Respir Crit Care Med* 2013, **187**(10):1143–1145.
11. Dardé ML: **Toxoplasma gondii, "new" genotypes and virulence.** *Parasite* 2008, **15**:366–371.
12. Demar M, Hommel D, Djossou F, Peneau C, Boukhari R: **Acute toxoplasmoses in immunocompetent patients hospitalized in an intensive care unit in French Guiana.** *Clin Microbiol Infect* 2012, **18**:E221–E231.
13. Nash G, Kerschmann RL, Herndier B, Dubey JP: **The pathological manifestations of pulmonary toxoplasmosis in the acquired immunodeficiency syndrome.** *Hum Pathol* 1994, **25**(7):652–658.
14. Jokelainen P, Vikøren T: **Acute fatal toxoplasmosis in a Great Spotted Woodpecker (Dendrocopos major).** *J Wildl Dis* 2014, **50**(1):117–120.
15. Stajner T, Vasiljević Z, Vujić D, Marković M, Ristić G, Mićić D, Pasić S, Ivović V, Ajzenberg D, Djurković-Djaković O: **Atypical strain of toxoplasma gondii causing fatal reactivation after hematopoietic stem cell transplantion in a patient with an underlying immunological deficiency.** *J Clin Microbiol* 2013, **51**(8):2686–2690.
16. Goodman PC, Schnapp LM: **Pulmonary toxoplasmosis in AIDS.** *Radiology* 1992, **184**(3):791–793.
17. Nunura J, Vásquez T, Endo S, Salazar D, Rodriguez A, Pereyra S, Solis H: **Disseminated toxoplasmosis in an immunocompetent patient from Peruvian Amazon.** *Rev Inst Med Trop Sao Paulo* 2010, **52**(2):107–110.

Intestinal current measurement versus nasal potential difference measurements for diagnosis of cystic fibrosis

Azadeh Bagheri-Hanson[†], Sebastian Nedwed[†], Claudia Rueckes-Nilges and Lutz Naehrlich[*]

Abstract

Background: Nasal potential difference (NPD) and intestinal current measurement (ICM) are functional *CFTR* tests that are used as adjunctive diagnostic tools for cystic fibrosis (CF). Smoking has a systemic negative impact on *CFTR* function. A diagnostic comparison between NPD and ICM and the impact of smoking on both *CFTR* tests has not been done.

Methods: The sweat chloride test, NPD, and ICM were performed in 18 patients with CF (sweat chloride >60 mmol/l), including 6 pancreatic sufficient (PS) patients, and 13 healthy controls, including 8 smokers. The NPD *CFTR* response to Cl-free and isoproterenol perfusion ($\Delta 0Cl^- + Iso$) was compared to the ICM *CFTR* response to forskolin/IBMX, carbachol, and histamine ($\Delta I_{sc,\ forskolin/IBMX+\ carbachol+histamine}$).

Results: The mean NPD *CFTR* response and ICM *CFTR* response between patients with CF and healthy controls was significantly different ($p < 0.001$), but not between patients with CF who were PS and those who were pancreatic insufficient (PI). Smokers have a decreased CFTR response measured by NPD ($p = 0.049$). For ICM there is a trend towards decreased CFTR response (NS). Three healthy control smokers had NPD responses within the CF-range. In contrast to NPD, there was no overlap of the ICM response between patients with CF and controls.

Conclusions: ICM is superior to NPD in distinguishing between patients with CF who have a sweat chloride > 60 mmol/l and healthy controls, including smokers. Neither NPD nor ICM differentiated between patients with CF who were PS from those who were PI. Smoking has a negative impact on *CFTR* function in healthy controls measured by NPD and challenges the diagnostic interpretation of NPD, but not ICM.

Keywords: (3–10): Cystic fibrosis, Nasal potential difference, Intestinal current measurement, Sweat chloride, Sweat test, Diagnosis, Smoking

Background

Cystic fibrosis (CF) is diagnosed based on a defined clinical phenotype and confirmation of *cystic fibrosis transmembrane regulator* (*CFTR*) dysfunction, commonly demonstrated by a sweat chloride value of ≥ 60 mmol/l and/or detection of two CF-causing mutations [1,2]. A small but increasing number of patients present with clinical symptoms characteristic of CF, an intermediate (30–60 mmol/l) or negative (≤29 mml/l) sweat test, and less than two CF-causing mutations [3-6]. For these query CF patients, a specific and sensitive *CFTR* functional test to exclude or confirm a *CFTR* functional defect characteristic of CF is needed [1,6]. *CFTR* modulating and correcting drugs have improved *CFTR*-function in cell cultures [7]. To test their effect in CF-patients, especially those with rare mutations, *CFTR*-functional tests with low variability and high reproducibility are needed [7].

In addition to sweat testing, two additional *CFTR* functional tests have been developed over the past 30 years; nasal potential difference (NPD) measurement [8] and intestinal current measurement (ICM) [9]. *CFTR* function is measured *in vivo* in the respiratory epithelium by NPD and *ex vivo* in superficial rectal biopsies by ICM. International standard operating procedures (SOPs) have been

* Correspondence: lutz.naehrlich@paediat.med.uni-giessen.de
[†]Equal contributors
Department of Pediatrics, Justus-Liebig-University Giessen, Feulgenstrasse 12, 35385 Giessen, Germany

established for both tests [8,10]. Both tests block epithelial sodium channels by amiloride and stimulate cAMP-mediated CFTR-mediated chloride transport in chloride-free solution and isoproterenol (NPD) or forskolin and IBMX (ICM). In addition, cholinergic chloride transport is tested by carbachol with ICM. The change after chloride-free and isoproterenol perfusion ($\Delta 0Cl^- + Iso$) with NPD [8] and the sum of the responses after carbachol, forskolin/IBMX ([11]) plus histamine ($\Delta I_{sc,\ forskolin/IBMX+carbachol+histamine}$) with ICM [12] has been proposed to be the best parameter of *CFTR* function. Both techniques can discriminate CF patients from healthy controls (NPD [13,14]; ICM [11,12,15,16]), but comparative clinical trials are lacking. Smoking has a systemic negative impact on CFTR-function [17,18], but the impact on the diagnostic aspects of NPD and ICM have not been investigated.

We performed NPD and ICM measurement in CF-patients and healthy controls to determine (1) the ability of these measurements to differentiate CF patients from healthy controls, and (2) the influence of smoking on CFTR function in healthy controls.

Methods

Between October 2012 and February 2013, 18 patients with CF and 13 healthy controls were recruited at the Justus-Liebig-University, Giessen, Germany. For this study, the diagnosis of CF was based on at least one clinical manifestation of CF, sweat chloride ≥60 mmol/l and the presence of two CF-causing mutations [1]. Pancreatic sufficiency (PS) was defined as fecal elastase >100 μg/g stool. Healthy controls had no clinical manifestation of CF and a sweat chloride value <60 mmol/l (Non-CF). Smoking was defined as any active or passive exposure to tobacco smoke. Exclusion criteria were participation in another medical clinical trial during the past 30 days, acute respiratory symptoms, intake of ivacaftor, known hemorrhoids, or bleeding diathesis. The ethics committee of the Justus-Liebig-Universität Giessen approved the protocol (AZ109/12). The study was performed in accordance with the declaration of Helsinki. Written informed consent was obtained from each participant aged 18 years and older. For participants younger than 18 years of age, written informed consent was obtained from each participant's parents or legal guardian, and age-appropriate consent was obtained from each participant. The sweat test, NPD, and ICM were performed on the same day for each subject.

The sweat test was performed according to Clinical and Laboratory Standards Institute guidelines [19]. For sweat stimulation and collection, the Macroduct® system (Wescor,

Table 1 Characteristics and CFTR response of pancreatic insufficient (CF-PI) and pancreatic sufficient (CF-PS) patients with CF and controls

	CF-PI (n = 12)	CF-PS (n = 6)	CF-all (n = 18)	Controls (n = 13)
Age, years	24.0 ± 6.1	23.3 ± 11.8	22.8 ± 8.0	30.6 ± 10.4
	22.0 (19.0 – 26.0)	16.0 (14.5 – 30.5)	20.5 (18.3 – 25.3)	25.0 (23.5 – 35.5)
Gender, females:males	3:9	5:1	8:10	7:6
Body mass index Z-score	−1.18 ± 0.80	−0.62 ± 1,41	−0.99 ± 1.03*	0.00 ± 0.65*
	−1.05 (−2.40 – 0.00)	1.41 (−0.20 – 0.70)	−0.90 (−2.60 – 0.70)	0.00 (−1.10 - 1.30)
Sweat chloride (mmol/l)	110 ± 13**	86 ± 14**	102 ± 17*	19 ± 8*
	106 (92 – 140)	90 (70 – 99)	104 (70 – 140)	19 (10 – 36)
NPD *CFTR* response average $\Delta 0Cl^- + Iso$ (mV)	4.6 ± 3.9	1.5 ± 4.1	3.6 ± 4.1*	−13.6 ± 8.5*
	5.1 (−3.0 -11.9)	1.5 (−3.2 – 6.23)	4.5 (−3.2 – 11.9)	−12.7 (−26.4 - -1.92)
ICM *CFTR* response average ΔIsc (μA/cm^{2}) (forskolin/IBMX + carbachol + histamine)	−0.3 ± 8.1	5.3 ± 10.9	1.6 ± 9.2*	77.8 ± 34.8*
	−0.6 (−12.6 – 17.9)	5.0 (−9.7 – 19.0)	0.1 (−12.6 – 19.0)	65.3 (39.6 -140.9)
Genotyping	F508/F508 (6×)	F508/R347P (2×)		148 T/R117H-7 T
	F508/G551D (2×)	F508/3849 + 10 kb C- > T (2×)		F508/–
	F508/G542X	F508/R334W		–/–
	F508/N1303K	F508/?		ND/ND (11)
	F508/1248 + 1G-A			
	F508/dele 14a,15,16,17a,17b			

Data are shown as ratios or the mean ± standard deviation incl. median (min – max). *p <0.001 (CF-all versus controls); **p = 0.003 (CF-PI versus CF-PS).

Inc., Logan, USA) was used. Chloride was measured by chloride titration. A sweat chloride level ≥60 mmol/l was interpreted as within the CF range, 30–60 mmol/l as equivocal, and ≤29 mmol as normal [1].

NPD was performed by one operator who was accredited by the Cystic Fibrosis Foundations' (CFF) Therapeutic Developments Network (TDN), and followed the CFF TDN SOP (version: January 2009) [8]. We used terbutaline as a substitute for isoproterenol in accordance with the SOP. The chloride-free and isoproterenol response ($\Delta 0Cl^- + Iso$) (NPD *CFTR* response) and the Wilschanksi score (defined as $e^{(\text{response to chloride-free and isoproterenol/response to amiloride})}$) [20] representing the *CFTR* response were calculated as the average or best result from both nostrils. The $\Delta 0Cl^- + Iso$ was interpreted as normal when < −12 mV, as in the CF range when > −7.7 mV, and as equivocal for results between −12 and −7.7 mV [6]. The Wilschanski score was interpreted as normal (<0.65), in the CF-range (>0.70), or equivocal (0.65–0.70) [20]. If the mean $\Delta 0Cl^- + Iso$ was > −7.7 mV in healthy controls, the NPD was repeated on a different day. Only the measurement with the highest $\Delta 0Cl^- + Iso$ was reported. If both measurements confirmed a $\Delta 0Cl^- + Iso$ in the CF range, *CFTR* genotyping (sequencing and multiplex ligation-dependent probe amplification) was offered as part of the participant's clinical care and reported as part of the baseline data. Genotyping of all healthy controls was not ethically approved.

The ICM followed the European Cystic Fibrosis Society-Therapeutic Development Network (ECFS-TDN) SOP (V2.7; Oct 26, 2011), which is based on the Rotterdam protocol. The tissues sliders (P2407C [1.5 mm diameter aperture slider; area 0,018 cm^2] or P2407B [1.2 mm diameter aperture slider; area 0.011 cm^2]; Physiologic Instruments, San Diego, USA) were mounted without tissue in the chambers (4-chamber system [EM-LVSYS-4; Physiologic Instrument, San Diego, USA]), which were filled on both sides with 2 ml Meyler buffer solution (10 mM Hepes; 0.3 mM Na_2HPO_4; 0.4 mM NaH_2PO_4; 1.0 mM $MgCl_2$; 1.3 mM $CaCl_2$; 4.7 mM KCl; 128 mM NaCl; 20.2 mM $NaHCO_3$; 10 mM D-Glucose; 0.01 mM indomethacin; pH 7.4; osmolarity 300 mOsm). PowerLab (4/30; ADInstruments Ltd., Dunedin, New Zealand) and Labchart® software (release 7.2; ADInstruments Ltd., Dunedin, New Zealand) were used for data acquisition. A stable open Potential Difference (PD) was ensured and an input offset to 0 mV was performed. Fluid resistance compensation was performed by applying short current pulses

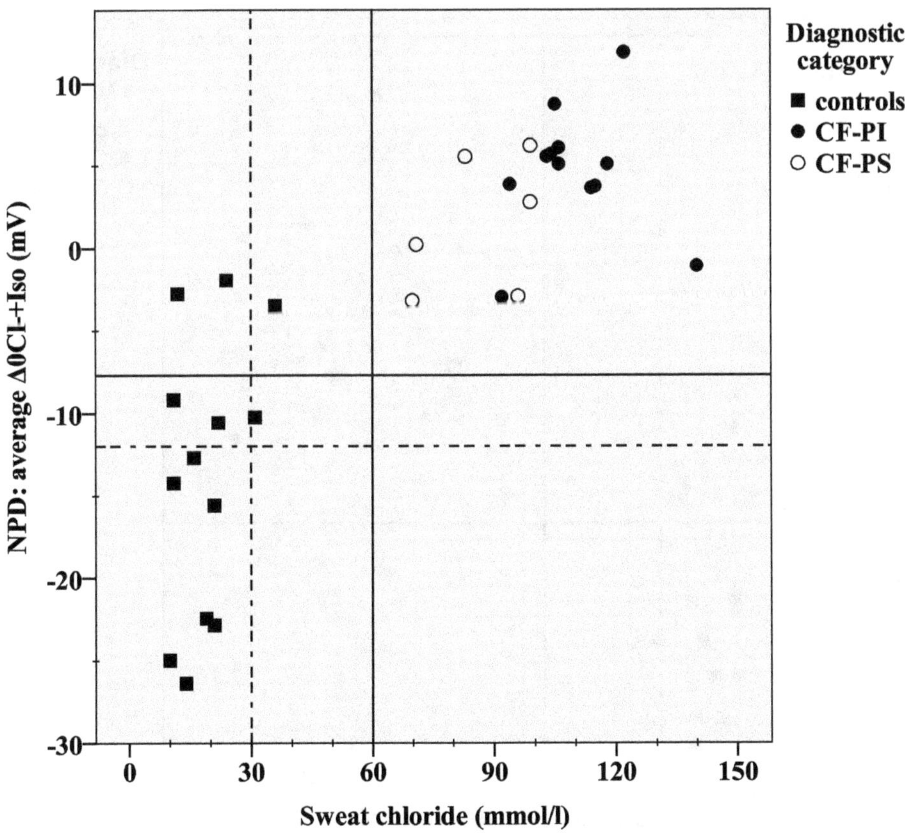

Figure 1 Correlation of average $\Delta 0Cl^- + Iso$ (NPD) and sweat chloride. The normal range is indicated for values below and left of the dotted lines, and the intermediate range is shown between the solid and dotted lines.

(15 μA) by the VCC MC4S Multi-Channel Voltage Current Clamp (Physiologic Instrument, San Diego, USA) and adjusting the fluid resistance.

For ICM, at least 4 superficial rectal biopsies were obtained by suction biopsies (aspiration biopsy instrument according to Wilital (UE7605); ulrich GmbH, Ulm, Germany) without prior bowel preparation. Biopsies were immediately stored in ice-cold buffer solution (Dulbecco's phosphate buffered saline and indomethacin, final concentration 10 μM) and mounted on adequate tissue sliders. After mounting the sliders in the heated and slightly sparged (95% O_2/5% CO_2) 4-chamber system, each basal resistance was measured by applying short current pulses (15 μA) and registering the corresponding change in V_t (typical range 15–30 Ohm × cm^2) with the VCC MC4S Multi-Channel Voltage Current Clamp (Physiologic Instrument, San Diego, USA). After that the voltage was clamped at 0 mV and the raw short circuit current ($_rI_{sc}$) was recorded from then on. Due to different sliders with different areas (P2407C [1.5 mm diameter aperture slider; area 0.018 cm^2] or P2407B [1.2 mm diameter aperture slider; area 0.011 cm^2]); Physiologic Instruments, San Diego, USA), the raw $_rI_{sc}$ was converted to I_{sc} (μA/cm^2). After applying 100 μM carbachol (which stimulates cholinergic Cl^- secretion by opening basolateral K^+ channels) to the serosal compartment, an I_{sc} response was evoked for quality control of the biopsy. After a 40-min equilibration in Meyler buffer, the basal I_{sc} was noted and 2 μl amiloride (to block amiloride-sensitive sodium channels) was added to the mucosal compartment. After 5 min or when the I_{sc} was stable, 10 μM forskolin and 100 μM IBMX (to stimulate cAMP-dependent CFTR-Cl^- transport) were added to the mucosal and serosal compartments ($\Delta I_{sc,\ forskolin/IBMX}$). After a minimum of 10 min, 10 μM genisteine (CFTR-potentiator) was added to both compartments. After a minimum of 5 min, 100 μM carbachol was added to the serosal compartment ($\Delta I_{sc,\ carbachol}$). After a minimum of 10 min, 200 μM 4,4′-Diisothiocyano-2,2′-stilbenedisulfonic acid (DIDS) (blocking non-CFTR-Cl^- channels) was added to the mucosal compartment. After 10 min, 500 μM histamine (to stimulate Ca^{2+} and proteinkinase C-mediated CFTR Cl^- secretion) was added to the serosal compartment ($\Delta I_{sc,\ histamine}$). In the open circuit, the final transepithelial voltage and final resistance were measured by applying short current pulses as in the beginning. Preliminary data suggested that the average $\Delta I_{sc,\ forskolin/IBMX+carbachol+histamine}$ is the best diagnostic ICM parameter for chloride secretory response (ICM CFTR response), but reference ranges have not been established [10].

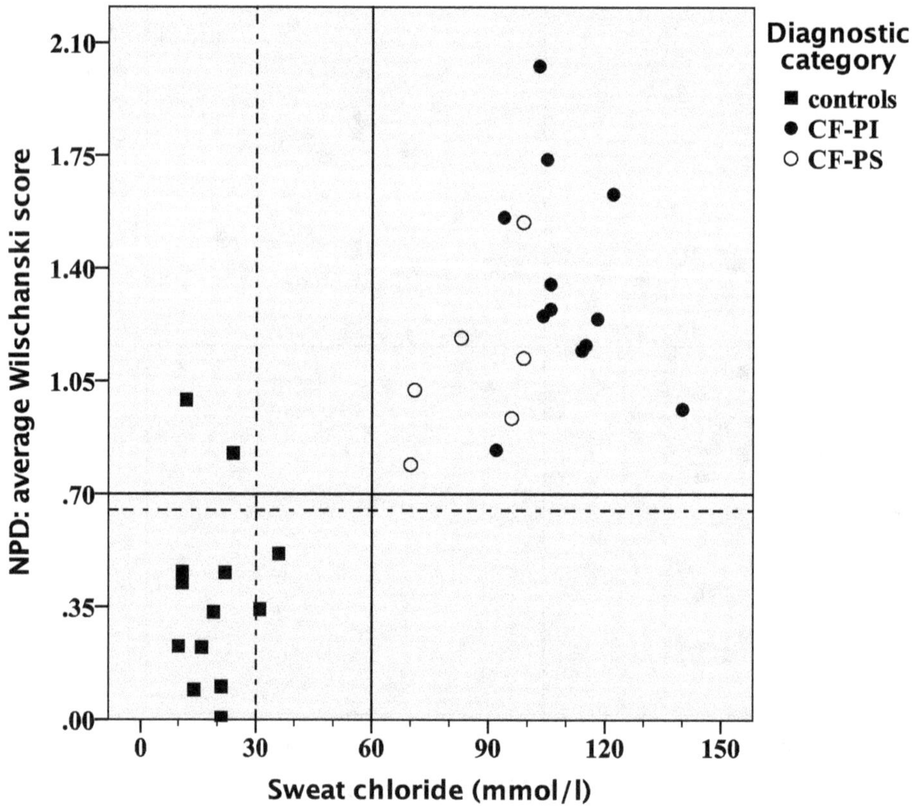

Figure 2 Correlation of the average Wilschanski score (NPD) and sweat chloride. The normal range is shown below and left of the dotted lines, and the intermediate range is shown between the solid and dotted lines.

Data are presented as the mean ± standard deviation (SD) (normally distributed variables), respective the median values, and 25th and 75th percentiles (non-normally distributed variables). Group comparisons were performed using the Student's t test or Mann–Whitney U test for normally or non-normally distributed variables, respectively. Statistical significance was defined as $p < 0.05$. All analyses were performed with IBM SPSS Statistics 21 (release 21; IBM, Armonk, USA).

Results

Our study included 18 patients with CF and 13 healthy controls with a median age of 20.5 and 25.0 years, respectively (NS) (Table 1). As consequence of our inclusion criteria, sweat chloride values distinguish patients with CF from healthy controls (p < 0.001). Although the mean sweat chloride differed between CF-PS and CF-PI patients (p = 0.003), an individual overlap occurs (Table 1, Figure 1). The mean NPD *CFTR* response significantly discriminated between CF patients and healthy controls (p <0.001), but not between patients with CF who were PS versus PI (Table 1). Four healthy controls had an average $\Delta 0Cl^- + Iso$ of > −7.7 mV. Three out of four controls had a repeatable average NPD CFTR response in the CF-range for $\Delta 0Cl^- + Iso > -7.7$ mV (23% of all healthy controls) (Figure 1), and two additional controls when using the Wilschanski score (15% of all healthy controls) (Figure 2). All these healthy controls were smokers. CFTR genotyping was offered to these three healthy controls as part of clinical routine and none had two CF-causing mutations (Table 1). For ICM a median of 6 (5–7) rectal biopsies were sampled per patient without severe adverse events. The mean ICM CFTR response was significantly different between CF patients and healthy controls (p <0.001), but not between patients with CF who were PS versus those who were PI (Table 1). We could not detect any age-dependency of the response to Isoproterenol/Forskolin. In contrast to NPD, there was no overlap between CF-patients and controls (Figures 3 and 4). Using the best instead of the average NPD, the *CFTR* response overlap did not change (Additional file 1). Using the best instead of the average ICM, the *CFTR* response resulted in one overlap (Additional file 2).

In healthy controls, smoking had no influence on sweat chloride (NS), but decreased *CFTR* function as measured by NPD (p = 0.049) (Table 2 and Figure 5),

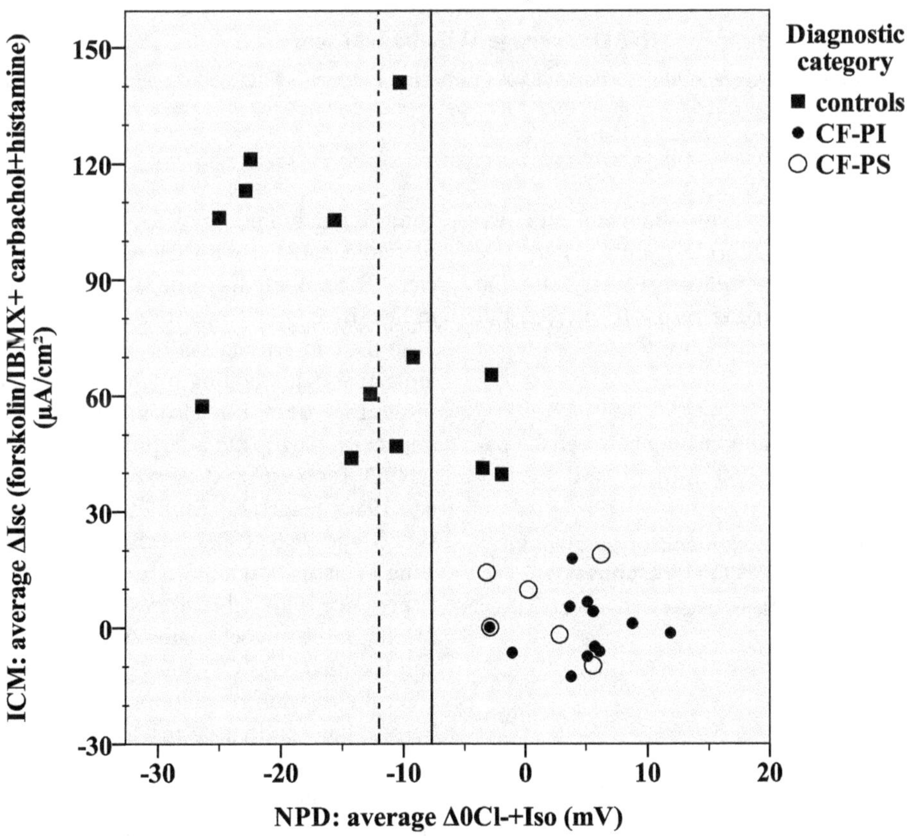

Figure 3 Correlation between the average ΔIsc (forskolin/IBMX + carbachol + histamine) (ICM) and average $\Delta 0Cl^-$ + Iso (NPD). The normal range is shown left of the dotted line. The intermediate range is shown between the solid and dotted lines. A higher ΔIsc (forskolin/IBMX + carbachol + histamine) represents a better CFTR response.

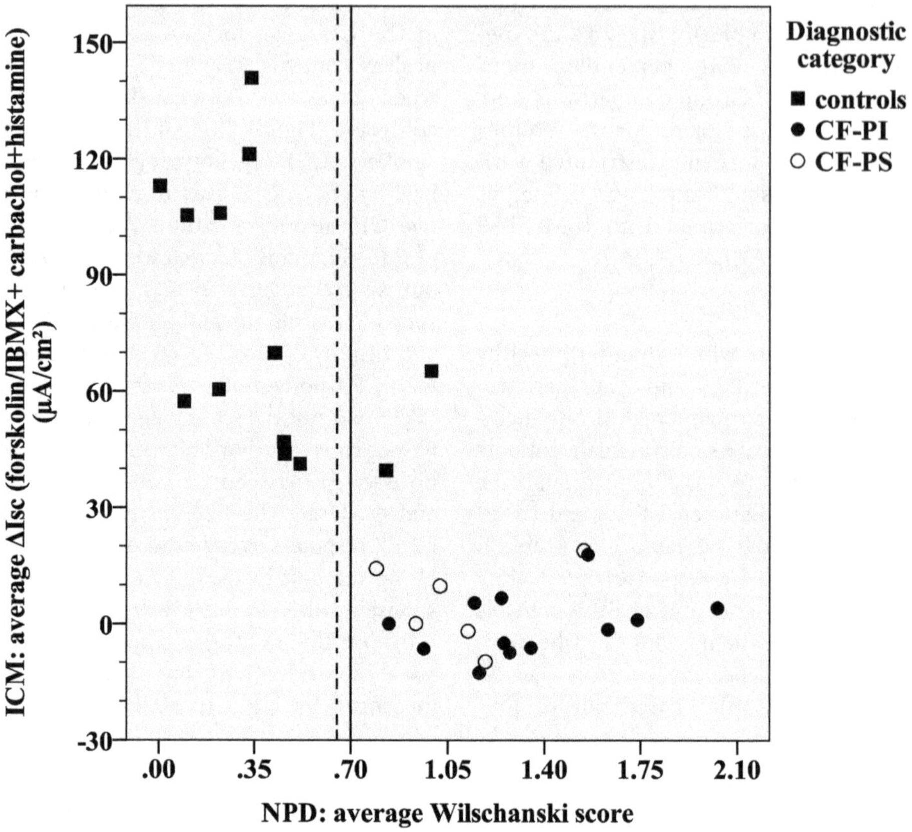

Figure 4 Correlation between the average ΔIsc (forskolin/IBMX + carbachol + histamine) (ICM) and average Wilschanski score (NPD). The normal range is shown left of the dotted line. The intermediate range is shown between the solid and dotted lines. A higher ΔIsc (forskolin/IBMX + carbachol + histamine) represents a better CFTR-response.

and resulted in intermediate or even abnormal NPD results, but not ICM or sweat chloride results. There is a trend in ICM measurements indicative that smoking might not only affect CFTR in the respiratory tract, but also in the intestine (Table 2 and Figure 6).

Discussion

ICM is superior to NPD for distinguishing between CF patients with a sweat chloride >60 mmol/l and healthy controls, including smokers. Neither NPD nor ICM differentiated patients with CF who were PS from those who were PI. Smoking has a negative impact on *CFTR* function in healthy controls measured by NPD, and challenges the diagnostic interpretation of NPD. There is a trend in ICM indicative that smoking might not only affect CFTR in the respiratory tract, but also in the intestine, which has no impact on diagnostic interpretation.

Table 2 Influence of smoking (active and/or passive) in healthy controls on NPD and ICM *CFTR* responses

	Nonsmokers n = 5	Smokers n = 8	*p-value*
Sweat chloride (mmol/L)	18 ± 8	20 ± 9	NS
NPD *CFTR* response Average $\Delta 0Cl^- + Iso$ (mV)	−19.3 ± 7.4	−10.1 ± 7.3	0.049
ICM *CFTR* response Average ΔIsc (μA/cm^2) (forskolin/IBMX + carbachol + histamine)	97.2 ± 37.1	65.7 ± 29.1	NS

All values are shown as the mean ± standard deviation.

NPD has been used as a diagnostic test for CF since the late 1980s [14,21,22]. Studies have shown 94.8–100% sensitivity and 96.5–100% specificity of $\Delta 0Cl^- + Iso$ for separating PI patients with CF from healthy controls [13,14,23]. Experience with a broader spectrum of patients with CF [24,25] and equivocal patients (sweat chloride <60 mmol/l and less than two CF-causing mutations) [20] described a clinically relevant overlap for $\Delta 0Cl^- + Iso$. Even in F508del homozygous patients, a residual *CFTR* NPD response with [26] or without [27,28] an observed clinical difference has been described. Some centers introduced an intermediate category for $\Delta 0Cl^- + Iso$ [6], interpret the highest NPD CFTR response [29], or use a composite score that includes sodium and chloride conductance [20,30]. Irrespective of the diagnostic criteria, our result showed a clinically

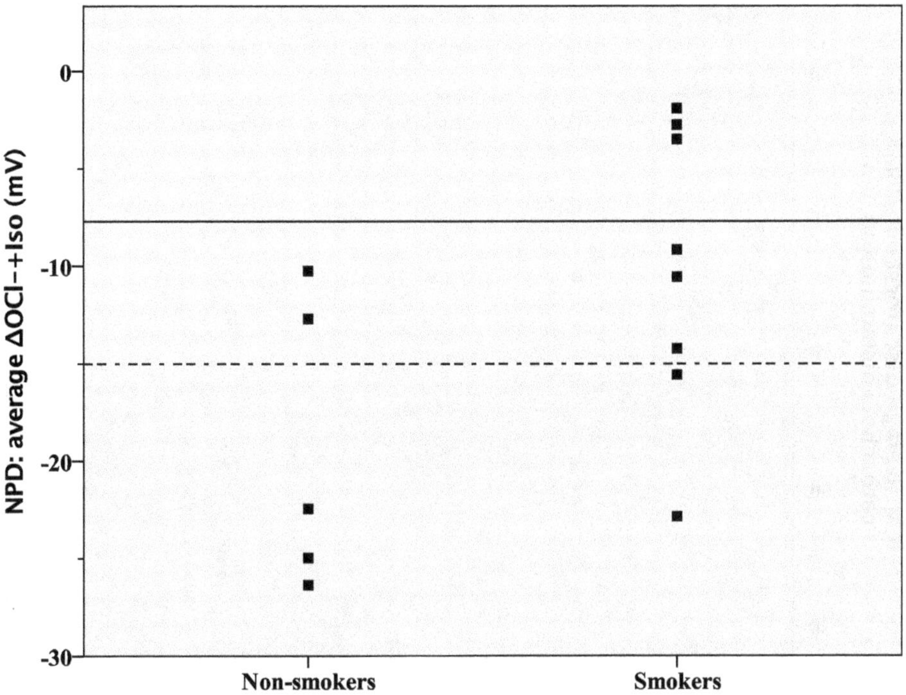

Figure 5 Average ΔOCl⁻ + Iso (NPD) in healthy controls according to smoking status. The normal range is shown below the dotted line and the intermediate range is shown between the solid and dotted lines.

relevant overlap between patients with CF and healthy controls. A normal average NPD *CFTR* response excludes CF, but an abnormal average NPD CFTR response could occur in healthy controls, especially in smokers, and can lead to a false-positive diagnosis of CF. A repeated measurement of a pathologic NPD response reduced the false-positive results in 1 out of 4 healthy controls in our cohort and should be recommended as a standard approach.

ICM was developed as a research tool for CFTR function in the 1990s [31] and has been used as a diagnostic test since the early 2000s [15,32]. Two different protocols are established; the Freiburg protocol [9] and the original [33] and adapted [34] Rotterdam protocol. We used the newest ECFS-ICM-SOP, which is an adapted Rotterdam protocol. The combination of cAMP-mediated Cl^- secretion, and the carbachol and histamine (Rotterdam protocol) responses separate patients with CF from those without CF [11,12,34], but not patients with CF who are PS from those who are PI [11,12], which is in accordance with our results. The 50% loss of CFTR protein in CF heterozygotes could not be detected by ICM [35] independent of the protocol [15,32]. For the Rotterdam protocol, De Jonge postulated that the ICM response is not proportional to the CFTR amount in the apical membrane of coloncytes except at a low level (<10–15%) and could therefore only detect an 80–85% loss of CFTR expression/function [32]. Therefore, mild mutations could result in a false-negative ICM. Interestingly, Derichs reported 8 patients with a sweat chloride >60 mmol/l, fewer than two CF-causing mutations after sequencing, and a normal ICM response who were judged as CF unlikely [12]. Our results with the new ECFS-ICM SOP confirm the high predictive value and practicability of this adapted ICM Rotterdam protocol.

Our data suggest that NPD is more likely to detect CFTR dysfunction in healthy controls than the ICM or sweat test. This could be explained by tissue specific differences in *CFTR* expression, alternative chloride channel expression, or extrinsic factors. Kälin et al. showed identical *CFTR* expression in the respiratory and intestinal tract of F508del-homozygous patients and healthy controls [36]. Highly variable CFTR expression in the nose [37] and colon [38] of F508del homozygous patients has been described, varying from 0–100% [37]. Therefore, in the respiratory and intestinal tract, individual *CFTR* expression seems to be more relevant than tissue specific expression. Alternative chloride channels could contribute to the chloride conductance, but have not been described in the distal colon [39]. Furthermore, previous infections [40], milder trauma [14], smoking [17], increased paracellular permeability [41], and decreased CFTR expression [42] and CFTR response [43]. With the exception of smoking, these extrinsic factors are relevant only for NPD, but not for rectal biopsies [44]. Smoking causes a decreased NPD response [17], but although a decreased systemic CFTR function mediated by acrolein [18]. Raju et al. demonstrated a 65% decrease in

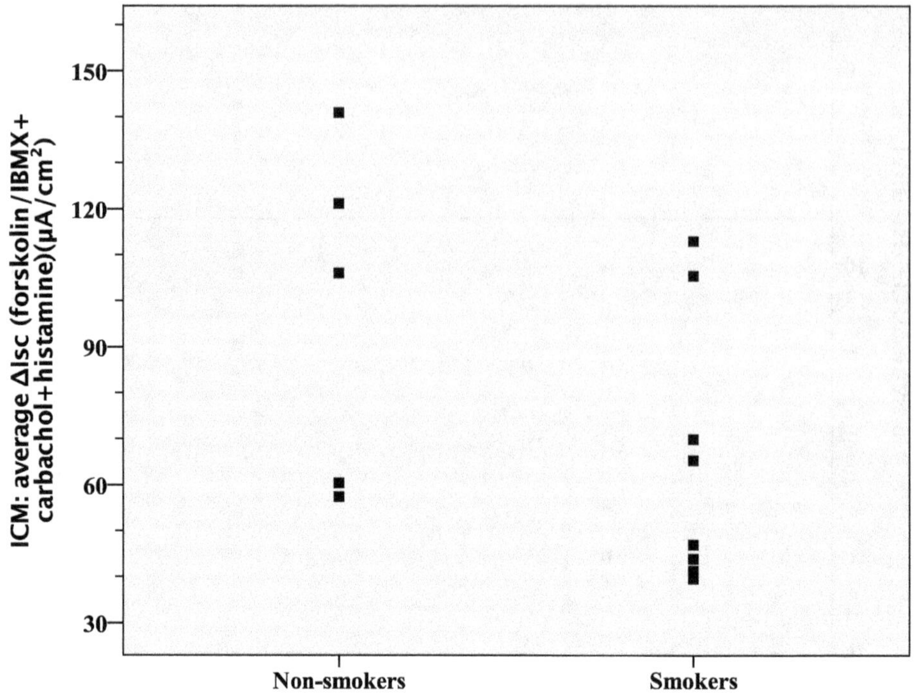

Figure 6 Average ΔIsc (forskolin/IBMX + carbachol + histamine) (ICM) in healthy controls according to smoking status. A higher ΔIsc (forskolin/IBMX + carbachol + histamine) represents a better CFTR response.

the ICM CFTR response in healthy smokers compared with non-smokers [18]. Our results confirm these findings. In contrast to NPD, smoking did not influence the diagnostic cut-off for ICM in our cohort. Therefore, ICM seems to be a more robust diagnostic test than NPD to distinguish primary from secondary *CFTR* dysfunction. This is important for the interpretation of NPD as an adjunctive diagnostic test in patients with query-CF who are exposed to smoking.

Limitations of our study include the small number of participants in each group, the lack of patients with CF with a sweat chloride value < 60 mmol/l, and patients with congenital bilateral absence of the vas deferens (CBAVD). The strength of our study is the genotyping of healthy controls with an abnormal CFTR NPD response, and the use of standardized protocols for sweat testing, NPD, and ICM.

Conclusions

From our results, a normal average NPD *CFTR* response excludes CF, but an intermediate or abnormal NPD *CFTR* response could be detected in healthy controls. NPD should be judged carefully, especially in patients with chronic rhinosinusitis and exposure to smoking. ICM combined with cAMP-mediated and cholinergic Cl secretion seems to be a practicable diagnostic test with an increased specificity compared with NPD. Discordant results of both *CFTR* functional tests could be detected and challenge the diagnostic interpretation. Larger study groups that include smokers and patients with CBAVD or CF with a sweat chloride between 30–60 mmol/l are needed to confirm our results.

Competing interests

The authors declare that they have no competing interests.

Authors' contributions

ABH recruited participants, performed the rectal biopsies, supported the NPD measurements, and helped draft the manuscript. SN recruited participants, performed the ICM measurements, and helped draft the manuscript. CRN supported the NPD measurements, performed the ICM measurements, and helped draft the manuscript. LN conceived the study, recruited participants, performed the rectal biopsies and statistical analysis, and drafted the manuscript. All authors read and approved the final manuscript.

Acknowledgements

The authors would like to thank the patients with CF and healthy controls; Kai Haus, Gießen, Germany, for technical support; Cornelia Kraus, Friedrich-Alexander University, Erlangen, Germany, for genotyping; and the Mukoviszidose Förderverein Gießen e.V, Gießen, Germany, for financial support.

References

1. De Boeck K, Wilschanski M, Castellani C, Taylor C, Cuppens H, Dodge J, Sinaasappel M: **Cystic fibrosis: terminology and diagnostic algorithms.** *Thorax* 2006, **61**(7):627–635.
2. Farrell PM, Rosenstein BJ, White TB, Accurso FJ, Castellani C, Cutting GR, Durie PR, Legrys VA, Massie J, Parad RB, Rock MJ, Campbell PW 3rd: **Guidelines**

for diagnosis of cystic fibrosis in newborns through older adults: cystic fibrosis foundation consensus report. *J Pediatr* 2008, **153**(2):S4–S14.
3. Gonska T, Choi P, Stephenson A, Ellis L, Martin S, Solomon M, Dupuis A, Dorfman R, Zielenski J, Ooi CY, Weiser W, Durie PR, Tullis E: **Role of cystic fibrosis transmembrane conductance regulator in patients with chronic sinopulmonary disease.** *Chest* 2012, **142**(4):996–1004.
4. Ooi CY, Dupuis A, Ellis L, Jarvi K, Martin S, Ray PN, Steele L, Kortan P, Gonska T, Dorfman R, Solomon M, Zielenski J, Corey M, Tullis E, Durie P: **Does extensive genotyping and nasal potential difference testing clarify the diagnosis of cystic fibrosis among patients with single-organ manifestations of cystic fibrosis?** *Thorax* 2014, **69**(3):254–260.
5. Segal I, Yaakov Y, Adler SN, Blau H, Broide E, Santo M, Yahav Y, Klar A, Lerner A, Aviram M, Ellis I, Mountford R, Shteyer E, Kerem E, Wilschanski M: **Cystic fibrosis transmembrane conductance regulator ion channel function testing in recurrent acute pancreatitis.** *J Clin Gastroenterol* 2008, **42**(7):810–814.
6. Ooi CY, Dupuis A, Ellis L, Jarvi K, Martin S, Gonska T, Dorfman R, Kortan P, Solomon M, Tullis E, Durie PR: **Comparing the American and European diagnostic guidelines for cystic fibrosis: same disease, different language?** *Thorax* 2012, **67**(7):618–624.
7. De Boeck K, Kent L, Davies J, Derichs N, Amaral M, Rowe SM, Middleton P, de Jonge H, Bronsveld I, Wilschanski M, Melotti P, Danner-Boucher I, Boerner S, Fajac I, Southern K, de Nooijer RA, Bot A, de Rijke Y, de Wachter E, Leal T, Vermeulen F, Hug MJ, Rault G, Nguyen-Khoa T, Barreto C, Proesmans M, Sermet-Gaudelus I: **CFTR biomarkers: time for promotion to surrogate end-point.** *Eur Respir J* 2013, **41**(1):203–216.
8. Rowe SM, Clancy JP, Wilschanski M: **Nasal potential difference measurements to assess CFTR ion channel activity.** *Methods Mol Biol* 2011, **741**:69–86.
9. Hug MJ, Derichs N, Bronsveld I, Clancy JP: **Measurement of ion transport function in rectal biopsies.** *Methods Mol Biol* 2011, **741**:87–107.
10. Derichs N, Pinders-Kessler L, Bronsveld I, Scheinert S, Rückes-Nilges C, de Jonge H, Nährlich L: **Multicenter European Standardization and reference values for intestinal current measurement in rectal biopsies.** *Pediatr Pulmonol* 2013, **48**(S36):300.
11. Sousa M, Servidoni MF, Vinagre AM, Ramalho AS, Bonadia LC, Felicio V, Ribeiro MA, Uliyakina I, Marson FA, Kmit A, Cardoso SR, Ribeiro JD, Bertuzzo CS, Sousa L, Kunzelmann K, Ribeiro AF, Amaral MD: **Measurements of CFTR-mediated Cl- secretion in human rectal biopsies constitute a robust biomarker for Cystic Fibrosis diagnosis and prognosis.** *PLoS One* 2012, **7**(10):e47708.
12. Derichs N, Sanz J, Von Kanel T, Stolpe C, Zapf A, Tummler B, Gallati S, Ballmann M: **Intestinal current measurement for diagnostic classification of patients with questionable cystic fibrosis: validation and reference data.** *Thorax* 2010, **65**(7):594–599.
13. Liu B, Hathorne H, Hill A, Cohen M: **J. B., Solomon MG, Calancy JP, Rowe SM: Normative values and receiver operating characteristics of NPD for diagnostic measurements.** *Pediatr Pulmonol* 2010, **303**(S33):307.
14. Knowles MR, Paradiso AM, Boucher RC: **In vivo nasal potential difference: techniques and protocols for assessing efficacy of gene transfer in cystic fibrosis.** *Hum Gene Ther* 1995, **6**(4):445–455.
15. Hirtz S, Gonska T, Seydewitz HH, Thomas J, Greiner P, Kuehr J, Brandis M, Eichler I, Rocha H, Lopes AI, Barreto C, Ramalho A, Amaral MD, Kunzelmann K, Mall M: **CFTR Cl- channel function in native human colon correlates with the genotype and phenotype in cystic fibrosis.** *Gastroenterology* 2004, **127**(4):1085–1095.
16. Cohen-Cymberknoh M, Yaakov Y, Shoseyov D, Shteyer E, Schachar E, Rivlin J, Bentur L, Picard E, Aviram M, Israeli E, Kerem E, Wilschanski M: **Evaluation of the intestinal current measurement method as a diagnostic test for cystic fibrosis.** *Pediatr Pulmonol* 2013, **48**(3):229–235.
17. Cantin AM, Hanrahan JW, Bilodeau G, Ellis L, Dupuis A, Liao J, Zielenski J, Durie P: **Cystic fibrosis transmembrane conductance regulator function is suppressed in cigarette smokers.** *Am J Respir Crit Care Med* 2006, **173**(10):1139–1144.
18. Raju SV, Jackson PL, Courville CA, McNicholas CM, Sloane PA, Sabbatini G, Tidwell S, Tang LP, Liu B, Fortenberry JA, Jones CW, Boydston JA, Clancy JP, Bowen LE, Accurso FJ, Blalock JE, Dransfield MT, Rowe SM: **Cigarette smoke induces systemic defects in cystic fibrosis transmembrane conductance regulator function.** *Am J Respir Crit Care Med* 2013, **188**(11):1321–1330.
19. Clinical and Laboratory Standards Institute: *Sweat Testing: Sample Collection and Quantitative Chloride Analysis; Approved Guideline-Third Edition*, Volume CLSI document C34-A3. Wayne, PA, USA: Clinical and Laboratory Standards Institute; 2009.
20. Wilschanski M, Famini H, Strauss-Liviatan N, Rivlin J, Blau H, Bibi H, Bentur L, Yahav Y, Springer H, Kramer MR, Klar A, Ilani A, Kerem B, Kerem E: **Nasal potential difference measurements in patients with atypical cystic fibrosis.** *Eur Respir J* 2001, **17**(6):1208–1215.
21. Alton EW, Currie D, Logan-Sinclair R, Warner JO, Hodson ME, Geddes DM: **Nasal potential difference: a clinical diagnostic test for cystic fibrosis.** *Eur Respir J* 1990, **3**(8):922–926.
22. Sauder RA, Chesrown SE, Loughlin GM: **Clinical application of transepithelial potential difference measurements in cystic fibrosis.** *J Pediatr* 1987, **111**(3):353–358.
23. Middleton PG, House HH: **Measurement of airway ion transport assists the diagnosis of cystic fibrosis.** *Pediatr Pulmonol* 2010, **45**(8):789–795.
24. Wilschanski M, Dupuis A, Ellis L, Jarvi K, Zielenski J, Tullis E, Martin S, Corey M, Tsui LC, Durie P: **Mutations in the cystic fibrosis transmembrane regulator gene and in vivo transepithelial potentials.** *Am J Respir Crit Care Med* 2006, **174**(7):787–794.
25. Walker LC, Venglarik CJ, Aubin G, Weatherly MR, McCarty NA, Lesnick B, Ruiz F, Clancy JP, Sorscher EJ: **Relationship between airway ion transport and a mild pulmonary disease mutation in CFTR.** *Am J Respir Crit Care Med* 1997, **155**(5):1684–1689.
26. Bronsveld I, Mekus F, Bijman J, Ballmann M, de Jonge HR, Laabs U, Halley DJ, Ellemunter H, Mastella G, Thomas S, Veeze HJ, Tummler B: **Chloride conductance and genetic background modulate the cystic fibrosis phenotype of Delta F508 homozygous twins and siblings.** *J Clin Invest* 2001, **108**(11):1705–1715.
27. Leal T, Fajac I, Wallace HL, Lebecque P, Lebacq J, Hubert D, Dall'Ava J, Dusser D, Ganesan AP, Knoop C, Cumps J, Wallemacq P, Southern KW: **Airway ion transport impacts on disease presentation and severity in cystic fibrosis.** *Clin Biochem* 2008, **41**(10–11):764–772.
28. Wallace HL, Barker PM, Southern KW: **Nasal airway ion transport and lung function in young people with cystic fibrosis.** *Am J Respir Crit Care Med* 2003, **168**(5):594–600.
29. Naehrlich L, Ballmann M, Davies J, Derichs N, Gonska T, Hjelte L, van Konigsbruggen-Rietschel S, Leal T, Melotti P, Middleton P, Tummler B, Vermeulen F, Wilschanski M: **Nasal potential difference measurements in diagnosis of cystic fibrosis: An international survey.** *J Cyst Fibros* 2014, **13**(1):24–28.
30. Sermet-Gaudelus I, Girodon E, Sands D, Stremmler N, Vavrova V, Deneuville E, Reix P, Bui S, Huet F, Lebourgeois M, Munck A, Iron A, Skalicka V, Bienvenu T, Roussel D, Lenoir G, Bellon G, Sarles J, Macek M, Roussey M, Fajac I, Edelman A: **Clinical phenotype and genotype of children with borderline sweat test and abnormal nasal epithelial chloride transport.** *Am J Respir Crit Care Med* 2010, **182**(7):929–936.
31. Veeze HJ, Halley DJ, Bijman J, de Jongste JC, de Jonge HR, Sinaasappel M: **Determinants of mild clinical symptoms in cystic fibrosis patients. Residual chloride secretion measured in rectal biopsies in relation to the genotype.** *J Clin Invest* 1994, **93**(2):461–466.
32. De Jonge HR, Ballmann M, Veeze H, Bronsveld I, Stanke F, Tummler B, Sinaasappel M: **Ex vivo CF diagnosis by intestinal current measurements (ICM) in small aperture, circulating Ussing chambers.** *J Cyst Fibros* 2004, **3**(Suppl 2):159–163.
33. Veeze HJ, Sinaasappel M, Bijman J, Bouquet J, de Jonge HR: **Ion transport abnormalities in rectal suction biopsies from children with cystic fibrosis.** *Gastroenterology* 1991, **101**(2):398–403.
34. Clancy JP, Szczesniak RD, Ashlock MA, Ernst SE, Fan L, Hornick DB, Karp PH, Khan U, Lymp J, Ostmann AJ, Rezayat A, Starner TD, Sugandha SP, Sun H, Quinney N, Donaldson SH, Rowe SM, Gabriel SE: **Multicenter intestinal current measurements in rectal biopsies from CF and non-CF subjects to monitor CFTR function.** *PLoS One* 2013, **8**(9):e73905.
35. Hogenauer C, Santa Ana CA, Porter JL, Millard M, Gelfand A, Rosenblatt RL, Prestidge CB, Fordtran JS: **Active intestinal chloride secretion in human carriers of cystic fibrosis mutations: an evaluation of the hypothesis that heterozygotes have subnormal active intestinal chloride secretion.** *Am J Hum Genet* 2000, **67**(6):1422–1427.
36. Kalin N, Claass A, Sommer M, Puchelle E, Tummler B: **DeltaF508 CFTR protein expression in tissues from patients with cystic fibrosis.** *J Clin Invest* 1999, **103**(10):1379–1389.

37. van Meegen MA, Terheggen-Lagro SW, Koymans KJ, van der Ent CK, Beekman JM: **Apical CFTR expression in human nasal epithelium correlates with lung disease in cystic fibrosis.** *PLoS One* 2013, **8**(3):e57617.
38. van Barneveld A, Stanke F, Tamm S, Siebert B, Brandes G, Derichs N, Ballmann M, Junge S, Tummler B: **Functional analysis of F508del CFTR in native human colon.** *Biochim Biophys Acta* 2010, **1802**(11):1062–1069.
39. Greger R: **Role of CFTR in the colon.** *Annu Rev Physiol* 2000, **62**:467–491.
40. Chilvers MA, McKean M, Rutman A, Myint BS, Silverman M, O'Callaghan C: **The effects of coronavirus on human nasal ciliated respiratory epithelium.** *Eur Respir J* 2001, **18**(6):965–970.
41. Yeo NK, Jang YJ: **Rhinovirus infection-induced alteration of tight junction and adherens junction components in human nasal epithelial cells.** *Laryngoscope* 2010, **120**(2):346–352.
42. Brezillon S, Dupuit F, Hinnrasky J, Marchand V, Kalin N, Tummler B, Puchelle E: **Decreased expression of the CFTR protein in remodeled human nasal epithelium from non-cystic fibrosis patients.** *Lab Invest* 1995, **72**(2):191–200.
43. Knowles M, Murray G, Shallal J, Askin F, Ranga V, Gatzy J, Boucher R: **Bioelectric properties and ion flow across excised human bronchi.** *J Appl Physiol* 1984, **56**(4):868–877.
44. Servidoni MF, Sousa M, Vinagre AM, Cardoso SR, Ribeiro MA, Meirelles LR, de Carvalho RB, Kunzelmann K, Ribeiro AF, Ribeiro JD, Amaral MD: **Rectal forceps biopsy procedure in cystic fibrosis: technical aspects and patients perspective for clinical trials feasibility.** *BMC Gastroenterol* 2013, **13**(1):91.

28

Comparative chest computed tomography findings of non-tuberculous mycobacterial lung diseases and pulmonary tuberculosis in patients with acid fast bacilli smear-positive sputum

Mei-Kang Yuan[1,2†], Cheng-Yu Chang[3†], Ping-Huang Tsai[2,4], Yuan-Ming Lee[5], Jen-Wu Huang[6] and Shih-Chieh Chang[2,4*]

Abstract

Background: Early diagnosis and treatment of nontuberculous mycobacterial lung diseases (NTM-LD) and pulmonary tuberculosis (PTB) are important clinical issues. The present study aimed to compare and identify the chest CT characteristics that help to distinguish NTM lung disease from PTB in patients with acid-fast bacilli (AFB) smear-positive sputum.

Methods: From January 2009 to April 2012, we received 467 AFB smear-positive sputum specimens. A total of 95 CT scans obtained from the 159 patients were analyzed, 75 scans were from patients with PTB and 20 scans from NTM-LD. The typical chest CT findings of mycobacterial diseases were analyzed.

Results: In patients with PTB, the prevalence of pleural effusion (38.7% vs. 15.0%; P =0.047), nodules < 10 mm in size (76.0% vs. 25.0%; P < 0.001), tree-in-bud pattern (81.3% vs. 55.0%; P =0.021), and cavities (31.1% vs. 5.0%; P =0.018) were significantly higher than patients with NTM. Of the 20 patients with NTM lung diseases, bronchiectasis and cystic changes were significantly higher than patients with PTB (20.0% vs. 4.0%; P = 0.034). In multivariate analysis, CT scan findings of nodules was independently associated with patients with diagnoses of PTB (odds ratio [OR], 0.07; 95% confidence interval [CI], 0.02-0.30). Presence of bronchiectasis and cystic changes in CT scans was strongly associated with patients with NTM-LD (OR, 33.04; 95% CI, 3.01-362.55).

Conclusions: The CT distinction between NTM-LD and PTB may help radiologists and physicians to know the most likely diagnoses in AFB-smear positive patients and avoid unnecessary adverse effects and the related costs of anti-TB drugs in endemic areas.

Keywords: Nontuberculous mycobacterial lung disease, Pulmonary tuberculosis, Acid-fast bacilli smear, Bronchiectasis and cystic changes

Background

The diagnosis and treatment of pulmonary diseases caused by mycobacterial infections are very important clinical issues. Among mycobacterial diseases, pulmonary tuberculosis (PTB) is the major entity and one of the world's leading infectious diseases. In 2012, 8.6 million people felt ill with TB and 1.3 million died from TB [1]. Isolation of Mycobacterium tuberculosis from respiratory specimens is recommended for the definite diagnosis of PTB [2]. Microscopic examination of sputum smears for acid-fast bacilli (AFB) is widely used and the most efficient procedure for the initial screening of PTB. The presence of AFB in the stained sputum (AFB smear-positive) indicates a preliminary diagnosis of pulmonary mycobacterial infection. However, positive AFB smear test is not specific for PTB [3-5]. AFB smear-positive sputum may represent mycobacterium tuberculosis, but it can also represent non-tuberculous mycobacteria (NTM) [6]. NTM are

* Correspondence: 11319@ymuh.ym.edu.tw
†Equal contributors
[2]Faculty of Medicine, School of Medicine, National Yang-Ming University, Taipei, Taiwan
[4]Department of Internal Medicine, National Yang-Ming University Hospital, #152, Xin-Min Road, Yilan City 260, Taiwan
Full list of author information is available at the end of the article

ubiquitous organisms and its radiographic abnormalities and clinical symptoms changes slowly as compared with PTB [7]. In endemic areas, it is not uncommon to administer empirical anti-TB drugs in clinically suspected PTB patients with AFB smear-positive sputum. The isolation prevalence of NTM has increased gradually, which raise the concerns of unnecessary adverse effect and costs of anti-TB drugs [8,9]. Therefore, additional diagnostic tools that help differentiate PTB and NTM is relevant in patients pending culture results. Radiological manifestations such as computed tomography (CT) features are useful to aid the diagnosis of PTB and NTM before definite mycobacterial culture because of its great availability and short examination time [10]. The aim of this study is to compare and identify the chest CT characteristics that help to distinguish NTM lung disease from PTB in patients with AFB smear-positive sputum.

Methods

Patients

From January 2009 to April 2012, we received 9,267 sputum specimens from 3,958 patients at the laboratory of National Yang-Ming University Hospital (a 512-bed regional teaching hospital in Yilan, Taiwan) and the Far Eastern Memorial Hospital (a 1050-bed tertiary medical center in Taipei, Taiwan). Of these sputum specimens, 467 from 236 patients were AFB stain-positive. Only 134 of the AFB stain-positive patients had proven pulmonary TB, and 25 patients proven NTM lung diseases. A total of 95 CT scans obtained from the 159 patients were analyzed, 75 scans were from patients with PTB and 20 scans from NTM lung disease. The study was approved by the Institutional Review Boards of the National Yang-Ming University Hospital and the Far Eastern Memorial Hospital. All participants gave written informed consent and agree of information collection in the study. All images of the participants were taken as part of standard patient care.

Diagnosis of pulmonary TB and NTM

All of the sputum specimens were treated with Ziehl-Neelsen staining. TB polymerase chain reaction (PCR) was performed with in-house IS6110-based PCR assays [11]. Mycobacterial cultures were performed using Löwenstein-Jensen medium [12]. Patients were diagnosed with pulmonary TB if M. tuberculosis was isolated from their sputum or tissue specimens. NTM was diagnosed according to mycobacterial cultures and the American Thoracic Society (ATS) guideline [13].

CT scanning methods

The CT scans were original films obtained from each institution. All CT examinations were performed within 3 months of AFB smear test. Conventional CT scans were performed with a 5 mm slice-thickness at 5 mm intervals by using multi-detector CT (Philips Brilliance 64). HRCT images were obtained with a 1 mm slice-thickness at 10 mm intervals. Scanning extended from the lung apices to below the costophrenic angles at maximum inspiration. The CT scans were reviewed independently by two experienced radiologists and pulmonary specialists blinded to the patient's microbiology results. The final decisions regarding the findings were determined by consensus.

Statistical analysis

All statistical analyses were conducted using SPSS software for Windows (v 20; IBM Corporation, Armonk, NY, USA). Data are presented as frequencies for categorical variables, and by mean ± standard deviation for numerical variables. Categorical variables were compared using a chi-square test or Fisher's exact test, and continuous variables were compared using an independent unpaired *t*-test. Univariate analysis was performed to evaluate the characteristic CT findings. Multivariate analysis was conducted using a logistic regression model to determine the independent predictive factors for patients with PTB and NTM infections. *P*-values of less than 0.05 were considered to be significant.

Table 1 Clinical characteristics of patients with pulmonary tuberculosis and NTM lung diseases

	Pulmonary tuberculosis n = 75	NTM lung disease n = 20	*P* value
Age, years	65.57 ± 18.20	67.60 ± 14.63	0.647
Male	58 (77.3)	11 (55.0)	0.047
Ever smoker	24 (32.0)	3 (15.0)	0.134
Diabetes mellitus	14 (18.7)	3 (15.0)	1.000
Malignancy	3 (4.0)	0 (0.0)	1.000
Autoimmune disease	2 (2.7)	1 (5.0)	0.512
COPD	9 (12.0)	4 (20.0)	0.463
Pneumoconiosis	1 (1.3)	1 (5.0)	0.378

Numbers in parentheses are percentages. *NTM*: non-tuberculosis mycobacterium; *COPD*: chronic obstructive pulmonary disease.

Results

The 75 patients with PTB included 58 men and 17 women with a mean age ± standard deviation of 65.6 years ±18.2 (range, 23–86 years). The 20 patients with NTM included 11 men and 9 women with a mean age ± standard deviation of 67.6 years ±14.6 (range, 30–92 years). The clinical data are summarized in Table 1. The CT findings were classified as presence or absence of pleural effusion, cavity formation, atelactasis, consolidation, nodules less than 10 mm in size, tree-in-bud pattern (branching centrilobular nodules), interlobular septal thickening, lung volume reduction, bronchiectasis, lymphadenopathy, calcified lymph nodes, as well as bronchiectasis and cystic changes. Of the 75 patients with PTB, 29 (38.7%) had pleural effusion vs. 3 (15.0%) in patients with NTM (P =0.047). 57 (76.0%) patients with PTB had nodules vs. 5 (25.0%) patients with NTM (P < 0.001). 61 (81.3%) patients with PTB had tree-in-bud opacities vs. 11 (55.0%) patients with NTM (P =0.021) (Figure 1). And 23 (31.1%) patients with PTB had cavities vs. 1 (5.0%) patient with NTM (P =0.018). Consalidation, lymphadenopathy and calcified lymph nodes were also more common in PTB patients. Of the 20 patients with NTM lung diseases, 4 (20.0%) had bronchiectasis and cystic changes vs. 3 (4.0%) patients with PTB; (P = 0.034) (Figures 2 and 3). Atelactasis, bronchiectasis without cystic changes and lung parenchymal volume reduction were more common in NTM lung diseases, but the univariate statistical results were not significant (Table 2). In multivariate analysis, CT scan findings of nodules was independently associated with patients with diagnoses of PTB (odds ratio [OR], 0.07; 95% confidence interval [CI], 0.02-0.30). Presence of bronchiectasis and cystic changes in CT scans was strongly associated with patients with NTM lung diseases (OR, 33.04; 95% CI, 3.01-362.55) (Table 3).

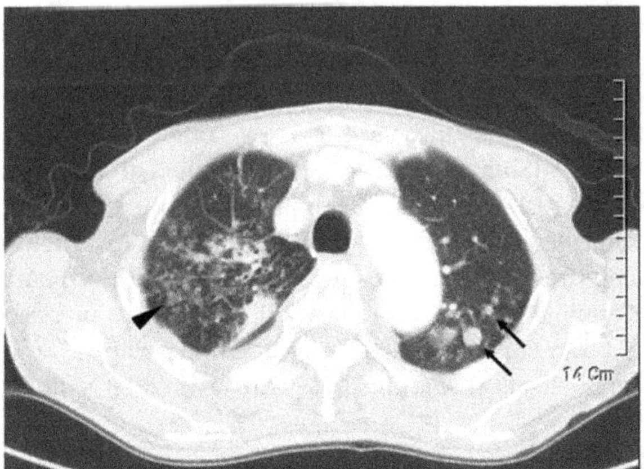

Figure 1 Thin section CT of a 72-year-old male with pulmonary tuberculosis demonstrating nodules (arrows) and tree-in-bud pattern (arrowhead); loculated pleural effusion at right lower lung zones.

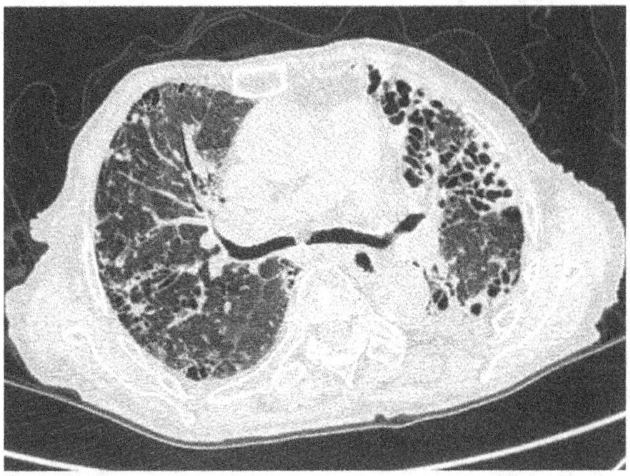

Figure 2 High resolution CT with 1 mm slice-thickness of a 92 - year-old female with NTM (*Mycobacterium avium complex*) lung disease demonstrating the bronchiectasis and cystic changes at left upper and lower lobes and at right lower lobe.

Discussion

The present study shows that chest CT findings could help to differentiate pulmonary TB from NTM lung diseases. Upon comparing CT features between PTB and NTM, pleural effusion, nodules are significantly more common in patients with PTB and bronchiectasis combined with cystic changes are significantly more common in patients with NTM infections. In multivariate analysis, presence of nodules is significantly associated with PTB, and bronchiectasis combined with cystic changes are strongly associated with NTM lung diseases.

The definite diagnosis of PTB still depends on PCR or mycobacterial culture from bronchial washing or sputum.

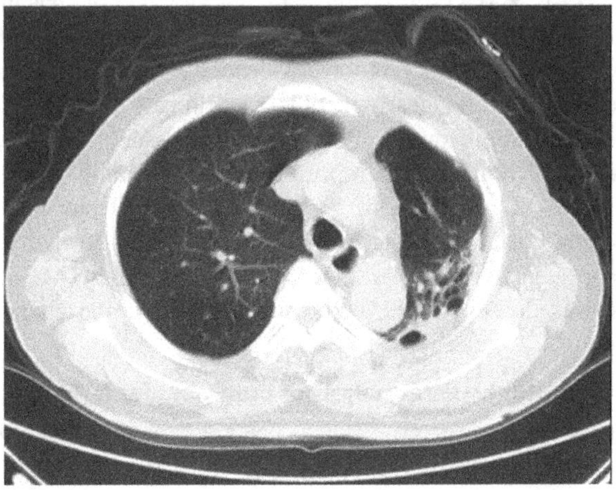

Figure 3 Thin section CT of an 86 -year-old male with NTM (*Mycobacterium avium complex*) lung disease demonstrating the bronchiectasis and cystic changes at left upper lobe.

Table 2 Comparative chest CT findings of non-tuberculous mycobacterial lung diseases and pulmonary tuberculosis

	Pulmonary tuberculosis n = 75	NTM lung diseases n = 20	*P* value
Chest CT findings			
Pleural effusion	29 (38.7)	3 (15.0)	0.047
Cavities	23 (31.1)	1 (5.0)	0.018
Atelectasis	41 (54.7)	12 (60.0)	0.670
Consolidation	41 (54.7)	9 (45.0)	0.442
Random nodules	57 (76.0)	5 (25.0)	<0.001
Interlobular septal thickening	67 (89.3)	17 (85.0)	0.694
Bronchiectasis	10 (13.3)	4 (20.0)	0.484
Lung volume reduction	7 (9.3)	4 (20.0)	0.236
Tree-in-bud pattern	61 (81.3)	11 (55.0)	0.021
Lymphadenopathy	18 (24.0)	1 (5.0)	0.066
Calcified lymph nodes	5 (6.7)	0 (0.0)	0.580
Bronchiectasis and cystic changes	3 (4.0)	4 (20.0)	0.034

Numbers in parentheses are percentages. *NTM* = non-tuberculous mycobacterium.
CT = computed tomography.

Clinical symptoms and image findings also play an important role in the diagnosis of TB. Typical radiological features of pulmonary TB include parenchymal diseases such as consolidation and cavities; pleural effusion, variable-sized nodules and lymphadenopathy are well documented and repeatedly reviewed in literatures. The CT findings in our study are mostly identical to the previously reported radiological findings of PTB. Familiar thin-section chest CT findings of nontuberculous mycobacterial infection include bronchiectasis, small and large nodules, centrilobular nodules, consolidation and fibrocavitary lesions [14,15]. Our study also demonstrates the common radiographic findings of bronchiectasis, tree-in-bud pattern, atelactasis and consolidation in patients with NTM lung diseases, but there are no significant differences as compared with the PTB patients. To our knowledge, the CT finding of bronchiectasis and cystic changes in NTM infection has not been emphasized in the previous studies. Although the radiological evidence of severe bronchiectasis and subsequent cystic changes, which is traditionally described as the honeycomb appearance, usually represents end-stage interstitial fibrosis, it is reported to be a dynamic process and may have different evolution [16,17]. In order to exclude the pre-existing bronchiectasis and cystic changes, the previous films of the four patients with NTM lung diseases demonstrating bronchiectasis and cystic changes were reviewed since the PACS implementation in our institutions from March 2004. Regarding the diagnosis of NTM, the isolation of NTM species from a respiratory sample is an insufficient evidence for the definite diagnosis of NTM lung disease. Some patients with positive NTM culture do not have evidences of pulmonary disease, and such infection may indicate colonization or transient infection. Therefore, the ATS issued diagnostic criteria for NTM lung diseases which not only rely on microbiological examinations, the clinical and radiographic evidences are also essential. Clinical researches have shown that disease attributable to NTM has a rising trend in many developed and developing countries [18,19]. In endemic areas, immediate and empirical treatment of mycobacterial diseases based on the result of AFB sputum smear has an important impact on disease transmission control. However, the administration of unnecessary empiric anti-TB treatment is not uncommon in real world practice and patients might suffer from the adverse effects of anti-TB drugs. Our colleagues (Shih-Chieh Chang, et al.) issued an article that revealed 40.4% of patients with positive sputum AFB stains did not have pulmonary TB in Taiwan [20]. According to Chang's results, among patients who had positive sputum AFB stains without pulmonary TB, 25.8% were prescribed anti-TB treatment and 44% of them developed various adverse effects (hepatitis: 32%; skin rash: 20%). Although

Table 3 Multivariate analysis of predictors for NTM lung diseases

CT findings	Odds ratio	95% CI	
Bronchiectasis and cystic changes	33.035	3.010-362.552	Favor NTM
Pleural effusion	0.198	0.038-1.031	Favor PTB
Random nodules	0.074	0.019-0.296	Favor PTB

CI = confidence interval; *PTB* = pulmonary tuberculosis; *NTM* = nontuberculous mycobacterium.

the adverse effects were usually not lethal, however, they did cause unnecessary harm. Our study provides radiographic evidence that chest CT finding of the bronchiectasis and cystic changes is statistically a strong indicator of NTM disease in patients with AFB smear-positive sputum. This characteristic CT feature is helpful to distinguish NTM from PTB in patients with equivocal clinical symptoms and pending culture results. Considering our results, physicians can make more precise decisions to initiate empiric anti-TB treatment and avoid unnecessary adverse effects on patients with final diagnoses of NTM lung diseases.

Our study had several limitations that are worth noting. Not all the AFB smear-positive patients with NTM lung diseases underwent chest CT. It was likely that the study was biased toward patients with severe infection who warranted further CT scans evaluation. In all cases, CT scans were obtained within 3 months of AFB smear tests. Some AFB smear-positive patients had received empirical anti-TB drugs. The CT findings in patients with actual PTB diagnoses might show improvement and somewhat not identical to the typical features of pulmonary TB. Finally, although there was a strong association of random nodules in PTB as well as bronchiectasis and cystic changes in NTM-LD statistically, the conclusions drawn by our statistical results needed a large-scale analysis to be confirmed.

Conclusions

Our results suggest that pulmonary tuberculosis and NTM lung diseases can usually be distinguished by assessing the CT findings of nodules in patients with PTB as well as bronchiectasis and cystic changes with NTM. The CT distinction between these two mycobacterial infections may help radiologists and physicians to know the most likely diagnoses in AFB-smear positive patients and avoid unnecessary adverse effects and costs of anti-TB drugs in endemic areas.

Competing interests

The authors declare that they have no competing interests.

Authors' contribution

MKY and CYC contributed equally to this work. MKY: study conception, design, and collection of data. CYC: drafting, submit and revise the manuscript. SCC: analysis and interpretation of data. PHT: study conception, design. Y-ML: acquisition and collection of data. JWH: acquisition and collection of data. All authors read and approved the final manuscript. All of the authors had access to the data and played a role in the writing this manuscript.

Author details

[1]Department of Radiology, National Yang-Ming University Hospital, Yilan, Taiwan. [2]Faculty of Medicine, School of Medicine, National Yang-Ming University, Taipei, Taiwan. [3]Department of Chest Medicine, Far Eastern Memorial Hospital, Taipei, Taiwan. [4]Department of Internal Medicine, National Yang-Ming University Hospital, #152, Xin-Min Road, Yilan City 260, Taiwan. [5]Department of Laboratory Medicine, National Yang-Ming University Hospital, Yilan, Taiwan. [6]Department of Surgery, National Yang-Ming University Hospital, Yilan, Taiwan.

References

1. World Health Organization: **Global tuberculosis report 2013.** http://www.who.int/tb/publications/global_report/en/.
2. Blumberg HM, Burman WJ, Chaisson RE, Daley CL, Etkind SC, Friedman LN, Fujiwara P, Grzemska M, Hopewell PC, Iseman MD, Jasmer RM, Koppaka V, Menzies RI, O'Brien RJ, Reves RR, Reichman LB, Simone PM, Starke JR, Vernon AA, American Thoracic Society, Centers for Disease Control and Prevention and the Infectious Diseases Society: **American Thoracic Society/ Centers for Disease Control and Prevention/Infectious Diseases Society of America: treatment of tuberculosis.** *Am J Respir Crit Care Med* 2003, **167**:603–662.
3. World Health Organization: *Treatment of tuberculosis: guidelines for national programmes.* 4th edition. http://www.who.int/tb/publications/tb_treatmentguidelines/en/.
4. Tuberculosis Division, International Union against Tuberculosis and Lung Disease: **Tuberculosis bacteriology-priorities and indications in high prevalence countries: position of the technical staff of the tuberculosis division of the International Union against Tuberculosis and Lung Disease.** *Int J Tuberc Lung Dis* 2005, **9**:355–361.
5. Maiga M, Siddiqui S, Diallo S, Diarra B, Traoré B, Shea YR, Zelazny AM, Dembele BP, Goita D, Kassambara H, Hammond AS, Polis MA, Tounkara A: **Failure to recognize nontuberculous mycobacteria leads to misdiagnosis of chronic pulmonary tuberculosis.** *PLoS One* 2012, **7**:e36902.
6. American Thoracic Society: **Diagnostic standards and classification of tuberculosis in adults and children.** *Am J Respir Crit Care Med* 2000, **161**:1376–1395.
7. Woodring JH, Vandiviere HM: **Pulmonary disease caused by nontuberculous mycobacteria.** *J Thorac Imaging* 1990, **5**:64–76.
8. Marras TK, Daley CL: **Epidemiology of human pulmonary infection with nontuberculous mycobacteria.** *Clin Chest Med* 2002, **23**:553–567.
9. Marras TK, Chedore P, Ying AM, Jamieson F: **Isolation prevalence of pulmonary non-tuberculous mycobacteria in Ontario, 1997–2003.** *Thorax* 2007, **62**:661–666.
10. Jeong YJ, Lee KS, Koh WJ, Han J, Kim TS, Kwon OJ: **Nontuberculous mycobacterial pulmonary infection in immunocompetent patients: comparison of thin-section CT and histopathologic findings.** *Radiology* 2004, **231**:880–886.
11. Sun JR, Lee SY, Perng CL, Lu JJ: **Detecting mycobacterium tuberculosis in bactec MGIT 960 cultures by inhouse IS6110-based PCR assay in routine clinical practice.** *J Formos Med Assoc* 2009, **108**:119–125.
12. Tarshis MS, Kinsella PC, Parker MV, Blood media for the cultivation of Mycobacterium tuberculosis: **VII: Comparison of blood agar-penicillin and lowenstein-jensen media under routine diagnostic conditions.** *J Bacteriol* 1953, **66**:448–452.
13. Diagnosis and treatment of disease caused by nontuberculous mycobacteria: **This official statement of the American Thoracic Society was approved by the Board of Directors, March 1997. Medical section of the American Lung Association.** *Am J Respir Crit Care Med* 1997, **156**:S1–S25.
14. Griffith DE, Aksamit T, Brown-Elliott BA, Catanzaro A, Daley C, Gordin F, Holland SM, Horsburgh R, Huitt G, Iademarco MF, Iseman M, Olivier K, Ruoss S, von Reyn CF, Wallace RJ Jr, Winthrop K, ATS Mycobacterial Diseases Subcommittee; American Thoracic Society; Infectious Disease Society of America: **An official ATS/IDSA statement: diagnosis, treatment, and prevention of non-tuberculous mycobacterial diseases.** *Am J Respir Crit Care Med* 2007, **175**:367–416.
15. Hollings NP, Wells AU, Wilson R, Hansell DM: **Comparative appearances of non-tuberculous mycobacteria species: a CT study.** *Eur Radiol* 2002, **12**:2211–2217.
16. Lee HY, Lee KS, Jeong YJ, Hwang JH, Kim HJ, Chung MP, Han J: **High-resolution CT findings in fibrotic idiopathic interstitial pneumonias with little honeycombing: serial changes and prognostic implications.** *AJR Am J Roentgenol* 2012, **199**:982–989.

17. Mineo G, Ciccarese F, Attinà D, Di Scioscio V, Sciascia N, Bono L, Rocca A, Stella F, Zompatori M: **Natural history of honeycombing: follow-up of patients with idiopathic pulmonary fibrosis treated with single-lung transplantation.** *Radiol Med* 2013, **118:**40–50.
18. Fowler SJ, French J, Screaton NJ, Foweraker J, Condliffe A, Haworth CS, Exley AR, Bilton D: **Nontuberculous mycobacteria in bronchiectasis: prevalence and patient characteristics.** *Eur Respir J* 2006, **28:**1204–1210.
19. Dailloux M, Abalain ML, Laurain C, Lebrun L, Loos-Ayav C, Lozniewski A, Maugein J, French Mycobacteria Study Group: **Respiratory infections associated with nontuberculous mycobacteria in non-HIV patients.** *Eur Respir J* 2006, **28:**1211–1215.
20. Chang CY, Hong JY, Yuan MK, Chang SJ, Lee YM, Chang SC, Hsu LC, Cheng SL: **Risk factors in AFB smear-positive patients who receive inappropriate antituberculous treatment.** *Drug Des Devel Ther* 2013, **7:**53–58.

Permissions

All chapters in this book were first published in PM, by BioMed Central; hereby published with permission under the Creative Commons Attribution License or equivalent. Every chapter published in this book has been scrutinized by our experts. Their significance has been extensively debated. The topics covered herein carry significant findings which will fuel the growth of the discipline. They may even be implemented as practical applications or may be referred to as a beginning point for another development.

The contributors of this book come from diverse backgrounds, making this book a truly international effort. This book will bring forth new frontiers with its revolutionizing research information and detailed analysis of the nascent developments around the world.

We would like to thank all the contributing authors for lending their expertise to make the book truly unique. They have played a crucial role in the development of this book. Without their invaluable contributions this book wouldn't have been possible. They have made vital efforts to compile up to date information on the varied aspects of this subject to make this book a valuable addition to the collection of many professionals and students.

This book was conceptualized with the vision of imparting up-to-date information and advanced data in this field. To ensure the same, a matchless editorial board was set up. Every individual on the board went through rigorous rounds of assessment to prove their worth. After which they invested a large part of their time researching and compiling the most relevant data for our readers.

The editorial board has been involved in producing this book since its inception. They have spent rigorous hours researching and exploring the diverse topics which have resulted in the successful publishing of this book. They have passed on their knowledge of decades through this book. To expedite this challenging task, the publisher supported the team at every step. A small team of assistant editors was also appointed to further simplify the editing procedure and attain best results for the readers.

Apart from the editorial board, the designing team has also invested a significant amount of their time in understanding the subject and creating the most relevant covers. They scrutinized every image to scout for the most suitable representation of the subject and create an appropriate cover for the book.

The publishing team has been an ardent support to the editorial, designing and production team. Their endless efforts to recruit the best for this project, has resulted in the accomplishment of this book. They are a veteran in the field of academics and their pool of knowledge is as vast as their experience in printing. Their expertise and guidance has proved useful at every step. Their uncompromising quality standards have made this book an exceptional effort. Their encouragement from time to time has been an inspiration for everyone.

The publisher and the editorial board hope that this book will prove to be a valuable piece of knowledge for researchers, students, practitioners and scholars across the globe.

List of Contributors

Sara Caldrer, Genny Verzè, Jan Johansson and Claudio Sorio
Department of Pathology and Diagnostics, General Pathology Section, University of Verona School of Medicine, Verona, Italy

Baroukh Maurice Assael, Paola Melotti, Chiara Angiari, Sara Caldrer and Genny Verzè
Cystic Fibrosis Center, Azienda Ospedaliera di Verona, Verona, Italy

Mario Buffelli
Department of Neurological Sciences, Physiology Section, University of Verona School of Medicine, Verona, Italy

Zhen Zhao, Li Jiang, Xiuming Xi, Qi Jiang, Bo Zhu and Meiping Wang
Intensive Care Unit, Fuxing Hospital affiliated with Capital Medical University, Beijing 100038, China

Jin Xing and Dan Zhang
Department of Ultrasonography, Fuxing Hospital affiliated with Capital Medical University, Beijing 100038, China

R M Schnabel, K van der Velden, A Osinski, P M H J Roekaerts and D C J J Bergmans
Department of Intensive Care Medicine, Maastricht University Medical Centre+, P. Debyelaan 25, 6202 AZ Maastricht, The Netherlands

G Rohde
Department of Respiratory Medicine, Maastricht University Medical Centre+, Maastricht, The Netherlands

Panayiotis Kouis, Stefania I. Papatheodorou and Panayiotis K. Yiallouros
Cyprus International Institute for Environmental & Public Health in Association with Harvard School of Public Health, Cyprus University of Technology, 95 Irenes Street, 3041 Limassol, Cyprus
Department of Pediatrics, Hospital "Archbishop Makarios III", Nicosia, Cyprus

Manabu Hayama, Norio Okamoto, Hidekazu Suzuki, Motohiro Tamiya, Takayuki Shiroyama, Ayako Tanaka, Takuji Nishida, Takashi Nishihara, Nobuko Uehara, Naoko Morishita and Tomonori Hirashima
Department of Thoracic Malignancy, Osaka Prefectural Medical Center for Respiratory and Allergic Diseases, 3-7-1, Habikino, Habikino City, Osaka 583-8588, Japan

Kunimitsu Kawahara
Department of Pathology, Osaka Prefectural Medical Center for Respiratory and Allergic Diseases, Osaka, Japan

Sara Piciucchi
Department of Radiology, Azienda USL Romagna, Ospedale GB Morgagni, Via C. Forlanini, Forlì FC 34-47121, Italy

Sara Tomassetti, Claudia Ravaglia, Christian Gurioli, Carlo Gurioli and Venerino Poletti
Department of Diseases of the Thorax, Azienda USL Romagna, Ospedale GB Morgagni, Forlì, Italy

Alessandra Dubini
Department of Pathology, Azienda USL Romagna, Ospedale GB Morgagni, Forlì, Italy

Angelo Carloni
Department of Radiology, Ospedale Santa Maria, Terni, Italy

Marco Chilosi
Department of Pathology and Diagnostics, University of Verona, Verona, Italy

Thomas V Colby
Department of Laboratory Medicine and Pathology, Mayo Clinic, Scottsdale, AZ, USA

Venerino Poletti
Department of Respiratory Diseases & Allergy, Aarhus University Hospital, Aarhus, Denmark

João Pedro Steinhauser Motta, Alexandre Pinto Cardoso, Marcos Eduardo Paschoal and José Roberto Lapa e Silva
Instituto de Doenças do Torax, Universidade Federal do Rio de Janeiro, Rua Professor Rodolpho Paulo Rocco, 255, 1 andar, sala 01D 58/60, Rio de Janeiro, RJ 21941-913, Brazil

Axel Tobias Kempa
Klinikum-Stuttgart, Kriegbergstrasse 60, 70174 Stuttgart, Germany

Ronir Raggio Luiz
Instituto de Estudos em Saúde Coletiva, Universidade Federal do Rio de Janeiro, Avenida HorácioMacedo, lha do Fundão - Cidade Universitária, 21941-598 Rio de Janeiro, RJ, Brazil

Franz Stanzel
Lungenklinik Hemer, Theo-Funccius-Straße 1, 58675 Hemer, NW, Germany

Takehiro Izumo, Yuji Matsumoto, Christine Chavez and Takaaki Tsuchida
Department of Endoscopy, Respiratory Endoscopy Division, National Cancer Center Hospital, 5-1-1, Tsukiji Chou-ku, Tokyo 104-0045, Japan

Chaosheng Deng, Dawen Wu, Haibo Ding, Xin Zhang and Qiaoxian Zhang
Division of Respiratory and Critical Care Medicine, First Affiliated Hospital of Fujian Medical University, Fuzhou 350005, Fujian, China

Yongquan Wu and Xiaoming Cao
Department of Respiratory Disease, First Hospital of Longyan City, 364000 Fujian, China

Ruixiong You and Qunlin Chen
Department of Medical Imaging, First Affiliated Hospital of Fujian Medical University, Fuzhou 350005, Fujian, China

Linying Chen
Department of Pathology, First Affiliated Hospital, Fujian Medical University, Fuzhou, Fujian Province, China

Martin Veaudor, Sébastien Couraud and Pierre-Jean Souquet
Service de Pneumologie Aigue Spécialisée et Cancérologie Thoracique, Centre Hospitalier Lyon Sud, Institut de Cancérologie des Hospices Civils de Lyon, 69495 Pierre Bénite, France

Virginie Avrillon, Martin Veaudor and Sébastien Couraud
Association PRUPET, Centre Hospitalier de Moulin Yzeure, Moulins, France

Sébastien Couraud
EMR 3738 Ciblage thérapeutique en oncologie, Faculté de médecine et de maïeutique Lyon Sud Charles Mérieux, Université Lyon 1, Villeurbanne, France

Sophors Chan, Chanraksmey Choun, Pisethmorokoth Keo and Chanty Ny
Service de pneumologie, Hôpital Preah Kossamak, Phnom Penh, Cambodia

Tsukasa Ishiwata, Kenji Tsushima, Kenichi Suzuki, Kosuke Hirota, Mitsuhiro Abe, Naoko Kawata, Jiro Terada and Koichiro Tatsumi
Department of Respirology, Graduate School of Medicine, Chiba University, 1-8-1, Inohana, Chuo-ku, Chiba 260-8670, Japan

Mai Fujie
Medical Equipment Control Center, Chiba University Hospital, 1-8-1, Inohana, Chuo-ku, Chiba 260-8670, Japan

Eef D. Telenga, Nick H. T. ten Hacken, Dirkje S. Postma and Maarten van den Berge
Department of Pulmonary Diseases, University of Groningen, University Medical Center Groningen, 9700 RB Groningen, The Netherlands
GRIAC Research Institute, University of Groningen, University Medical Center Groningen, Groningen, The Netherlands

Matthijs Oudkerk, Peter M. A. van Ooijen and Rozemarijn Vliegenthart
Center for Medical Imaging North East Netherlands, University of Groningen, University Medical Center Groningen, Groningen, The Netherlands

Peter M. A. van Ooijen and Rozemarijn Vliegenthart
Department of Radiology, University of Groningen, University Medical Center Groningen, The Netherlands

Yasuhiro Norisue
Department of Pulmonary and Critical Care Medicine, Tokyo Bay Urayasu-Ichikawa Medical Center, 3-4-32 Toudaijima, Urayasushi, Chiba 279-0001, Japan

Yasuharu Tokuda
Japan Community Healthcare Organization, 3-22-12, Takanawa, Tokyo 108-0074, Japan

Mayrol Juarez
Mercy Hospital, 1235 E Cherokee St, Springfield, MO 65804, USA

Ryo Uchimido
Beth Israel Deaconess Medical Center, 330 Brookline Ave, Boston, MA 02215, USA

Shigeki Fujitani
Department of Emergency and Critical Care Medicine, St. Marianna University Hospital, 2-16-1, Miyamae, Kawasaki, Kanagawa, Japan

David A. Stoeckel
Division of Pulmonary, Critical Care and Sleep Medicine, Saint Louis University, 1402S. Grand Avenue, Saint Louis, MO 63104-1004, USA

Sandeep J. Khandhar
Inova Health System, Fairfax Hospital, Falls Church, VA, USA

Mark R. Bowling
East Carolina University, Greenville, NC, USA

Javier Flandes
Pulmonary Department, IIS-Fundacion Jimenez Diaz University Hospital, CIBERES, Madrid, Spain

Thomas R. Gildea
Department of Pulmonary, Allergy and Critical Care Medicine and Transplant Center, Cleveland Clinic, Cleveland, OH, USA

Jennifer J. Wolvers and Kristin L. Hood
Medtronic, Minneapolis, MN, USA

William S. Krimsky
Pulmonary and Critical Care Associates of Baltimore, Baltimore, MD, USA

Douglas J. Minnich
Division of Cardiothoracic Surgery, University of Alabama at Birmingham, Birmingham, AL, USA

Septimiu D. Murgu
Interventional Pulmonology Fellowship Program, The University of Chicago Medicine, Chicago, IL, USA

Michael Pritchett
Pulmonary Department, Pinehurst Medical Clinic and First Health Moore Regional Hospital, Pinehurst, NC, USA

Eric M. Toloza
Department of Thoracic Oncology, Moffitt Cancer Center, Tampa, FL, USA
Department of Surgery and Department of Oncologic Sciences, University of South Florida Morsani College of Medicine, Tampa, FL, USA

Momen M. Wahidi
Department of Medicine, Duke University Medical Center, Durham, NC, USA

Erik E. Folch
Division of Pulmonary and Critical Care Medicine, Massachusetts General Hospital, Harvard Medical School, 55 Fruit Street, Bulfinch 148, Boston, MA 02114, USA

Douglas J. Minnich
Present Address: Princeton Baptist Medical Center, Birmingham, AL, USA

Joseph Jacob, Anne Laure Brun and David M. Hansell
Department of Radiology, Royal Brompton Hospital, Royal Brompton and Harefield NHS Foundation Trust, London, UK

Brian J. Bartholmai
Division of Radiology, Mayo Clinic Rochester, Rochester, MN, USA

Ryoko Egashira
Department of Radiology, Faculty of Medicine, Saga University, 5-1-1 Nabeshima, Saga-City, Japan

Ronald Karwoski and Srinivasan Rajagopalan
Department of Physiology and Biomedical Engineering, Mayo Clinic Rochester, Rochester, MN, USA

Athol U. Wells and Maria Kokosi
Interstitial Lung Disease Unit, Royal Brompton Hospital, Royal Brompton and Harefield NHS Foundation Trust, London, UK

Seher Raza Zaidi, Andrea M. Collins, Elena Mitsi, Jesús Reiné, Angela D Wright, Jessica Owugha, Daniela Mulari Ferreira and Jamie Rylance
Respiratory Infection Group, Liverpool School of Tropical Medicine, Pembroke Place, Liverpool L3 5QA, UK

Richard Fitzgerald, Amitava Ganguli, Jamie Rylance, Kayleigh Davies, Seher Raza Zaidi, Andrea M. Collins and Angela D Wright
Respiratory Research Group, Royal Liverpool and Broadgreen University Hospital NHS Trust, Liverpool L7 8XP, UK
Clinical Research Network, Northwest Coast, Liverpool, UK

Stephen B Gordon
Malawi-Liverpool-Wellcome Trust Clinical Research Programme, Blantyre, Malawi

Yan-Bing Wu†, Li-Li Xu, Xiao-Juan Wang, Zhen Wang, Jun Zhang, Zhao-Hui Tong and Huan-Zhong Shi
Department of Respiratory and Critical Care Medicine, Beijing Institute of Respiratory Medicine and Beijing Chaoyang Hospital, Capital Medical University, Beijing, China

Changjiang Xue, Na Wu, Meihua Qiu, Xuqin Du and Qiao Ye
Department of Occupational Medicine and Toxicology, Clinical Center for Interstitial Lung Diseases, Beijing Chao-Yang Hospital, Capital Medical University, 8 Gongren Tiyuchang Nanlu, Chao-Yang District, Beijing 100020, China

Xue Li
Department of Pathology, Beijing Chao-Yang Hospital, Capital Medical University, 8 Gongren Tiyuchang Nanlu, Chao-Yang District, Beijing 100020, China

Mario Silva, Nicola Sverzellati, Davide Colombi and Gianluca Milanese
Department of Medicine and Surgery (DiMeC), Section of Radiology, Unit of Surgical Sciences, University of Parma, Padiglione Barbieri, Via Gramsci 14, 43126 Parma, Italy

Ugo Pastorino
Department of Thoracic Surgery, Fondazione IRCCS Istituto Nazionale dei Tumori, Milan, Italy

Carlotta Galeone and Carlo La Vecchia
Department of Clinical Sciences and Community Health, University of Milan, Milan, Italy

Alfonso Marchianò
Department of Radiology and Radiotherapy, Fondazione IRCCS Istituto Nazionale dei Tumori, Milan, Italy

Akifumi Uchida, Takuya Samukawa, Tomohiro Kumamoto, Masahiro Ohshige, Keiko Mizuno, Ikkou Higashimoto and Hiromasa Inoue
Department of Pulmonary Medicine, Graduate School of Medical and Dental Sciences, Kagoshima University, 8-35-1 Sakuragaoka, Kagoshima 890-8520, Japan

Kazuhito Hatanaka
Department of Pathology, Tokai University School of Medicine, 143 Shimokasuya, Isehara, Kanagawa, Japan

Masami Sato and Yoshihiro Nakamura
Department of General Thoracic Surgery, Graduate School of Medical and Dental Sciences, Kagoshima University, 8-35-1 Sakuragaoka, Kagoshima, Japan

Beomsu Shin
Department of Internal Medicine, Yonsei University Wonju College of
Medicine, Wonju, South Korea

Boksoon Chang
Department of Pulmonary and Critical Care Medicine, Kyung Hee University Hospital at Gangdong, School of Medicine, Kyung Hee University, Seoul, South Korea

Hojoong Kim and Byeong-Ho Jeong
Division of Pulmonary and Critical Care Medicine, Department of Internal Medicine, Samsung Medical Center, Sungkyunkwan University School of Medicine, 81 Irwon-ro, Gangnam-gu, Seoul 06351, South Korea

Pongdhep Theerawit
Division of Critical Care Medicine, Department of Medicine, Faculty of Medicine Ramathibodi Hospital, Mahidol University, Bangkok, Thailand

Charn Kiatboonsri, Sumalee Kiatboonsri, Dararat Eksombatchai and Yuda Sutherasan
Division of Pulmonary and Pulmonary Critical Care Medicine, Department of Medicine, Faculty of Medicine Ramathibodi Hospital, Mahidol University, Bangkok, 270 Rama 6 Road, Thung Phaya Thai, Ratchathewi, Bangkok 10400, Thailand

Thitiporn Suwatanapongched
Department of Diagnostic and Therapeutic Radiology, Faculty of Medicine Ramathibodi Hospital, Mahidol University, Bangkok, Thailand

Trieu-Nghi Hoang-Thi, Marie-Pierre Revel, Charlotte Martin and Guillaume Chassagnon
Radiology Department, Groupe Hospitalier Cochin-Hôtel Dieu, AP-HP, Université Paris Descartes - Sorbonne Paris Cité, Paris, France

Pierre-Régis Burgel and Isabelle Honoré
Pulmonary Department, Groupe Hospitalier Cochin-Hôtel Dieu, AP-HP, Université Paris Descartes - Sorbonne Paris Cité, Paris, France

Bernard Maitre and Laurence Bassinet
Service de Pneumologie et de Pathologie Professionnelle, DHU A-TVB, Centre Hospitalier Intercommunal de Créteil, Université Paris Est Créteil, Créteil, France

Thong Hua-Huy
Physiology Department, Groupe Hospitalier Cochin-Hôtel Dieu, AP-HP, Université Paris Descartes - Sorbonne Paris Cité, Paris, France

Guillaume Chassagnon
Center for Visual Computing, CentraleSupelec, Gif-sur-Yvette, France

Trieu-Nghi Hoang-Thi
Department Diagnostic Imaging, Vinmec International Hospital - Central Park, Ho Chi Minh City, Vietnam

Li-Li Xu, Yuan Yang, Zhen Wang, Xiao-Juan Wang, Zhao-Hui Tong and Huan-Zhong Shi
Department of Respiratory and Critical Care Medicine; Beijing Institute of Respiratory Medicine and Beijing Chaoyang Hospital, Capital Medical University, 8 Gongti Nanlu, Chaoyang District, Beijing 100020, China

Gülmisal Güder, Berna DL Broekhuizen, Arno W Hoes and Frans H Rutten
Julius Center for Health Sciences and Primary Care, University Medical Center Utrecht, Utrecht, The Netherlands

Susanne Brenner, Stefan Störk and Gülmisal Güder
Department of Internal Medicine I, Cardiology, University Hospital Würzburg, Oberdürrbacherstr. 6, D-97080 Würzburg, Germany
Comprehensive Heart Failure Center, University of Würzburg, Würzburg, Germany

Matthias Held
Medical Mission Hospital, Department of Internal Medicine, Respiratory Medicine and Cardiology, Würzburg, Germany

Jan-Willem J Lammers
Department of Respiratory Medicine, University Medical Center Utrecht, Utrecht, The Netherlands

Karina de Souza Giassi
Radiology Division, Hospital Sírio-Libanês, R. Dona Adma Jafet, 91, Bela Vista, SP 01308-050, Brazil
Radiology Institute (InRad), University of São Paulo Medical School (FMUSP), Av. Dr. Enéas de Carvalho Aguiar, 44, Consolação, SP 05403-900, Brazil

Ronaldo Adib Kairalla, Andre Apanavicius, Caio Julio Cesar Fernandes, Andre Nathan Costa and Fernando Bin Teixeira
Pulmonary Division, Hospital Sírio-Libanês, R. Dona Adma Jafet, 91, Bela Vista, SP 01308-050, Brazil
Pulmonary Division, Heart Institute (InCor), University of São Paulo Medical School (FMUSP), Av. Dr. Enéas de Carvalho Aguiar, 44, 2nd floor, block 1, Consolação, SP 05403-900, Brazil

Azadeh Bagheri-Hanson, Sebastian Nedwed, Claudia Rueckes-Nilges and Lutz Naehrlich
Department of Pediatrics, Justus-Liebig-University Giessen, Feulgenstrasse 12, 35385 Giessen, Germany

Mei-Kang Yuan
Department of Radiology, National Yang-Ming University Hospital, Yilan, Taiwan

Ping-Huang Tsai and Shih-Chieh Chang
Faculty of Medicine, School of Medicine, National Yang-Ming University, Taipei, Taiwan
Department of Internal Medicine, National Yang-Ming University Hospital, #152, Xin-Min Road, Yilan City 260, Taiwan

Cheng-Yu Chang
Department of Chest Medicine, Far Eastern Memorial Hospital, Taipei, Taiwan

Yuan-Ming Lee
Department of Laboratory Medicine, National Yang-Ming University Hospital, Yilan, Taiwan

Jen-Wu Huang
Department of Surgery, National Yang-Ming University Hospital, Yilan, Taiwan

Index

www.ingramcontent.com/pod-product-compliance
Lightning Source LLC
LaVergne TN
LVHW080808220926
848485LV00011B/427